ADVANCES IN **SPORT** AND **EXERCISE** SCIENCE SERIES

Exercise Physiology in **Special Populations**

For Elsevier:

Commissioning Editor: Dinah Thom/Claire Wilson
Development Editor: Catherine Jackson
Project Manager: Elouise Ball
Designer: Stewart Larking
Illustration Manager: Kirsteen Wright
Illustrator: Richard Morris

ADVANCES IN **SPORT** AND **EXERCISE** SCIENCE SERIES

Exercise Physiology in Special Populations

Edited by

John P Buckley BPE MSc PhD BASES Accr

Senior Lecturer, Centre for Exercise & Nutrition Science, University of Chester; Founding Managing Partner, Lifestyle Exercise & Physiotherapy Centre, Shrewsbury, UK

Series Editors

Neil Spurway MA PhD

Emeritus Professor of Exercise Physiology, University of Glasgow, Glasgow, UK

Don MacLaren BSc MSc PhD CertEd

Professor of Sports Nutrition, School of Sport and Exercise Sciences, Liverpool John Moores University, Liverpool, UK

Foreword by
Dr Ann Redgrave & Sir Steven Redgrave

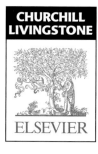

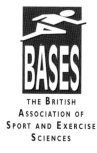

THE BRITISH
ASSOCIATION OF
SPORT AND EXERCISE
SCIENCES

EDINBURGH LONDON NEW YORK OXFORD PHILADELPHIA ST LOUIS SYDNEY TORONTO 2008

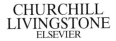

CHURCHILL
LIVINGSTONE
ELSEVIER

ISBN: 978 0 443 10343 8

British Library Cataloguing in Publication Data
A catalogue record for this book is available from the British Library.

Library of Congress Cataloging in Publication Data
A catalog record for this book is available from the Library of Congress.

Note
Knowledge and best practice in this field are constantly changing. As new research and experience broaden our knowledge, changes in practice, treatment and drug therapy may become necessary or appropriate. Readers are advised to check the most current information provided (i) on procedures featured or (ii) by the manufacturer of each product to be administered, to verify the recommended dose or formula, the method and duration of administration, and contraindications. It is the responsibility of the practitioner, relying on their own experience and knowledge of the patient, to make diagnoses, to determine dosages and the best treatment for each individual patient, and to take all appropriate safety precautions. To the fullest extent of the law, neither the Publisher nor the Editor assumes any liability for any injury and/or damage to persons or property arising out of or related to any use of the material contained in this book.

The Publisher

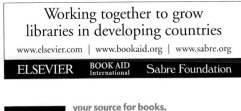

ELSEVIER   your source for books, journals and multimedia in the health sciences

www.elsevierhealth.com

The publisher's policy is to use **paper manufactured from sustainable forests**

Printed in China

Contents

Dedications vii

Contributors ix

Foreword xi

Preface xiii

1. Introduction 1
   John P Buckley and Adrienne R Hughes

2. Obesity and diabetes 21
   David Stensel

3. Cardiac disease and dysfunction 51
   John P Buckley and Patrick J Doherty

4. Lung disease and dysfunction 97
   Alison McConnell

5. Arthritis and low back pain 119
   Alan Leigh, Helen Mitchell and Paul Firth

6. Ageing and older people 161
   Dawn A Skelton and Susann M Dinan-Young

7. Bone health 225
   Jacky J Forsyth and Rachel C Davey

8. The exercising female 249
   Karen M Birch and Joseph I Esformes

9. Neurological and neuromuscular disorders, a guide to pathological processes and primary symptoms 269
   Helen Dawes

10. Spinal cord injury 309
    Nick Webborn and Victoria Goosey-Tolfrey

Index 335

Dedications

I would like to dedicate this book to:

Fiona Buckley, for her patience in helping me find the time to write and edit this book.

The cardiac rehabilitation team at the University Hospital of North Staffordshire (Dr JD, Alan, Lynn, Phil, Sue, Alison, Liz and Chris); a special group of people who have influenced my understanding of key aspects of specialist clinical rehabilitation and patient care.

All the patients, clients and staff, who have made working in this area highly rewarding, including those at The Lifestyle Exercise & Physiotherapy Centre (Shrewsbury), The Royal Shrewsbury Hospital, The North Staffordshire Hospital, The Oswestry Orthopaedic Hospital, The Countess of Chester Hospital, The School of Health and Rehabilitation, Keele University and The Centre for Exercise & Nutrition Science, University of Chester.

Contributors

Karen M Birch, BSc(Hons) PhD
Senior Lecturer in Exercise Physiology, Centre for Sport and Exercise Sciences, Institute of Membranes and Systems Biology, University of Leeds, UK

John P Buckley, BPE MSc PhD BASES Accr
Senior Lecturer, Centre for Exercise & Nutrition Science, University of Chester; Founding Managing Partner, Lifestyle Exercise & Physiotherapy Centre, Shrewsbury, UK

Rachel C Davey, BSc MMedSci PhD
Professor of Physical Activity for Public Health, Centre for Sport and Exercise Research, University of Staffordshire, Stoke-on-Trent, UK

Helen Dawes, MCSP MMedSci PhD
Reader, Movement Science Group, School of Life Sciences, Oxford Brookes University and Associate Research Fellow, Department of Clinical Neurology, University of Oxford, Oxford, UK

Susann M Dinan-Young, BEd MSc
Senior Research Fellow, Primary Care and Population Sciences, Royal Free and University College, Medical School, London; School of Health Informatics, University of Derby, UK

Patrick J Doherty, MCSP PhD
Professor of Rehabilitation, Faculty of Health and Life Sciences, York St John University, York, UK

Joseph I Esformes, BSc MSc PhD CSCS FHEA
Lecturer in Exercise Physiology, Discipline Director for Sport Conditioning, Rehabilitation, and Massage, Cardiff School of Sport, University of Wales Institute, Cardiff, UK

Paul Firth, BSc(Hons)
Exercise Physiologist, Lifestyle Exercise & Physiotherapy Centre, Shrewsbury, UK; Head of Clinical Education (Physiotherapy), Keele University, Staffs, UK

Jacky J Forsyth, BA(Hons) QTS MPhil PhD
Senior Lecturer, Exercise Physiology, Centre for Sport and Exercise Research, University of Staffordshire, Stoke-on-Trent, UK

Victoria Goosey-Tolfrey, BSc(Hons) PhD
Senior Lecturer in Exercise Physiology, School of Sport and Exercise Sciences, Loughborough University, UK

Adrienne R Hughes, BSc(Hons) PhD
Lecturer in Physical Activity and Health, Department of Sports Science, University of Stirling, UK

Alan Leigh, MSc OMT (NZ) MCSP
Managing Partner and Senior Physiotherapist, Lifestyle Exercise & Physiotherapy Centre, Radbrook Professional Centre, Shrewsbury, UK

Alison McConnell, BSc MSc PhD FACSM BASES Accr
Professor of Applied Physiology, Centre for Sports Medicine and Human Performance, Brunel University, Uxbridge, UK

Helen Mitchell, MSc
Exercise Physiologist, Lifestyle Exercise & Physiotherapy Centre, Shrewsbury, UK

Dawn A Skelton, BSc PhD
Reader in Ageing and Health, HealthQWest, Glasgow Caledonian University, Glasgow; Scientific Co-ordinator of ProFaNE (Prevention of Falls Network Europe), School of Nursing, Midwifery and Social Work, University of Manchester, UK

David Stensel, BA(Hons) PGCE MSc PhD
Senior Lecturer in Exercise Physiology, School of Sport and Exercise Sciences, Loughborough University, UK

Nick Webborn, MB BS FFSEM FACSM FISM MSc Dip Sports Med
Medical Director, The Sussex Centre for Sport and Exercise Medicine, University of Brighton, UK

Foreword

It is well documented that the lifespan of man in many different modern social cultures is considerably longer than it was in the last century. It was not so long ago that you were considered old at the age of fifty, but now it is not uncommon for a person to live in excess of one hundred years – twice the lifespan. Why you may ask. Is it because we are now able to treat a lot of conditions that used to kill us off? Is it that we are able to diagnose these problems earlier and apply more appropriate interventions? Or is it an influence of diet and better general living? The debate could go on. Of relevance to this text though, is that alongside the increasing lifespan there is a greater need for exercise prescription in people over the age of fifty; people who need to maintain mobility to keep good health; people who have medical conditions that need specific advice in exercise; and people whose medication can be reduced if appropriate exercise is taken.

Beyond retirement there is an increasing population who are challenging exercise and healthcare professionals to help establish good exercise practice and principles based on science, not myth. Having been successful during their working life, they are searching for personal challenges which increasingly require a higher level of fitness than sometimes they have ever had in their lives before – expeditions to the North or South Pole, climbing Everest, running the London Marathon, to name but a few, the list goes on.

Conversely in the same population we are witnessing a reduction in the fitness of our children and teenagers. The advancement in technology, especially computers, has made childhood more sedentary, and this, combined with the reducing requirements of the National Curriculum for Physical Education in schools, and repeated security scares covered almost daily by the media, mean the youth of today (-) that is, the elderly of tomorrow (-) have a diminishing level of baseline fitness and increasing prevalence of conditions such as diabetes, obesity, hypertension and cardiac pathology.

The challenge is the same whether the individual wishing to exercise is an elite athlete, a child wishing to play soccer or an elderly person wanting to fight the functional decline of old age. The healthcare or exercise professional needs to ascertain what the baseline fitness is, define where the individual is aiming to take their fitness, and work out a plan to achieve this change.

This textbook is a welcome breath of fresh air. It looks in depth at a number of relevant medical conditions, assesses the influence of the condition on the exercising individual, provides research evidence to verify what is being said, and clearly lays out a practical approach to exercising with specific conditions. It does not claim to have all the answers, and, in fact, points out where science still needs to progress.

Individual conditions are considered by experts in their field who draw on their many years of experience.

During my own medical work in elite international sport, there have been two notable occasions when I was confronted by significant medical conditions which I had not previously had much exposure to. One was ulcerative colitis, newly diagnosed 16 weeks before the 1992 Olympic Games in Barcelona Spain. The other was diabetes mellitus.

Of course I had a basic knowledge of the conditions but this was not sufficient to provide reassurance to an aspiring Olympic medallist. I needed to understand how the illness would affect the body, and the body's response to exercise. I needed to understand whether continuing to train would be detrimental or beneficial. I needed so many answers. This textbook would have been invaluable and I congratulate all who have contributed to its publication. It will I am sure become the bible for sports physicians and exercise professionals across the World.

Dr Ann Redgrave 2008

Preface

It has been an honour to edit this new textbook on two counts. The first honour is to have been invited by two of the UK's most notable exercise physiologists, Professors Don McLaren and Neil Spurway, to head up this project. The second honour is to have been able to be associated with so many of the UK's leading authorities on the specialist topics found within each of the chapters.

The book is aimed at two main groups of readers: i. Students studying the health and rehabilitative aspects of exercise physiology at upper undergraduate or postgraduate level; and ii. Healthcare and rehabilitation specialists requiring a reference source in order to provide their clients and patients with exercise guidance based on the best evidence.

In reading this book, there is a general framework for most of the chapters. This framework includes an initial review of the epidemiology of each disease or condition, which has either been strongly influenced by a history of physical inactivity and low fitness or other poor health habits that influence low levels of activity and fitness. After the epidemiology section the reader will find a review of the pathophysiology and aetiology of the specific condition before moving onto exercise guidance for each condition, either as a means of primary or secondary (rehabilitative) healthcare and performance. Within the exercise guidance sections, the various forms of exercise will be explored, including aerobic endurance, muscular strength and endurance, flexibility, and balance and coordination, and the evidence related to these components for each of the chapter's specific health conditions. There are a few chapters which obviously do not have an initial section on physical inactivity and its influence on epidemiology, including lung disease, the female participant, certain acquired neurological conditions, spinal cord injury and ageing.

Chapter 1

Introduction

John P Buckley and Adrienne R Hughes

CHAPTER CONTENTS

Increasing and maintaining physical
  activity 4
  Client-centred approach 5
  Stages of change 6
  Decisional balance 6
  Overcoming barriers to activity 7
  Social support 8
  Goal-setting and self-monitoring 8
  Enhancing self-efficacy 9
  Preventing relapse 9
  Psychological effects of physical
    activity 10
Misperceptions about physical
  activity 10

Monitoring the exercise dose 11
Physical activity monitoring and
  guidance 11
Relative versus absolute intensity of
  physical activity 12
Aerobic exercise 12
Muscular strength and endurance 14
  Establishing the strength training
    prescription 15
Flexibility 15
Balance/coordination/proprioception
  and movement control 16
Summary 17
References 17

This text on exercise physiology in special populations aims to cover a number of the prevalent health conditions that are linked to an inactive lifestyle or whose effects can be ameliorated by increasing physical activity and physical fitness. Throughout the text the terms physical activity, exercise and fitness will be used. It is therefore important at this point to first define the assumed meanings of these three terms. Following this, the concepts of physical activity behaviour and the various measurement parameters used by exercise professionals or healthcare practitioners to either monitor or prescribe exercise will be reviewed.

Physical activity is considered to be any muscular movement occurring above resting levels. It is an all-encompassing concept that includes any physical movements occurring within free daily living or planned leisure pursuits (exercise and sport). As will be mentioned in a number of chapters, the prevalence of some diseases is greater in those who expend less than 1500 kilocalories per week above their basal metabolic rate. The arguments highlighted in the Chief Medical Officer's (CMO) report for England and Wales (Department of Health 2004) tend to suggest that declines in health which are related to inactivity (hypokinesis) and obesity are due more to the loss of physical activity in free daily living than to the debatable reduction in the population's participation in organized exercise and sport (Cordain et al

1998, Eaton & Eaton 2003). One only has to look at the increased number of sports and fitness centres that have been built in the UK in the last decade to realize that there is certainly not a decline in those already engaged in organized sport and exercise. The reduction in energy expenditure in normal daily life, especially in non-sporty/ exercise participants, has greatly increased in the last two decades (Department of Health 2004). This is a result of the increased preference for sedentary leisure pursuits and decreases in the physicality of daily domestic-occupational tasks and transportation.

The discussion thus far focuses on the correlation between inactivity and the increased prevalence of chronic diseases. However, a number of chapters within this text consider exercise in individuals with conditions acquired by poor nutrition or smoking, an accident, or an unfortunate health event, including pulmonary disease, osteoporosis, Parkinson's disease, multiple sclerosis, arthritis or spinal injury. These conditions can lead to declines in physical activity that contribute to an inactive life-style, thus putting the sufferers at risk of chronic diseases such as coronary heart disease and diabetes. In these cases, exercise can be used as a means of combating the future potential ills of inactivity as well as a therapeutic intervention in helping the individual cope better in living with the physiological and psychosocial challenges that lie ahead.

Exercise is typically a planned and/or structured physical activity which has an aim. The aim is usually to satisfy either a physical, psychological or social need, or often a mixture of all three. Exercise was traditionally used as a means of preparing soldiers for battle but in the last 50 years has become prominent in enhancing sporting performance, physical health and personal 'body image'. Sports performance targets provide a natural motivation for maintaining exercise training. One's self-image, as promoted through the popular press, often relates to promoting shorter-term targets such as looking good in a holiday swimsuit or for a large social event such as a wedding or important party. The benefit of regular and sustained participation in health-promoting activity is less easy to quantify than athletic performance as the true health outcomes may only be observed after years of participation. Enhancing social and enjoyment aspects of participation in health-based exercise becomes a very important aspect of sustaining any regimen (Biddle & Mutrie 2001). More frequent bouts (≥ 3 times per week) of more intense activity provide a training threshold at which physiological fitness adaptations occur (i.e. enhanced cardiorespiratory fitness, improved blood lipid profile, glucose control and reduced insulin resistance) (ACSM 1998).

Physical *fitness* has seven components, which indicate the ability to perform a given task or physical activity. The benefits of improving fitness for health are twofold:

1. Being able to sustain an active life in order to contribute to one's personal needs and/or roles within family, community and society.
2. Improved fitness is inversely linked with the incidence of morbidity of a variety of diseases and all-cause mortality.

Whether exercising for health or sport performance, the seven components of fitness are the same (summarized below and in Fig. 1.1), namely:

1. *Aerobic (cardiorespiratory) power*, typically described as $\dot{V}O_2$max. This is the maximal amount of oxygen the body can take in and utilize. It is influenced by three factors: the lungs' ability to oxygenate the blood, the cardiovascular system's ability to deliver the oxygenated blood to the exercising muscles and the muscles' ability to extract and utilize the oxygen to produce energy for sustained contractions.

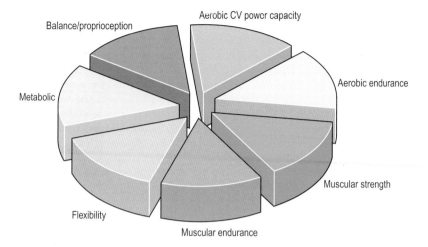

Figure 1.1   The components of physical fitness.

Inactivity and/or disease impair one or a combination of these three systems and hence reduce an individual's ability to function.

2. *Aerobic (cardiorespiratory) endurance* is the highest proportion of $\dot{V}O_2$max at which an individual can sustain >20 minutes' activity. It is closely allied to the lactate thresholds described in standard exercise physiology texts, the point at which muscular fatigue begins to be hastened. Elite endurance athletes can sustain activity typically at greater than 80% of their aerobic power, whereas sedentary or diseased individuals may only be able to sustain activity at 40–50% of aerobic power. What this means is that the inactive or diseased person not only has a reduced capacity but also cannot utilize as much of whatever capacity they possess compared with the more active or fitter individual.

3. *Metabolic function* from a health perspective relates to the ability to control blood sugar levels better and from an exercise performance perspective the ability to deal with or buffer exercise-related changes in muscle and blood pH. The latter demonstrates that the more active individual is also able to tolerate and deal with higher levels of metabolites, prolonging the time before muscular fatigue sets in.

4. *Muscular strength* is the absolute amount of force that can be generated for one maximal voluntary contraction. It also needs to be considered that movement strength is a product of both the force produced by individual muscles and the coordinated effect of a group of muscles. Strength is often represented by a one-repetition-maximum lift known as a '1-REP max'. As described in the next fitness component, muscular endurance, maintaining or increasing strength is functionally advantageous to older individuals. There are also metabolic and cardiovascular benefits from increased muscular strength. The stronger and larger muscle has a greater number of blood vessels. Theoretically, on exertion, possessing a greater number of blood vessels means a reduced rise in systolic blood pressure, compared to a smaller muscle, and a resultant reduced workload on the heart, and reduced sympathetic stimulation of the respiratory system. As discussed in a number of the chapters, reduced exertion-related symptoms provide both real and perceived enhancements to movement in daily living.

5. *Muscular endurance* relates to the anaerobic power of an individual and the ability to sustain the highest level of muscular contractions for periods between 30 seconds and 2 minutes. The older individual, whose life consists of short bouts of activity, is often limited more by a lack of strength and muscular endurance than by inadequate aerobic fitness.
6. *Flexibility* is the range of motion through which a joint or group of joints can be moved. It is a function of the flexibility of the soft tissues in and around a joint (tendons, ligaments and cartilage) plus the ability of the muscle's neurological unit to relax. All movement requires a given amount of flexibility and regardless of the strength or endurance capabilities an individual has, flexibility can be a key limiting factor to function and performance.
7. *Coordination/balance/proprioception* is the ability of an individual to perform a sequence of movements and their awareness of joint positions within space. For sports that involve dynamic skill (typically ball sports) and for those with neurological disease (e.g. stroke, Parkinson's, multiple sclerosis, head injury), this becomes the limiting factor in functional performance movement, regardless of strength, endurance and flexibility.

Within each of the chapters that follow, the discussions will often focus on the amount of exercise necessary to bring about some health benefit from simple increases in daily physical activity or by an improvement in any one of the above seven components of fitness (Fig. 1.2). With some conditions, the enhancement of one or a number of these seven components will become the focus of the evidence that relates to either decreases in morbidity and mortality or increased quality of life for individuals with a given health condition. For example, increased muscular strength and endurance and enhanced balance and coordination are primary outcome benefits for the older person (for instance in preventing falls) or an individual with osteoporosis.

INCREASING AND MAINTAINING PHYSICAL ACTIVITY

For the individual studying sport and exercise science/medicine there is much focus on the technical, biological or biomechanical measures that can be learned and researched. Yet these are of no value unless factors influencing an individual's behaviour of being physically active within free daily living and structured exercise are

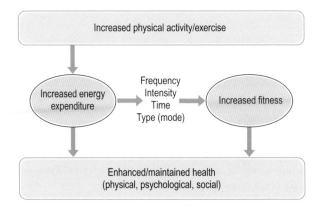

Figure 1.2   The relationship between health and physical activity/fitness.

seriously addressed by the exercise professional or healthcare practitioner. If physical activity is not maintained, then any related physical or psychological health gains will eventually be lost (Biddle & Mutrie 2001). In other words the benefits of increased physical activity cannot be 'banked' for the long term. For example, in the context of a structured exercise session (typically offered in a leisure, fitness or rehabilitation centre) it is important to acknowledge the overall psychological (cognitive and behavioural) milieu surrounding physical activity participation. Long-term maintenance of a physically active life is greatly influenced by the psychosocial environment of non-athletic individuals. Such a setting needs to ensure that the exercise is enjoyable, non-inhibiting, and promotes confidence and success. Most people do not engage in adequate amounts of physical activity to benefit health and approximately 50% of adults who begin an exercise programme drop out within 6 months. Therefore, encouraging people to initiate and sustain a physically active lifestyle is a difficult and challenging task for exercise professionals and healthcare practitioners.

Health professionals need to understand the key psychosocial factors influencing participation in physical activity and know how to address these factors in order to improve participation. In addition, understanding exercise issues specific to the client's medical condition is required, such as the dose needed to produce benefits, contraindications to exercise and the appropriate exercise prescription. The aim is to develop an exercise prescription/activity plan that is tailored to the individual's motivation, health status, lifestyle, activity and fitness levels, taking into account key psychosocial factors such as barriers to exercise and self-efficacy to ensure that clients adopt and maintain an active lifestyle in the long term.

A number of psychological and social factors have been shown to have a strong influence on participation in physical activity and exercise in both non-clinical and clinical populations (Trost et al 2002, Woodward et al 2001). These include self-efficacy, enjoyment of activity, social support, perceived benefits of activity and perceived barriers to activity. Therefore, targeting these factors can assist individuals with behaviour change. Furthermore, several theoretical models of behaviour change have been used to understand physical activity behaviour and interventions based on these models have successfully increased and maintained physical activity in the general population and client groups (Biddle & Mutrie 2001, Khan et al 2002). The following section describes key cognitive behavioural strategies that can be used to help clients adopt and sustain a physically active lifestyle. These strategies are guided by evidence-based models of behaviour change and target the key factors influencing participation in physical activity and exercise. The strategies can be applied to all client groups and include the stages of change, decisional balance, self-monitoring, goal-setting, enhancing self-efficacy and relapse prevention training. Healthcare professionals can use these techniques in consultations with individual clients but could also incorporate them into small-group-based exercise programmes.

Client–centred approach

Consultations about behaviour change are more effective if practitioners actively engage clients in the behaviour change process rather than persuading or telling them what to do (Rollnick et al 2005). Therefore, clients should be encouraged to accept responsibility for the behaviour change, to elicit their own reasons for change and set their own goals for change. The practitioner's task is to guide the client through the process by helping them weigh up the value of change and ensure realistic goals are set (Loughlan & Mutrie 1995, Rollnick et al 2005). Core interpersonal skills required to achieve a client-centred approach include good verbal and non-verbal communication, active listening and expressing empathy. For further information on the client-centred approach see Rollnick et al (2005) and Loughlan & Mutrie (1995).

Stages of change

The stages of change are part of the transtheoretical model (TTM), which has been used to understand and modify a broad range of health behaviours including physical activity (Biddle & Mutrie 2001). The TTM proposes that individuals attempting to change their physical activity behaviour progress through five stages. The stages differ according to an individual's motivation and behaviour, and have been labelled:

- precontemplation (inactive and no intention to change)
- contemplation (inactive, but intending to change in the next 6 months)
- preparation (engaging in some activity, but not regularly)
- action (regularly physically active, but only began in the past 6 months)
- maintenance (regularly active for more than 6 months).

Individuals progress through these stages at varying rates and often relapse back to an earlier stage when attempting behaviour change (Marcus & Simkin 1994). The model proposes that strategies to encourage change should be matched to the individual's stage or motivation (described in Table 1.1). Interventions based on the TTM have been effective in promoting and maintaining physical activity in several populations including people with type 2 diabetes and coronary heart disease (CHD) (Hughes et al 2007, Kirk et al 2004, Marcus et al 1998). Exercise practitioners can use the stages of change to assess an individual's motivation to become more active and then select appropriate stage-matched strategies to promote and maintain behaviour change. For further information on the TTM within the context of physical activity see Biddle & Mutrie (2001).

Decisional balance

The ability to weigh up the pros and cons of becoming more physically active has been significantly correlated with whether individuals do indeed become more physically active (Trost et al 2002, Woodward et al 2001). Decisional balance, a component of the TTM, involves a comparison of the perceived pros (benefits) and cons (costs) of

Table 1.1   Appropriate strategies to use in each stage of change (adapted from Biddle & Mutrie 2001)

Stage of change	Suggested strategies
Precontemplation	Raise awareness of the benefits of activity and risks of inactivity
Contemplation	Decisional balance (perceived pros and cons of activity), overcome barriers to activity
Preparation	Decisional balance, overcome barriers, set goals for increasing activity, seek support
Action	Set goals for regular activity, seek support, relapse prevention
Maintenance	Vary activities to prevent boredom, seek support, relapse prevention

increasing activity (Biddle & Mutrie 2001). Through this process, clients are asked to consider the personal benefits of becoming more active. Examples include increased fitness, improved well-being, increased confidence and better weight management. Health professionals may need to help clients understand the benefits of physical activity in relation to their medical condition (Biddle & Mutrie 2001). For example, a client with CHD may not realize that participation in regular physical activity will improve cardiac symptoms. The perceived cons (costs) of increasing activity should also be explored. Examples include having to make time for exercise and not liking to walk in inclement weather. It is likely that some perceived costs will be related to the client's medical condition. The exercise practitioner should help the client find ways to overcome or cope with perceived cons, for example having an alternative indoor activity to do when it is raining. The aim of the decisional balance is to help individuals realize that the pros of becoming active outweigh the cons. This is an important strategy for individuals in the contemplation and preparation stages of change because the perceived costs of exercise are likely to equal or outweigh the perceived benefits (Marshall & Biddle 2001).

Overcoming barriers to activity

A significant relationship between perceived barriers and involvement in exercise and physical activity has been demonstrated in several groups (Trost et al 2002, Woodward et al 2001). Therefore, identifying barriers to physical activity and devising ways to overcome these barriers is a useful strategy to increase activity (Biddle & Mutrie 2001). Some of the individual's barriers to activity will be similar to their perceived cons discussed previously. Common barriers to activity include time constraints, low fitness level, lack of energy and inclement weather. Possible solutions to these barriers are described in Box 1.1. It is likely that clinical groups will experience particular barriers to activity as a result of their medical condition and will need support from the exercise practitioner to overcome these barriers (Biddle & Mutrie 2001). For example, an individual with type 2 diabetes may fear that exercise will cause hypoglycaemia; therefore education on how to avoid this situation during and after exercise will be required. Perceived barriers to exercise among individuals with osteoporosis include fear of falling and concern that exercising will increase the risk of fracture. These anxieties could be alleviated by providing guidance on appropriate exercises. Many clients do not feel confident in their ability to engage in exercise, so reassurance that the exercise prescription will be tailored to the individual's abilities and disease state, and utilizing strategies to enhance confidence (see 'Enhancing self-efficacy' below) may address this barrier. Exercise practitioners

---

Box 1.1 Strategies to overcome barriers

- Lack of time: incorporate activity into daily living (e.g. walk part of the journey to work, walk at lunchtime) instead of having to take 'time out' of daily life to participate in structured exercise sessions.
- Low fitness: tailor the exercise prescription to the individual's physical ability and fitness level and very gradually increase the frequency, duration and/or intensity.
- Lack of energy: engage in moderate activities or accumulate activity in short bouts (e.g. 10 minutes), which require less effort than exercising vigorously or continuously.

should understand the specific barriers to exercise among the client group with whom they are working and be able to provide advice and reassurance about these barriers.

Social support

Social support has a major influence on participation in physical activity and exercise in clinical and non-clinical settings (Trost et al 2002, Woodward et al 2001). Sources of support include friends, family members, neighbours, exercise leaders and other participants, co-workers and health professionals. Different types of social support may be required, such as having a 'buddy' to go walking with, receiving encouragement and praise for achieving an activity goal, obtaining information and advice from an exercise practitioner on appropriate types of activity, and having someone to make it easier to be active (e.g. to look after the children so that the client can attend an exercise class). Joining an appropriate group exercise programme can provide a supportive environment for some individuals but choice of the programme is paramount; sometimes it can have the opposite effect on confidence and self-esteem from that intended.

Goal-setting and self-monitoring

Throughout this text, there will be specific physiological doses, targets or thresholds that need to be achieved in relation to the frequency, intensity, duration and type of activities performed. It must be remembered that each individual needs to be psychologically ready to cope with such targets, even if they are physiologically capable. Initially therefore the activity dose may need to be progressed from levels below the actual physiological target threshold, until such time as the client clearly has the self-efficacy to achieve it and the various social barriers have been overcome.

Goal-setting and self-monitoring are frequently used in physical activity interventions to increase and maintain people's motivation for behaviour change (Biddle & Mutrie 2001). The acronym SMARTER (specific, measurable, acceptable, realistic, time-phased, enjoyable and recorded) can be used to ensure effective goals are set (Biddle & Mutrie 2001). Specific goals (e.g. brisk walk for 15 minutes on 3 days per week) are more effective than vague, such as 'to be more active'. Goals should be acceptable and realistic in order to enhance confidence and ensure success. Individuals should be encouraged to make small, progressive changes to their physical activity behaviour by setting short-, intermediate- and long-term goals (Table 1.2). Participants should choose activities that they enjoy and they should receive a copy of their goals for future reference. Keeping a written record of physical activity patterns

Table 1.2   Effective goal-setting

2-week goal	2-month goal	4-month goal
Brisk walk for 15 minutes on 2 days	Increase brisk walking to 20 minutes on 3 days	Increase brisk walking to 30 minutes on 4 days
Use the stairs instead of the lift at work	Continue to use the stairs at work	Continue to use the stairs at work
		One swim session each week for 15 minutes

(i.e. self-monitoring) allows the individual to evaluate progress towards their goals. Individuals should set their own goals; however, the exercise practitioner should assist with goal-setting to ensure they follow SMARTER principles (Loughlan & Mutrie 1995, Rollnick et al 2005). Goals should be tailored to the individual's motivation, baseline levels of activity and fitness, lifestyle and health status and take into account other psychosocial factors such as barriers to activity and self-efficacy to ensure long-term adherence to exercise and physical activity.

Enhancing self–efficacy

Self-efficacy is an important component in a number of theoretical models including the TTM and has a very strong influence on the adoption and maintenance of physical activity in non-clinical and clinical settings (Trost et al 2002, Woodward et al 2001). Self-efficacy is defined as a person's confidence in their ability to perform a specific behaviour (Bandura 1977) and can have different forms including a person's confidence in their ability to participate in regular physical activity in certain situations (e.g. when they are tired after a hard day at work or when it is raining). It can also relate to a person's confidence in their ability to overcome typical barriers to exercise, to achieve an activity goal (e.g. walking continuously for 30 minutes daily) or to perform a specific activity (e.g. going to an aerobics class).

Self-efficacy can be enhanced by targeting the main sources of self-efficacy: mastery experiences, verbal persuasion, modelling and interpretation of physiological states (Biddle & Mutrie 2001). The experience of performing a task successfully (i.e. mastery experience) has a strong positive influence on self-efficacy. This can be achieved by dividing a challenging goal (e.g. walking continuously for 30 minutes daily) into manageable components (e.g. walking for 10 minutes three times daily) that individuals feel confident they can achieve; successfully mastering the smaller goal will increase their confidence in their ability to set and master more challenging goals. Verbal persuasion can build confidence through the provision of encouragement and praise from important others, for example an exercise practitioner praising a client for achieving an activity goal. Clients observing other people of similar age, physical characteristics or abilities successfully engaging in physical activity (known as modelling) can increase self-efficacy. This could be achieved by grouping people of similar abilities together in an exercise class, encouraging a client to attend an exercise class to observe others or providing examples of how similar clients have successfully increased physical activity. Self-efficacy can also be enhanced by having a plan to overcome barriers to exercise. Novice exercisers often view the normal physiological responses to exercise (i.e. increased heart rate and breathing, perspiration and muscle soreness) with some anxiety or discomfort, which can adversely affect self-efficacy. Therefore, exercise practitioners should teach participants how to monitor and positively interpret the body's response to activity.

High levels of self-efficacy are needed both to become regularly active *and* to maintain an active lifestyle in the long term (Marshall & Biddle 2001). Thus, an individual's self-efficacy for exercise and activity should be assessed and then developed using appropriate strategies.

Preventing relapse

Relapse prevention training is an effective strategy to encourage individuals to maintain regular physical activity in the long term (Biddle & Mutrie 2001, King et al 1988). Relapse is a breakdown or setback in a person's attempt to change a target behaviour.

The relapse prevention model was first developed to understand relapse from addictive behaviours such as alcoholism and smoking (Marlatt & Gordon 1985), but has since been applied to exercise and physical activity. The model proposes that relapse may result from an individual's inability to cope with situations that pose a risk of return to the previous behaviour. Common high-risk situations relevant to exercise and physical activity include bad weather, an increase in work commitments, boredom, change in routine or illness. Therefore, developing a plan to cope with high-risk situations will help to avoid relapse. For example, increased work commitments could be overcome by rescheduling an activity session or engaging in a shorter bout of activity. In addition, teaching individuals that a lapse from exercising (e.g. missing a few days of planned activities) need not lead to a relapse (missing planned activity sessions for an extended period) can help to improve adherence. If relapse is unavoidable, for example as a result of illness, then a gradual restart in activity is recommended. Overall, relapse prevention training involves helping individuals to identify high-risk situations that may cause a lapse or a relapse and helping them acquire strategies to cope with these high-risk situations.

Psychological effects of physical activity

This text focuses on managing the physiological and metabolic effects of exercise in a range of chronic diseases. However, participation in regular physical activity can also produce substantial psychological benefits in a range of clinical conditions (Department of Health 2004). These benefits include increased quality of life, improved mood, reduced anxiety and depression, and increased social opportunities. All of these factors impact on participation in physical activity. These benefits are important because many people with the medical conditions described throughout this text also have an impaired quality of life and reduced psychological well-being. There is evidence that the psychological effects of exercise may be just as important as the physiological effects among people with medical conditions (Biddle & Mutrie 2001, Oldridge et al 1988). Furthermore, it is the psychological effects of exercise that appear to motivate people to be physically active and continue participation in the long term (Biddle & Mutrie 2001).

MISPERCEPTIONS ABOUT PHYSICAL ACTIVITY

A possible reason for low levels of physical activity in the population may be a misperception that health benefits can only be achieved by participation in continuous, high-intensity exercise or sport (Biddle & Mutrie 2001). Many people may not realize that performing moderate amounts of physical activity can improve health and instead believe that they must exercise at a hard level to gain benefit. These perceptions are partly caused by the traditional exercise guideline (ACSM 1990), which recommended engaging in at least 20 minutes of continuous, vigorous exercise on 3 days per week to improve fitness. However, most people failed to achieve these recommendations and common reasons given for not exercising included not being the sporty type, lack of time, too much effort required and dislike of vigorous exercise (Biddle & Mutrie 2001). People are more likely to adopt and maintain moderate-intensity activity than high-intensity exercise (Trost et al 2002). It is now known that lower levels of physical activity than the amount required to improve fitness can produce substantial health benefits. New guidelines were published in 1995 which recommend accumulating 30 minutes of moderate physical activity on most days of the week to produce health benefits (Pate et al 1995). This recommendation is more acceptable for sedentary individuals and clinical groups who are likely to have low fitness levels and functional limitations, and may be more appealing to those who dislike vigorous exercise. It should be noted, however, that this recommendation is intended to complement the 1990 traditional exercise guideline. It is much easier for sedentary individuals to incorporate small bouts of moderate activity into their daily routine rather than engaging in structured, planned programmes of vigorous exercise. However, individuals who are moderately active will gain additional health and fitness benefits by increasing the duration and/or intensity of their activities. The American Heart Association and the American College of Sports Medicine have published a joint update on the appropriate doses of physical activity that positively influence health (Haskell et al 2007).

MONITORING THE EXERCISE DOSE

Physiological health and fitness benefits are a function of the total volume of physical activity performed. The components of the physical activity volume include the *frequency, intensity, duration* and *type of activity* (FITT) performed. This premise holds true for attaining improvement in each of the seven components of fitness (aerobic power, aerobic endurance, muscular strength, muscular endurance, flexibility, metabolic control, or balance/coordination). The debates continue on the 'optimal dose' required for health gain or fitness performance gain, where at one end of the spectrum is low-intensity activity with frequent bouts throughout the day and week and at the other end is higher-intensity activity performed in shorter bouts as little as one to two times per week (McFarlane et al 2006, *Medicine and Science in Sports and Exercise* 2001, Swain 2005).

PHYSICAL ACTIVITY MONITORING AND GUIDANCE

Measuring physical activity reliably and validly is far more difficult than measuring fitness. Fitness can be measured in a very controlled testing situation. However, physical activity is a measure which needs to be assessed throughout the hours and days of typical weeks within an individual's daily life. Within structured or controlled physical activity settings and environments (e.g. exercise classes, sports play, playground activity) it is now possible to accurately observe and measure energy expenditure, but the activities of a person's free daily living still pose a challenge to gaining an accurate measure of energy expenditure (Cordain et al 1998, Eaton & Eaton 2003).

The two gold standards for measuring physical activity within free daily living (not in a controlled laboratory) are doubly labelled water and accelerometry. In the *doubly labelled water technique*, participants are given a known volume of water which contains 'marker isotopes'. Over a period of days or weeks, samples of body water (from saliva, urine or blood plasma) are assessed for the elimination of these isotopes, which occurs through the body's metabolism. There is a direct correlation between energy expenditure and the amount of carbon dioxide and metabolic water produced. The changes in the isotopes in the body water over time are linked to oxygen usage and carbon dioxide production, both of which are main biochemical components of energy metabolism (Schoeller & van Santen 1982). The use of *accelerometers* involves placement of monitors on different parts of the body that aggregate recorded total motion activity of these different body segments over hours, days and weeks (Chen & Bassett 2005).

In addition to the high cost, the limitation of the doubly labelled water technique or accelerometry is that they do not give a good indication of the physiological intensity involved in the physical activities being monitored. Heart rate monitoring has been added into accelerometry devices in order to gain information on intensity and thus provide a better picture of the volume of activity being performed (Brage et al 2006).

It is important to determine whether the health gains from increases in activity levels include significant increases in fitness above and beyond the benefits of daily increases in caloric energy expenditure. Williams (2001) reported that when increased physical activity resulted in increased fitness, the health gains were significantly greater as compared to when daily energy expenditure was increased without gains in fitness. There were, however, definite health gains with increased daily physical activity even when improved fitness was not achieved.

Within health promotion and health-based physical activity, the practical and inexpensive alternative measures to doubly labelled water and accelerometry include physical activity diaries, questionnaires and pedometers. If questionnaire protocols or pedometers are being used they need to have been validated against either doubly labelled water, laboratory measures of energy expenditure and/or accelerometry. It is important, when evaluating the reliability and validity of the evidence for measuring energy expenditure, that one is aware of the benefits and drawbacks of the mode or device used to evaluate the volume of physical activity; much concern has been expressed about the use of self-report questionnaires and diaries on their own (Shephard 2003).

RELATIVE VERSUS ABSOLUTE INTENSITY OF PHYSICAL ACTIVITY

Throughout this text, beneficial levels of physical activity and exercise will be described either in absolute terms (e.g. speed, resistance, metabolic equivalents, heart rate) or in relative terms (e.g. percentage of maximal strength, maximal heart rate or maximal oxygen uptake). The health promotion message in Europe, the UK and the USA is for individuals to accumulate 30 minutes of moderate physical activity on most days of the week, with the option of allowing for this to be achieved in 10-minute bouts of activity (Department of Health 2004). One of the issues with this is deciding what constitutes 'moderate-intensity' activity? For the less fit, sedentary, older or clinical populations, the recommended 'absolute' walking pace of 3 miles per hour that qualifies for 'moderate intensity' (Lee et al 2001) could in fact qualify in 'relative' terms as vigorous activity; it is possible for this intensity in such individuals to be greater than 70% of maximal aerobic capacity. It is therefore important when reading the literature to see how moderate has been defined; is it in relative (e.g. percentage of one's maximum) or in absolute terms (e.g. a given walking speed, metabolic equivalent or, more recently, metabolic-equivalent-hours)?

AEROBIC EXERCISE

Typically the intensity of aerobic exercise is described as a percentage of one's maximal aerobic power ($\%\dot{V}O_2max$). In clinical or scientific settings a participant's $\dot{V}O_2max$ will be measured using a maximal testing protocol that involves the collection of pulmonary gas exchange responses to the exercise being performed. In conjunction with this will be measures of heart rate, blood pressure and blood lactate, ECGs, and ratings of perceived exertion (RPE) that can then be correlated with various proportions of an individual's $\dot{V}O_2max$. From the correlations between these measures a very accurate exercise prescription can be given. It is of importance to note when testing clinical populations that they may not meet the criteria for attaining a $\dot{V}O_2max$ (see guidelines from ACSM (2006) or the British Association of Sport and Exercise Sciences (Winter et al 2006)). They may have a clinical perturbation

Box 1.2 Example

An older or clinical-population individual will typically have a $\dot{V}O_2$max of 20 mL·kg^{-1}·min^{-1}. Assuming a resting $\dot{V}O_2$ is 3.5 mL·kg^{-1}·min^{-1}, they will have a $\dot{V}O_2$ reserve of 16.5 mL·kg^{-1}·min^{-1}. If they exercised at 65% of $\dot{V}O_2$max (13 mL·kg^{-1}·min^{-1}) this would require using 79% of $\dot{V}O_2$ reserve. For a younger to middle-aged individual, typically with a $\dot{V}O_2$max of 35 mL·kg^{-1}·min^{-1} and thus a $\dot{V}O_2$ reserve of 31.5 mL·kg^{-1}·min^{-1}, exercising at 65% of $\dot{V}O_2$max (22.8 mL·kg^{-1}·min^{-1}) would require using 72% of $\dot{V}O_2$ reserve. For the same %$\dot{V}O_2$max the older/clinical individual is actually using more of their $\dot{V}O_2$ reserve than the younger/fitter individual.

during the test or a co-morbidity that prevents them from attaining a true physiological maximum. In this instance test results reported in the evidence may often use the term $\dot{V}O_2$ peak. More recent evidence, especially when dealing with lower fitness populations, makes use of the $\dot{V}O_2$ reserve method (shown in Box 1.2), which takes into account the difference between resting and maximal oxygen uptake.

The ACSM recommendation for increasing aerobic capacity is to activate large muscle groups in a rhythmical manner for at least 20 minutes three times per week at an intensity greater than 50% of $\dot{V}O_2$max or 40% $\dot{V}O_2$ reserve (ACSM 1998). A period of at least 8 to 12 weeks is often cited as the length of time over which a significant change occurs. For some individuals who are very sedentary or fall within a clinical population, the ACSM recommendations give intensities as low as 40% $\dot{V}O_2$max as being an adequate physiological stimulus to bring about change. Where aerobic fitness is low due to a clinical condition, the minimum 20 minutes of exercise may be achieved through an interval approach giving participants periods of lower-intensity active recovery in between bouts of moderate-to-vigorous exercise.

In more advanced clinical settings or research work, aerobic exercise intensity is established using actual $\dot{V}O_2$max measures. However, in many practical settings, exercise intensity will be set using surrogates of $\dot{V}O_2$ and %$\dot{V}O_2$max (or %$\dot{V}O_2$ reserve); these include: heart rate, ratings of perceived exertion (RPE) and estimated metabolic equivalents (METs). It has long been established that heart rate is closely linked to $\dot{V}O_2$ (Åstrand et al 2003), which is why it provides the best indirect indication of $\dot{V}O_2$. This association includes the fact that $\dot{V}O_2$max and maximum heart rate coincide, maximum heart rate being estimated by subtracting the person's age from 220 (Robinson 1939). However, the error of this estimation is on average ±10 beat·min^{-1} (ACSM 2006). Heart rate reserve and % heart rate reserve maximum similarly provide a practical correlate for $\dot{V}O_2$ reserve. Determining heart rate reserve is typically known as the Karvonen method (Karvonen et al 1957), which is described in most standard exercise physiology texts and clinical exercise guidelines.

Borg's RPE scales are the most widely cited scales, and have been validated against relative physiological correlates (e.g. % maximum heart rate, blood lactate, %$\dot{V}O_2$max) during numerous modes of exercise in healthy, athletic and clinical populations (Borg 1998, Noble & Robertson 1996). They have become commonplace in exercise laboratories and exercise centres. As with any measurement tool, for it to be valid and reliable, these scales must be 'calibrated' properly with each user (see Buckley & Eston 2006 and Borg 1998 for guidance on appropriate use). Scale ratings between 12 and 15 on Borg's 6–20 scale or 3 and 4 on Borg's CR-10 scale relate to the level of lung and muscular sensations corresponding to the training thresholds described above; these scale points are linked to the anaerobic, lactate or ventilatory

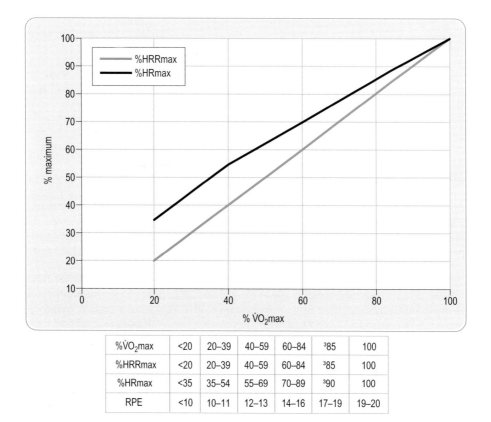

%$\dot{V}O_2$max	<20	20–39	40–59	60–84	³85	100
%HRRmax	<20	20–39	40–59	60–84	³85	100
%HRmax	<35	35–54	55–69	70–89	³90	100
RPE	<10	10–11	12–13	14–16	17–19	19–20

Figure 1.3   Summary of the relationship between the percentages of maximal aerobic power ($\dot{V}O_2$max), maximal heart rate reserve (%HRRmax), maximal heart rate (%HRmax) and Borg's rate of perceived exertion (RPE). (Adapted from ACSM 2006, Noble & Robertson 1996.)

thresholds typically described in the exercise physiology literature. A summary of the relationship between $\dot{V}O_2$, heart rate and RPE is presented in Figure 1.3.

MUSCULAR STRENGTH AND ENDURANCE

Muscular strength and endurance training that focuses on exercising specific muscle groups falls under one of three traditional categories:

- Swedish remedial/medical gymnastics for health and rehabilitation (Kleen 1921)
- 'body building' for purely aesthetic goals (Chapman 1994)
- athletic performance enhancement (Kraemer et al 2002; www.nsca-lift.org).

It is beyond the remit of this text to delve into the specific physiological and bio-mechanical principles of muscular strength and endurance training. The reader may be required to review, from other texts, some underpinning elements that relate to the evidence and its application to specific populations. The three main types of muscular contraction used in strength and endurance training are of specific note: iso-tonic, isometric and isokinetic. Some biomechanists may actually question the theoretical constructs of each of these types of contraction but from a practical perspective they are adequate to describe the type of exercise being performed. Typically *isotonic activity* involves using a fixed amount of weight (e.g. a dumbbell or barbell). In this case, the challenge of moving this given amount of resistance will be dependent upon the angle of the joint(s), which in turn affects the length and tension of the muscle at its tendons. *Isometric activity* indicates the presence of a muscular contraction where no joint movement occurs. *Isokinetic activity* refers to muscular work where velocity (linear, or more often, angular) is kept constant throughout the movement. This requires that the resistance changes with the joint angle, which is achieved by employing a device, machine or apparatus. All three types of muscular activity are used in health- and rehabilitation-based exercise.

It is important to remember that improved movement and functionality, rather than muscular strength/endurance, is the most important outcome of any training or rehabilitation programme. Often the evidence reports an improvement in muscular strength but this is only of value if it translates into enhanced functioning or performance. The movement power which can be generated by a person is not just a function of the size and strength of a muscle. It is also significantly influenced by the neurological motor coordination, dynamic balance, stability and ultimately the amount of muscular discomfort an individual is willing to tolerate in producing the given movement. For example, in the chapters on pulmonary and cardiac disease, evidence is presented that increased muscular strength, independent of aerobic exercise training, can enhance walking endurance. The potential mechanisms include improved movement efficiency as a result of improved dynamic stability of the ankle, knee, hip and pelvic-lumbar joints, and the ability to tolerate higher levels of muscle fatigue.

Establishing the strength training prescription

The standard reference point for muscular strength and endurance training is the one repetition maximum (1-RM) (www.nsca-lift.org). This is a practical surrogate measure for the physiological standard of the maximal voluntary contraction (MVC). The MVC requires accurate measurement devices whereas the 1-RM is determined using the exercise resistance equipment used within the training regimen. As with $\dot{V}O_2$max, in health and rehabilitation populations it may not be advisable, safe or even necessary to determine a 1-RM from which to establish an exercise prescription. If a weight causes a muscle to fatigue in 8 or fewer repetitions then the individual is likely to be working at >80% 1-RM, whereas for a weight which allows between 8 to 15 repetitions to be completed, the individual will be working at ~65% 1-RM (Kraemer et al 2002; www.nsca-lift.org).

For untrained individuals, older or clinical populations, strength gains can be attained by working at 50% 1-RM for 12–15 repetitions but this must be progressed towards higher intensities in the range of 8–12 repetitions (Kraemer et al 2002). With regard to populations covered in this text, the recommended training dose is a frequency of two to three times per week, at an intensity of >50% 1-RM, for a duration of 8 to 15 repetitions and involving 8 to 10 major muscle groups (ACSM 1998, Kraemer et al 2002, Pollock et al 2000). When the number of repetitions exceeds 15, then the resulting training adaptations are more likely to be increased metabolic endurance with smaller amounts of strength gain.

FLEXIBILITY

Performing flexibility exercises (e.g. stretching) pre- and post-training or sports performance has taken on almost a ritual status for most recreational exercisers or competitive and elite participants (Herbert & Gabriel 2007). The two aims of flexibility exercises are either preventing muscle/joint aches or injury, or improving joint flexibility to enhance movement capability or performance (Thacker et al 2004). There is a continuing debate on the effectiveness of pre- and post-event stretching as a means of preventing injury (Hart 2005, Thacker et al 2004). There is, however, consensus that flexibility exercises performed regularly two to three times per week lead to increased range of joint motion by improving the viscoelastic properties of the muscle tendons and joint ligaments (ACSM 1998). For individuals with joint trauma, this may increase amounts of pain-free movement.

The ACSM (1998) recommend one of three modes of training: static stretching, proprioceptive neuromuscular facilitation stretching (PNF) or ballistic stretching. The two latter techniques are recommended to be used only under expert supervision and with healthy athletic populations. Static stretching would seem the most prudent mode of stretching for health-based training within the general population or in non-athletic and clinical populations. The static stretch is recommended to be held for 10 to 30 seconds (no added benefit for holding for longer durations) and repeated four times for each muscle group, two to three times per week.

There again is a problem with finding practical means of accurately measuring changes in joint range of movement. The standard measurement technique within the evidence base is electrogoniometry (Gerhardt & Rondinelli 2001). From a clinical perspective, client feedback on incidence of symptoms or enhancements in movement performance is always the most important element and goal for both the practitioner and client.

BALANCE/COORDINATION/PROPRIOCEPTION AND MOVEMENT CONTROL

In many exercise physiology recommendations and documents, this area of health-related balance/coordination/proprioception and movement (discussed subsequently as movement control) is often overlooked. It rarely features officially as a component of fitness and yet much evidence is published on the 'trainability' of the neuromuscular interface. Typically it is included in the area of skill acquisition related to sport performance. However, it does not seem to feature highly within mainstream research or practice guidelines of health-related sports medicine and exercise science even though the evidence confirms that skill acquisition relates clearly to improved functional performance (or improved performance of everyday activities) and confidence. The three chapters in this text which exemplify the area of movement control are those concerned with exercise in spinal injury, neurological disorders and the ageing process. A good example of its importance can be drawn from people who suffer a stroke or a brain/head injury. The effects in some individuals may mean that their muscles may well have power but due to a loss of motor control of this power, simple functional movements are impaired or lost.

Within Western society, the average age of the population is increasing and the integration of balance and strength into exercise programming is gaining prominence as a key component of fitness related to maintaining functional independence and quality of life. At present, the majority of the population in Western society are under the age of 60 years and this goes some way to explaining why the present health promotion (primary prevention) focus is more on aerobic and metabolic health and fitness; both of these have strong links with the chronic diseases that consume much of the present day health service resources and influence general economic productivity (cardiovascular disease, diabetes, obesity, cancer and back pain). As the population ages, however, the potential of exercise to maintain and restore capacity in order to have a good quality of life will become more prominent as a result. It will be interesting to see in the future how health is perceived by a population dominated by older people. Will they be interested in issues of extending life beyond the age of 85 years or will more interest be placed on the 'quality of life'? So much of the present science related to healthcare focuses on adding 'years to life' as opposed to adding 'life to years'.

Due to the lack of prominence of exercise prescription guidelines for maintaining motor control throughout the lifespan, there is a paucity of reviews and published 'consensus statements' in this area. The chapter on older people in this book goes a long way to fulfilling much of this need. Unlike measuring levels of cardiorespiratory, muscular strength, and metabolic fitness, more specific tools to measure movement control are still to be developed for use in health promotion and exercise settings. At present, these assessment tools are restricted to use within secondary care settings by medical and therapy professionals. As health promotion work increases (e.g. to prevent falls) with frailer older people, it would be helpful for these assessment tools to be used as a means of risk screening and prevention, as opposed to waiting until an individual has an 'event' (e.g. a fall) before such tools are employed.

SUMMARY

A fully integrated approach to applying principles of exercise physiology, either for research or for practice, must include all seven components of fitness that have been discussed. A balance between attempts to enhance each of these seven components must then be integrated into a needs analysis that dovetails with the client's personal psychological and social motivations and limitations. Each of the chapters to follow will cover, in varying degrees, the evaluation and application of the seven components of fitness for each of the special conditions.

References

American College of Sports Medicine (ACSM) 1990 The recommended quality and quantity of exercise for developing and maintaining cardiorespiratory and muscular fitness in healthy adults. Medicine and Science in Sports and Exercise 22:265–274

American College of Sports Medicine 1998 Position stand on the recommended quantity and quality of exercise for developing and maintaining cardiorespiratory and muscular fitness, and flexibility in adults. Medicine and Science in Sports and Exercise 30:975–991

American College of Sports Medicine 2006 Guidelines for exercise testing and prescription. Lippincott Williams & Wilkins, Baltimore

Åstrand P, Rodahl K, Dahl H, Stromme S 2003 Textbook of work physiology: physiological bases of exercise. Human Kinetics, Champaign, IL

Bandura A 1977 Towards a unifying theory of behaviour change. Psychological Review 84:191–215

Biddle S J H, Mutrie N 2001 Psychology of physical activity: determinants, well-being and interventions. Routledge, London

Borg G A V 1998 Borg's rating of perceived exertion and pain scales. Human Kinetics, Champaign, IL

Brage S, Brage N, Ekelund U et al 2006 Effect of combined movement and heart rate monitor placement on physical activity estimates during treadmill locomotion and free-living. European Journal of Applied Physiology 96:517–524

Buckley J P, Eston R G 2006 Perceived exertion. In: Winter E, Jones A, Davison R C et al (eds) Sport and exercise physiology testing guidelines. Volume II: Exercise and clinical testing. Routledge, London

Chapman L 1994 Sandow the Magnificent: Eugene Sandow and the beginnings of bodybuilding. University of Illinois Press, Urbana, IL

Chen K Y, Bassett D R 2005 The technology of accelerometry-based activity monitors: current and future. Medicine and Science in Sports and Exercise 37(11 Suppl):S490–S500

Cordain L, Gotshall R W, Eaton S B, Eaton S B 1998 Physical activity, energy expenditure and fitness: an evolutionary perspective. International Journal of Sports Medicine 19:328–335

Department of Health 2004 At least five a week: evidence on the impact of physical activity and its relationship to health. A report from the Chief Medical Officer. Department of Health, Physical Activity, Health Improvement and Prevention, London

Eaton S B, Eaton S B 2003 An evolutionary perspective on human physical activity: implications for health. Comparative Biochemistry and Physiology. A. Molecular and Integrative Physiology 136:153–159

Gerhardt J J, Rondinelli R D 2001 Goniometric techniques for range-of-motion assessment. Physical Medicine and Rehabilitation Clinics of North America 12:507–527

Hart L 2005 Effect of stretching on sport injury risk: a review. Clinical Journal of Sports Medicine 15:113

Haskell W L, Lee I M, Pate R R et al 2007 Physical activity and public health. Update recommendation for adults from the American College of Sports Medicine and the American Heart Association. Medicine and Science in Sports and Exercise 39:1423–1434

Herbert R, Gabriel M 2007 Stretching to prevent or reduce muscle soreness after exercise: Cochrane Database of Systematic Reviews Issue 3. The Cochrane Collaboration, Wiley, London

Hughes A R, Mutrie N, MacIntyre P 2007 Effect of an exercise consultation on maintenance of physical activity after completion of phase III exercise-based cardiac rehabilitation. European Journal of Cardiovascular Prevention and Rehabilitation 14:114–121

Kahn E B, Ramsey L T, Brownson R C, Heath G W et al 2002 The effectiveness of interventions to increase physical activity. American Journal of Preventive Medicine 22:73–107

Karvonen M J, Kentala E, Mustala O 1957 The effects of training on heart rate; a longitudinal study. Annales Medicinae Experimentalis Biologiae Fenniae 35:307–315

King A C, Taylor C B, Haskell W L, DeBusk R F 1988 Strategies for increasing early adherence to and long-term maintenance of home-based exercise training in healthy middle-aged men and women. American Journal of Cardiology 61:628–632

Kirk A F, Mutrie N, MacIntyre P D, Fisher B M 2004 Promoting and maintaining physical activity in people with type 2 diabetes. American Journal of Preventive Medicine 27:289–296

Kleen A G 1921 Massage and medical gymnastics, 2nd edn. J A Churchill, London

Kraemer W J, Ratamess N A, French D N 2002 Resistance training for health and performance. Current Sports Medicine Reports 1(3):165–171

Lee I-M, Rexrode K M, Cook N R et al 2001 Physical activity and coronary heart disease in women: is 'no pain, no gain' passé? JAMA 285:1447–1454

Loughlan C, Mutrie N 1995 Conducting an exercise consultation: Guidelines for health professionals. Journal of the Institute of Health Education 33:78–82

Macfarlane D J, Taylor L H, Cuddihy F T 2006 Very short intermittent vs continuous bouts of activity in sedentary adults. Preventive Medicine 43:332–336

Marcus B H, Simkin L R 1994 The transtheoretical model: applications to exercise behaviour. Medicine and Science in Sports and Exercise 26:1400–1404

Marcus B H, Bock B C, Pinto B M et al 1998 Efficacy of an individualized, motivationally-tailored physical activity intervention. Annals of Behavioral Medicine 20:174–180

Marlatt G A, Gordon J R 1985 Relapse prevention: maintenance strategies in the treatment of addictive behaviors. Guilford Press, New York

Marshall S J, Biddle S J H 2001 The transtheoretical model of behavior change: A meta-analysis of applications to physical activity and exercise. Annals of Behavioral Medicine 23:229–246

Medicine and Science in Sports and Exercise 2001 Supplement: Dose-response issues concerning physical activity and health: an evidence-based symposium. Medicine and Science in Sports and Exercise 33(6):S345–S641

Noble B J, Robertson R J 1996 Perceived exertion. Human Kinetics, Champaign, IL

Oldridge N B, Guyatt G H, Fischer M E, Rimm A A 1988 Cardiac rehabilitation after myocardial infarction: combined experience of randomized clinical trials. JAMA 260:945–950

Pate R R, Pratt M, Blair S N et al 1995 Physical activity and public health. A recommendation from the Centers for Disease Control and Prevention and the American College of Sports Medicine. JAMA 273:402–407

Pollock M L, Franklin B A, Balady G J et al 2000 AHA Science Advisory. Resistance exercise in individuals with and without cardiovascular disease: benefits, rationale, safety, and prescription: An advisory from the Committee on Exercise, Rehabilitation, and Prevention, Council on Clinical Cardiology, AHA. Position paper endorsed by the ACSM

Robinson S 1939 Experimental studies of physical fitness in relation to age. arbeitsphysiologie 10:251–323

Rollnick S, Butler C, McCambridge J et al 2005 Consultations about changing behaviour. BMJ 331:961–963

Schoeller D A, van Santen E 1982 Measurement of energy expenditure in humans by doubly labeled water method. Journal of Applied Physiology 53:955–959

Shephard R J 2003 Limits to the measurement of habitual physical activity by questionnaires. British Journal of Sports Medicine 37:197–206

Swain D P 2005 Moderate or vigorous intensity exercise: Which is better for improving aerobic fitness? Preventive Cardiology 8:55–58

Thacker S B, Gilchrist J, Stroup D F, Kimsey C D 2004 The impact of stretching on sports injury risk: a systematic review of the literature. Medicine and Science in Sports and Exercise 36:371–378

Trost S G, Owen N, Bauman A E, Sallis J F 2002 Correlates of adults' participation in physical activity: review and update. Medicine and Science in Sports and Exercise 34:1996–2001

Williams P T 2001 Physical fitness and activity as separate heart disease risk factors: a meta-analysis. Medicine and Science in Sports and Exercise 33:754–761

Winter E, Jones A, Davison R et al 2006 Sport and exercise physiology testing guidelines. Volume II: Exercise and clinical testing. The British Association of Sport and Exercise Sciences Guide, Routledge, London

Woodward M C, Berry M J 2001 Enhancing adherence to prescribed exercise: structured behavioural interventions in clinical exercise programs. Journal of Cardiopulmonary Rehabilitation 21:201–209

Chapter 2

Obesity and diabetes

David Stensel

CHAPTER CONTENTS

Learning objectives   21
Introduction   22
Aetiology of obesity and diabetes   22
   Obesity   22
   Diabetes   25
Prevalence of obesity and diabetes   27
   Obesity   27
   Diabetes   29
Evidence that physical activity reduces
   the risk of obesity and diabetes   30
   Obesity   30
   Diabetes   32
Role of physical activity in managing
   obesity and diabetes   35
   Obesity   35
   Diabetes   36

Exercise prescription for the
   prevention and management of
   obesity and diabetes   38
   Obesity   38
   Diabetes   39
Co-morbidities   40
   Obesity   40
   Diabetes   40
Gaps in the evidence and
   practical issues   41
   Obesity   41
   Diabetes   41
Key points   41
References   42
Further reading   49

LEARNING OBJECTIVES

After studying this chapter, you should be able to:

1. Explain the energy balance equation and describe how obesity develops.
2. Identify some of the hormones involved in appetite regulation and describe the significance of these for obesity.
3. Explain how obesity is defined in children and adults.
4. Distinguish between type 1 and type 2 diabetes.
5. Understand the underlying causes of type 1 and type 2 diabetes.
6. Explain the link between obesity and type 2 diabetes.
7. Highlight literature indicating that the prevalence of obesity and type 2 diabetes is increasing in children and adults.
8. Critically evaluate the strengths and limitations of the evidence linking physical activity with the prevention of obesity and type 2 diabetes.

9. Critically evaluate the strengths and limitations of the evidence suggesting that physical activity is beneficial in the management of obesity and type 2 diabetes.
10. Make recommendations regarding the prescription of exercise for preventing obesity and type 2 diabetes and explain the rationale for these recommendations.
11. Make recommendations regarding the prescription of exercise for managing obesity and type 2 diabetes and explain the rationale for these recommendations.
12. Explain the co-morbidities associated with obesity and diabetes.
13. Suggest avenues for future research in the areas of obesity and diabetes.

INTRODUCTION

The focus of this chapter is on the relationship between physical activity, obesity and type 2 diabetes. Type 1 diabetes is occasionally mentioned in this chapter but the predominant focus is on obesity and type 2 diabetes. There is currently great interest in these areas for several reasons: (1) the prevalence of obesity and type 2 diabetes has increased in many countries in recent years both in adults and in children, (2) there is evidence to suggest that these trends are related in part to a general decline in physical activity levels amongst the inhabitants of developed countries, (3) several hormones have been discovered recently which have enhanced understanding of the mechanisms underlying obesity and diabetes and (4) there is evidence that changes in lifestyle – including increased levels of physical activity – are effective in preventing and managing obesity and type 2 diabetes.

AETIOLOGY OF OBESITY AND DIABETES

Obesity

Obesity is a condition involving an excessive accumulation of body fat such that health is endangered. Obesity is often defined using the body mass index (BMI), which is calculated by dividing weight (in kilograms) by height (in metres) squared, i.e. kg/m^2. A BMI $\geq 30\ kg/m^2$ is usually used as a cut-off point to indicate obesity and a BMI $\geq 25\ kg/m^2$ is usually used to indicate overweight. However, there are some issues with using the BMI as an indicator of obesity and these will be discussed later in the chapter.

It is generally accepted that obesity is caused by an imbalance between energy intake (food) and energy expenditure (physical activity). Thus, if energy consumption exceeds energy expenditure weight gain will occur and if this pattern continues over months and years then obesity will follow. Put simply, obesity is due to too much food and too little exercise. The validity of this 'model' has been questioned recently (see Gard & Wright 2005, pp. 37–67) but there does not seem to be a plausible alternative to this explanation. The situation is more complex than appears, however, since some of the energy consumed in food may be excreted instead of being absorbed into the body (Jacobsen et al 2005) and measurements of energy intake do not take this into account. Similarly, energy can be expended in 'non-purposeful' activities such as fidgeting (Levine et al 2000) and many of the methods used to estimate energy expenditure do not assess this.

A notable example of the influence of reduced food intake on bodyweight comes from a case report of a 27-year-old man who fasted under medical supervision for 382 days. The man initially weighed 207 kg and by the end of the fast his weight was reduced to 82 kg. Moreover, 5 years after undertaking the fast his weight was still relatively low at 89 kg (Stewart & Fleming 1973). Although this is an extreme example (which apparently made it into the Guinness Book of Records in 1971 as the longest recorded fast) it does illustrate clearly that weight loss occurs when food intake is reduced or absent. That the reverse is also true (i.e. weight gain occurs with overeating) has been demonstrated in an elegant experiment involving 12 pairs of monozygotic (identical) twins (Bouchard et al 1990). These twins were overfed by 4.2 MJ per day, 6 days per week for a total of 84 days during a 100-day period. This resulted in an excess energy intake of 353 MJ and an average weight gain of 8.1 kg (range 4.3 to 13.3 kg).

In addition to showing that overeating causes weight gain, the study of Bouchard and colleagues (1990) demonstrated that weight gain is dependent to some extent on genetic factors since there was about three times more variance in the amount of weight gain between twin pairs than within twin pairs. Other studies confirm that there is a genetic influence on weight gain. An interesting example is a study of 540 adult Danish adoptees. Despite the fact that 90% of these adoptees had been transferred to their adoptive homes within the first year of life there was a strong relationship between the weight class of the adoptees (thin, median weight, overweight and obese) and the BMI of their biological parents and no relationship between the weight class of the adoptees and the BMI of their adoptive parents (Stunkard et al 1986). These findings suggest that genetic influences are more important determinants of bodyweight (and presumably body fatness) than child-hood family environment.

Although evidence consistently indicates obesity has a strong genetic component this does not rule out overeating and inactivity as major causes of obesity. What is suggested is that some individuals are more susceptible to overeating and inactivity than others. Precisely why this should be remains elusive. With respect to overeating one likely cause is a variation in hormonal regulation of appetite. A clear example of this is leptin deficiency. This is associated with extreme obesity due to hyperphagia (overeating) and leptin therapy is effective in treating this disorder (Box 2.1, Table 2.1, Fig. 2.1). Some other hormones involved in appetite regulation that may be involved in the development of obesity are included in Table 2.2.

Leptin deficiency is a clear example of a monogenic (single gene) obesity syn-drome. Several other monogenic obesity syndromes have been identified and these

Box 2.1 Leptin

Leptin is a hormone secreted from adipocytes. Leptin acts as a long-term regulator of appetite via the hypothalamus. Leptin secretion is positively associated with the fat content of adipocytes. Thus, when the fat content of adipocytes is high leptin secretion is increased and hunger is suppressed. Conversely, if the fat content of adipocytes is low then leptin secretion will be low and hunger will be enhanced.

The discovery of leptin (in the mid-1990s) brought hope of a cure for obesity. It was thought that injections of leptin would suppress appetite in obese individuals and prevent them from overeating. It was subsequently discovered, however, that most obese individuals are not deficient in leptin – rather they have elevated levels but are insensitive to the appetite-suppressing effects of leptin (Considine et al 1996).

In a handful of cases humans have been identified who are leptin deficient. In these individuals, daily subcutaneous injections of leptin are highly effective in reducing bodyweight and fat mass as indicated in Table 2.1.

Table 2.1   Mean values for body mass, fat mass, fat-free mass and percentage body fat in three leptin-deficient patients who received daily subcutaneous injections of leptin for 18 months

	Baseline	18 months
Body mass (kg)	125.0	66.3
Fat mass (kg)	58.5	15.6
Fat-free mass (kg)	66.5	50.8
Body fat (%)	47.1	22.9

Data are from Licino et al (2004).

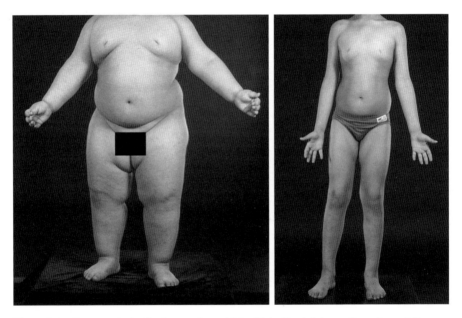

Figure 2.1   Response to leptin therapy in a child with leptin deficiency. From Farooqi & O'Rahilly (2005) with permission.

'dispel the notion that obesity represents an individual defect in behaviour with no biological basis' (Farooqi & O'Rahilly 2005). However, these syndromes are rare and they do not explain a large percentage of obesity cases. Other cases of obesity are likely to be polygenic and involve defects in several genes which influence both food intake and physical activity. The effects of these genes are only likely to be seen when the environmental conditions are conducive, i.e. when there is an abundant food supply and limited necessity for physical activity.

Table 2.2   Some of the hormones involved in appetite regulation and obesity

Hormone	Site of release	Action	Cause of obesity
Leptin	Adipocytes	Suppresses appetite via the hypothalamus	Yes – in a few cases (Farooqi et al 1999, Licino et al 2004)
PYY	Intestine	Suppresses appetite via the hypothalamus	Some evidence of deficiency in obese adults (Batterham et al 2003) and in obese children (Roth et al 2005)
CCK	Small intestine	Satiety signal. Slows gastric emptying. Delays transit time of food through the small intestine	Uncertain
Ghrelin	Stomach and duodenum	Enhances appetite via the hypothalamus	Uncertain, but ghrelin levels are increased after weight loss (Cummings et al 2002), encouraging weight regain
PP	Pancreas	Satiety signal	Uncertain
GLP-1	Intestine	Satiety signal	Uncertain
Oxyntomodulin	Small intestine	Satiety signal. Increases energy expenditure	Uncertain, but oxyntomodulin administration reduces food intake and increases energy expenditure in humans (Wynne et al 2006)
Obestatin	Stomach and duodenum?	Opposes the action of ghrelin	Recent discovery (Zhang et al 2005), too early to tell

PYY: Peptide YY; CCK: cholecystokinin; PP: Pancreatic polypeptide, GLP-1: Glucagon-like peptide 1.

Diabetes

Diabetes mellitus (sugar diabetes) refers to a group of metabolic disorders characterized by chronic hyperglycaemia (elevated blood glucose concentrations). Early warning signs of diabetes mellitus are excessive thirst and frequent urination. This is due to glucose being filtered out of the blood in the kidneys and then excreted in urine. Hence the term 'diabetes' (meaning 'siphon') 'mellitus' (meaning 'sweet'). There is another form of diabetes called diabetes insipidus which is also characterized by excessive thirst and frequent urination but in this case the urine is watery and non-sweet. Diabetes insipidus is caused by a low secretion of vasopressin (antidiuretic hormone, ADH) from the pituitary gland and thus a low reabsorption of water from the kidneys (Frayn 2003). This is a rare disease and will not be discussed further. Henceforth the term diabetes will be used when referring to diabetes mellitus.

There are two main forms of diabetes, termed type 1 and type 2. Type 1 diabetes is also known as juvenile onset diabetes because it usually begins in youth whereas type 2 diabetes is sometimes referred to as adult (or maturity) onset diabetes because it usually (though not always) begins in adulthood. Although hyperglycaemia is a feature of both forms of diabetes the underlying cause of this differs. Type 1 diabetes involves an insulin deficiency due to an autoimmune destruction of the insulin-producing β-cells in the pancreas whereas type 2 diabetes is characterized by insulin resistance (although insulin production may also be impaired).

Insulin deficiency and insulin resistance are a problem because insulin acts as a signal for liver cells, muscle cells and adipocytes to take up and store glucose. Left untreated, insulin deficiency and insulin resistance will lead to hyperglycaemia which is associated with damage to blood vessel walls and to nerves. This leads to a variety of complications and to premature mortality – most notably from cardiovascular disease. The only way to prevent hyperglycaemia in type 1 diabetes is by using insulin injections. Hence type 1 diabetes is also known as insulin-dependent diabetes mellitus (IDDM). In type 2 diabetes insulin resistance can be managed using diet and exercise as well as drugs to enhance insulin sensitivity. Insulin injections may be unnecessary with type 2 diabetes and because of this it is sometimes referred to as non-insulin-dependent diabetes mellitus (NIDDM).

Type 2 diabetes is the most prevalent form of diabetes, accounting for 90–95% of all cases (Krentz & Bailey 2001). An important determinant of type 2 diabetes risk is obesity. This has been demonstrated by the Health Professionals Follow-Up Study, which involved 27 270 men and 13 years of follow-up (Wang et al 2005). During the follow-up period 884 cases of type 2 diabetes emerged and there was a 'dose–response' relationship between BMI and risk of diabetes. Age-adjusted relative risk of diabetes for those in quintile 5 for BMI (27.2–54.2 kg/m^2) was 7.9 compared with those in quintile 1 for BMI (14.2–22.8 kg/m^2). Moreover, the association between waist circumference (a marker for abdominal obesity) and diabetes risk was higher than that between BMI and diabetes risk (Fig. 2.2). Some studies have found even stronger associations between obesity and type 2 diabetes risk. In the Nurses Health

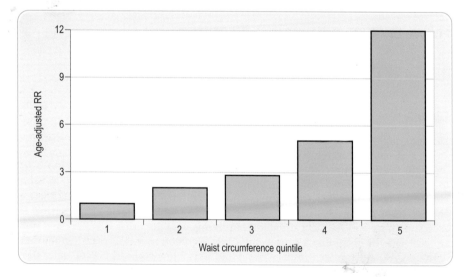

Figure 2.2 The association between waist circumference and relative risk (RR) of type 2 diabetes in the Health Professionals Follow-Up Study. Waist circumference values (cm) for each quintile are as follows: 1 (73.7–86.4), 2 (87.0–91.4), 3 (92.1–95.9), 4 (96.5–101.0), 5 (101.6–157.5). Figure drawn from data in Wang et al (2005).

Study, for example, women with a BMI $\geq 35 \text{ kg}/\text{m}^2$ were 60 times more likely to develop type 2 diabetes than women with a BMI $<22 \text{ kg}/\text{m}^2$ (Colditz et al 1990).

The mechanism by which obesity causes type 2 diabetes has not been conclusively established but obesity is associated with insulin resistance, which potentially decreases glucose uptake into adipocytes, muscle and the liver. This may be overcome by increased insulin secretion from the pancreas and some obese individuals manage to cope in this way without developing diabetes. For others, however, the pancreas cannot sustain high rates of insulin secretion indefinitely; in these individuals insulin secretion eventually declines and blood glucose concentration rises. Ironically, a contributing factor to hyperglycaemia in this latter group is increased endogenous glucose output from the liver (Weyer et al 1999).

Recent research suggests that a variety of proteins secreted by adipose tissue may play a role in obesity-associated insulin resistance and diabetes (Lazar 2005). One such protein is the hormone resistin (Steppan et al 2001). Resistin is a signalling molecule secreted from adipocytes. It is sometimes referred to as an adipocytokine, i.e. an adipocyte-derived cytokine (signalling protein). In mice, blood concentrations of resistin are elevated with obesity and the influence of resistin is antagonistic to that of insulin, i.e. increases in resistin concentration lead to reductions in glucose uptake into tissues. This may be due to a disruption of the insulin signalling mechanism within the cells (hence the name 'resistin', which means 'resistance to insulin'). In humans, however, the evidence linking resistin to diabetes and obesity is less clear (Berggren et al 2005).

Another potential link between obesity, insulin resistance and type 2 diabetes is adiponectin. Like resistin, adiponectin is released from adipocytes and is considered an adipocytokine. In contrast to resistin, however, a high concentration of adiponectin is associated with improved glucose tolerance and enhanced insulin sensitivity. Adiponectin concentration is reduced in obesity and type 2 diabetes (Weyer et al 2001) and there is some evidence that low adiponectin concentrations predict future risk of type 2 diabetes (Lindsay et al 2002).

PREVALENCE OF OBESITY AND DIABETES

Obesity

Surveys in many countries throughout the world have indicated that the prevalence of obesity has risen in recent years (British Heart Foundation 2005). This trend is occurring in both developed and developing countries (Mendez et al 2005). In the UK the prevalence of obesity (BMI $>30 \text{ kg}/\text{m}^2$) increased from 7% to 23% in men and from 12% to 23% in women between 1986 and 2003. This rate of increase is one of the highest in the world (British Heart Foundation 2005); higher in fact than the USA where data from the Behavioural Risk Factor Surveillance System indicated a nationwide prevalence (again based on a BMI $>30 \text{ kg}/\text{m}^2$) of 20% in 2000 (Mokdad et al 2001). A more recent report, however, states that the prevalence of obesity among adults in the USA has now risen to 32% (Ogden et al 2006). Table 2.3 shows the prevalence of obesity in selected countries worldwide.

Some writers have questioned the obesity prevalence figures due to legitimate concerns regarding the use of the BMI for assessing obesity (Gard & Wright 2005). A major concern is that the BMI does not distinguish between fat mass and fat-free mass. Thus, predictions of body fat may be inaccurate. This is particularly true for an individual with a BMI under $25 \text{ kg}/\text{m}^2$ but it can apply to those with higher BMIs also. Thus, it is argued that the widespread use of the BMI may be leading to artificially high estimates of the prevalence of overweight and obesity. Although there

Table 2.3 Obesity prevalence (BMI $\geq$30 kg/m^2) in selected countries worldwide. Data are from the British Heart Foundation (2005) except data for the USA which are from Ogden et al (2006)

Country	Year	Males (%)	Females (%)
Australia	1995	17.9	16.7
Canada	1996	13.3	11.8
China	1993	0.7	0.7
Finland	1997	20.1	19.2
Germany	1990–1	17.2	19.3
India	1995–6	0.3	0.6
Japan	1993	1.8	2.6
Jordan	1994–6	32.7	59.8
Netherlands	1996–8	6.5	9.1
New Zealand	1997	14.7	19.2
Samoa	1991	46.8	66.1
South Africa	1998	9.1	29.4
Spain	1989–94	11.5	15.2
UK	2003	23.0	23.0
USA	2003–4	31.1	33.2

may be some validity to this argument with respect to the prevalence of overweight (BMI between 25 and 30 kg/m^2) it seems less likely to be true for obesity. Moreover, among middle-aged adults, BMI is usually strongly correlated with fat mass measured using densitometry (Willett et al 1999).

Another concern with using the BMI is the extent to which it predicts future ill health. Again this is a legitimate concern as illustrated by the findings of the INTER-HEART case-control study, which examined the link between obesity and risk of myocardial infarction (MI) in 52 countries (Yusuf et al 2005). This study found only a 'modest' association between BMI and MI risk (the odds ratio for MI was 1.44 in the top quintile compared with the bottom quintile for BMI), leading to the suggestion that the BMI is 'obsolete' as a measure of obesity (Kragelund & Omland 2005). Measures of abdominal obesity (waist circumference, waist-to-hip ratio) were more closely associated with MI risk than BMI in the INTERHEART study but still the risk ratio for MI was less than 3 between those in the lowest and highest quintiles for each abdominal obesity marker. This is much lower than the risk ratio for lung cancer in smokers compared with non-smokers, which may be as high as 30. As noted earlier, however, the association between type 2 diabetes and obesity is stronger – particularly if waist circumference is used to indicate obesity.

Despite the limitations of using BMI for assessing obesity it has also been used to assess obesity prevalence in children. Centile curves have now been established for obesity by sex for each age group (0 to 18 years). These curves indicate the BMI for a given age which would pass through a BMI of 25 and 30 kg/m^2 respectively at age 18 (Cole et al 2000). For example, a BMI of 24 kg/m^2 in a 10-year-old boy would indicate a likely BMI of 30 kg/m^2 when this boy reaches 18 years of age. Using these centile curves, Chinn & Rona (2001) observed that although the prevalence of obesity increased in British children (aged 4 to 11 years) from 1984 to 1994, the overall prevalence was relatively low (2–3%). However, by 2002–2003 the estimated prevalence of obesity had risen to 6% in English boys and 6.6% in English girls aged 5 to 10 years (Stamatakis et al 2005).

Another study in England has examined obesity prevalence in very young children aged 2.9 to 4 years (Bundred et al 2001). In this study obesity was diagnosed by a BMI value above the 95th centile standardized for age and sex using British growth reference charts. Obesity prevalence increased from 5.4% to 9.2% between 1989 and 1998. The study also detected a significant increase in weight and BMI in children between these years but no significant change in height. Finally, a study involving 11- to 16-year-old children in England examined trends in waist circumference between 1977 and 1997 and observed that increases in waist circumference have 'greatly exceeded' those in BMI. The study concluded that the BMI is a poor proxy for central fatness and that the use of the BMI has systematically underestimated the prevalence of obesity in young people (McCarthy et al 2003).

Britain is not the only country experiencing an increase in the prevalence of childhood obesity. Childhood and adolescent obesity prevalence is increasing in the USA (Ogden et al 2006, Strauss & Pollack 2001) and in many other countries (Speiser et al 2005). This is a cause for concern because obesity in childhood increases the risk of obesity in later life (Whitaker et al 1997). Moreover, despite the frequently cited limitations of the BMI a recent study in adolescents found that BMI values were highly correlated with adiposity assessed using dual-energy X-ray absorptiometry (Steinberger et al 2005) and two recent reviews have concluded that BMI for age is a valid measure of both adiposity and morbidity risk in children (Must & Anderson 2006, Reilly 2006). In the future, however, it is likely that BMI measurements will be replaced or at least supplemented by direct assessments of adiposity in children. To this end body fat reference curves for children have been established (McCarthy et al 2006). In addition, measurement of waist circumference is likely to play a more prominent role in the assessment of childhood and adolescent obesity in future.

Diabetes

According to the International Diabetes Federation (2003) there are currently more than 194 million people (5.1% in the adult population) with diabetes worldwide and it is estimated that this figure will increase beyond 333 million (6.3% in the adult population) by 2025 if current trends continue. The International Diabetes Federation (2003) estimates that at least 50% of all people with diabetes are unaware of their condition and in some countries this figure may be as high as 80%. The prevalence of diabetes varies between countries. In some parts of the world the prevalence of diabetes is less than 2% (e.g. Vietnam), in others it is as high as 30% (i.e. Nauru in the Western Pacific). The prevalence of diabetes also varies between ethnic groups. For example, among Indian men in Singapore the prevalence of diabetes is over 20% whereas the national prevalence of diabetes in Singapore is around 12% (International Diabetes Federation 2003).

In 2003 the prevalence of diagnosed diabetes in England was 4% for men and 3% for women (type 2 diabetes accounts for 90% of these cases). Based on these figures it is estimated that 1.9 million adults have diagnosed diabetes in the UK (British Heart Foundation 2005). When this figure is combined with the estimated prevalence of undiagnosed diabetes in adults (600 000 men and women) it gives a total of 2.5 million adults in the UK with diabetes (British Heart Foundation 2005). The proportion of people with diabetes increases with age. Thus, in the 65 to 74 years age group, nearly 12% of men and over 8% of women in the UK have diabetes. It is interesting to note that approximately 30% of men and women in this age group have a BMI >30 kg/m^2. Such associations have also been noted in the USA. In the year 2000, for example, Mississippi had the highest rates of obesity (24.3%) and diabetes (8.8%) of any state in the USA (Mokdad et al 2001).

Consistent with the findings in adults, increases in diabetes prevalence have also been noted in children in many countries. Although type 1 diabetes accounts for a minority of diabetes cases in adults it is the predominant form of diabetes in children. In 2003, the prevalence of type 1 diabetes in children (aged 0 to 14 years) was estimated at 0.02% (430 000 cases worldwide). Furthermore, the estimated overall annual increase in type 1 diabetes is currently 3% (International Diabetes Federation 2003). The cause of this increase is unknown.

An emerging trend in recent years is the prevalence of type 2 diabetes in children. Pinhas-Hamiel & Zeitler (2005) provide an informative review of this area. The first cases of type 2 diabetes in children were reported in the late 1970s and early 1980s among Native Americans and Canadian First Nations people, who were known to be genetically susceptible. Since then there have been reports of type 2 diabetes in black and Hispanic American children, Japanese children and white American children. More recently cases have been reported in Europe (Pinhas-Hamiel & Zeitler 2005).

In the UK the first published report on type 2 diabetes in young people concerned children from the West Midlands and Leicester (Ehtisham et al 2000). Eight girls were identified with type 2 diabetes, aged 9–16 years. These girls were of Pakistani, Indian or Arabic origin. All of the girls were overweight and all had a family history of diabetes in at least two generations. Subsequently a report from Drake et al (2002) identified four obese white adolescents (three females and one male) aged 13 to 15 years who had type 2 diabetes. More recently it has been reported that the number of people aged 0 to 18 years admitted to hospital with type 2 diabetes has risen by 44% between 1996–1997 and 2003–2004 from 18 per million to 26 per million (Aylin et al 2005). Although this is a large increase in percentage terms it should be noted that the overall number of cases is low (498 patients aged 18 and under were admitted to English hospitals for type 2 diabetes in 2003–2004). Moreover, it is unclear at present whether this increase is real or is due to a better recognition and recording of type 2 diabetes in children. Nevertheless, these trends give cause for concern since they possibly 'represent only a small fraction of an increasing population of young people affected by … type 2 diabetes' (Aylin et al 2005).

EVIDENCE THAT PHYSICAL ACTIVITY REDUCES THE RISK OF OBESITY AND DIABETES

Obesity

Many observational studies have indicated that there is a relationship between physical inactivity and obesity (for reviews of these see Hill & Wyatt 2005, Wareham et al 2005). These studies have used a variety of techniques to assess physical activity including motion picture sampling (Bullen et al 1964), accelerometers (Ekelund et al 2002, Levine et al 2005), doubly labelled water (Esparza et al 2000, Weinsier et al 2002) and indirect calorimetry (Levine et al 2000) (see Frayn 2003, pp. 306–310, for an explanation of the assessment of energy expenditure using doubly labelled water and indirect calorimetry). Questionnaires have also been used to quantify leisure time physical activity (Haapanen et al 1997, Kahn et al 1997, Williamson et al 1993) and the physical activity involved in commuting to/from work (Lahti-Koski et al 2002). Other studies have used surrogate markers of physical inactivity (such as car ownership and television viewing) when attempting to determine the causes of obesity (Hancox et al 2004, Ludwig & Gortmaker 2004, Prentice & Jebb 1995). Although there are exceptions, there is general agreement among these studies that overweight and obese individuals are less physically active than non-obese individuals.

One recent study has confirmed an association between physical inactivity and obesity by studying changes in posture and movement associated with the routines of daily life (the investigators termed this non-exercise activity thermogenesis or NEAT). This study used inclinometers and triaxial accelerometers to measure NEAT in 10 obese and 10 lean subjects. Data were collected 120 times each minute over a 10-day period and the findings revealed that obese individuals were seated for an average of 2 hours longer each day than lean individuals. The investigators argued that posture allocation was biologically determined because it did not change when non-obese individuals gained 4 kg or when obese individuals lost 8 kg. It was concluded that obese individuals might expend an additional 350 kilocalories (1470 kJ) per day if they adopted the NEAT-enhanced behaviours of their lean counterparts (Levine et al 2005). Other research from this group suggests that the energy expenditure of 'fidgeting-like and low-grade activities' may differ markedly between individuals (Levine et al 2000) and that NEAT varies between people by up to 2000 kilocalories (8400 kJ) per day (Levine et al 2006).

Three recent questionnaire-based studies have confirmed a relationship between physical inactivity and age-related weight gain by examining the activity expended in recreational/sporting exercise (Littman et al 2005, Williams & Pate 2005, Williams & Wood 2006). Littman and colleagues examined the association between physical activity over the previous 10 years and weight change after age 45 in 15 500 participants aged 53 to 57 years. Both the amount (MET-hours) and frequency of activity were inversely related to weight gain after age 45 years. Associations were stronger for women than for men and for obese compared with normal weight individuals (Table 2.4). It was concluded that physical activity prevented some of the weight gain associated with ageing. These findings are supported by the findings of two studies examining the association between age and adiposity in runners (Williams & Pate 2005, Williams & Wood 2006). However, these studies also concluded that even among those most active, BMI and waist circumference increase with age.

Recent studies have also confirmed an association between physical inactivity and weight gain in childhood and adolescence. One notable example is a study of 1152 black and 1135 white girls from the USA, who were followed up prospectively from ages 9 or 10 to 18 or 19 years. Height, weight and skinfold thickness (at three sites) were assessed annually whereas habitual physical activity was assessed (via questionnaire) at years 1, 3, 5, and 7–10. The findings revealed smaller increases in BMI and sum of skinfolds in girls classed as active versus girls classed as inactive. At ages 18 or 19 years, BMI differences between active and inactive girls were 2.98 kg/m^2 for black girls and 2.10 kg/m^2 for white girls (Kimm et al 2005).

Table 2.4 Weight gain after age 45 years in obese (BMI $\geq$30 kg/m^2) men and women aged 53 to 57 years grouped by weekly frequency of physical activity over the previous 10 years. Values are adjusted for six potential confounding factors. Data are from Littman et al (2005)

Men					
Frequency (per week)	None	>0–1.4	1.5–3.4	3.5–6.1	6.2–25
Weight change (kg)	6.5	5.0	4.0	0.2	0.3
Women					
Frequency (per week)	None	>0–1.2	1.2–2.7	2.8–5.2	5.3–23
Weight change (kg)	6.5	5.8	3.7	2.5	−0.2

Another interesting study published recently involved Old Order Mennonites, a religious group who are resistant to social and technological changes and therefore live a traditional agrarian lifestyle. Physical activity was examined in children aged 8–13 years from this group using accelerometers. Health-related physical fitness was determined from measurements of triceps skinfold, grip strength, push-ups, partial curl-ups, and aerobic fitness (using a step test). The findings were compared with results from similar tests conducted in children from urban and rural Saskatchewan. Old Order Mennonite children were found to be leaner, stronger and more active than urban and rural dwelling children living a contemporary Canadian lifestyle. This was despite the fact that the Old Order Mennonite children were of low socio-economic status (a known correlate of obesity) and had no physical education classes or institutionalized sport (Tremblay et al 2005).

Physical inactivity is not a strong predictor of overweight and obesity in all paediatric studies, however. The Stockholm Weight Development Study (SWEDES) examined the association between physical activity and body composition in 445 (190 male, 255 female) 17-year-old adolescents. Physical activity was not significantly related to fatness in girls and explained $<4\%$ of the variance in body fatness in boys (Ekelund et al 2005, Styne 2005). Moreover, although a recent prospective cohort study found that children who watched more than 8 hours of television per week at 3 years of age were at increased risk of obesity at age 7, the strongest determinants of risk were obesity in both parents and very early (by 43 months) BMI or adiposity rebound (after an increase in the first year of life, BMI declines until the age of around 4 to 6 years after which it increases again – this is termed the adiposity rebound) (Reilly et al 2005). Furthermore, a recent systematic review identified being big and growing fast in infancy as risk factors for obesity in later life. This led the authors to conclude that strategies for the prevention of childhood and adult obesity might need to focus on the period before and during infancy (Baird et al 2005).

A limitation of all of the studies mentioned here is that they are observational and therefore they do not prove cause and effect. It is possible, for example, that overweight/obesity precedes inactivity in these studies and that inactivity is a consequence rather than a cause of obesity. Support for this suggestion comes from the finding that there is no difference in the physical activity levels (assessed by doubly labelled water measurement and by heart rate monitoring) of children aged 6–8 years who are or are not at risk of obesity based on the BMI values of their parents (Rennie et al 2005). Therefore, although the evidence from observational studies is fairly consistent in suggesting a role of physical inactivity in the development of obesity, randomized controlled trials are required to provide definitive evidence. Only a few trials of this nature have been completed and for various methodological reasons the conclusions are uncertain (Wareham et al 2005).

Diabetes

To the author's knowledge there is no evidence that physical activity reduces the risk of developing type 1 diabetes. There is, however, strong evidence that physical activity reduces the risk of developing type 2 diabetes. What follows is a brief review of some of this evidence. More extensive coverage of the evidence linking physical activity to the prevention of type 2 diabetes can be found elsewhere (Bassuk & Manson 2005, Hardman & Stensel 2003, Hawley 2004, LaMonte et al 2005).

Some of the earliest evidence suggesting a link between physical inactivity and the development of type 2 diabetes came from studies showing an increase in the prevalence of type 2 diabetes in societies that had abandoned a 'traditional' lifestyle in favour of a 'modern' (Westernized) lifestyle. One such group are the Pima Indians living in the USA. The presumption here is that 'traditional' lifestyles involve higher amounts of physical activity than modern lifestyles and that the decline in physical activity accompanying the adoption of a modern lifestyle is related to an increase in diabetes prevalence. Support for this proposition comes from the findings of migration studies that demonstrate an increased prevalence of type 2 diabetes in those who migrate to Westernized environments in comparison to their counterparts who remain in less urban/Westernized areas (Abate & Chandalia 2003, Albright et al 2000, Hawley 2004).

The findings from these early studies stimulated more rigorous investigation in this area in the form of observational epidemiological studies. These studies have consistently found an inverse association between physical activity and risk of type 2 diabetes. One example is the Nurses Health Study, which involved 84 941 nurses in the USA who were followed from 1980 to 1996. The relative risk of diabetes was 0.71 in those who reported 7 or more hours per week of moderate to vigorous physical activity (requiring an energy expenditure of 3 METs or more per hour) in comparison with those who reported less than 0.5 hours of weekly exercise. This indicated a 29% lower risk in the most active group compared with the least active group. These findings are similar to those of the Physicians' Health Study, which demonstrated an inverse association between the frequency of vigorous physical activity (enough to work up a sweat) and the relative risk of diabetes in male physicians (Manson et al 1992).

In addition to examining physical activity, the Nurses Health Study examined other lifestyle-related factors including diet, BMI, smoking status and daily alcohol consumption. Nurses classified as low risk by all five of these factors were found to have a relative risk of only 0.09 in comparison to nurses classified as high risk for all five factors. This corresponds to a 91% lower risk of developing type 2 diabetes in the 3.4% of nurses who were classified as low risk for all five factors (Hu et al 2001a). These findings emphasize the importance of a holistic approach when making recommendations with respect to diabetes prevention.

A few studies have examined the association between physical fitness and the risk of type 2 diabetes. One example is a study of 4747 Japanese men employed by the Tokyo Gas Company (Sawada et al 2003). These men were aged 20 to 40 years at baseline (in 1985) and were followed for 14 years (to 1999) during which time 280 cases of type 2 diabetes emerged. Cardiorespiratory fitness was estimated in this study using a submaximal cycle ergometer test and the Åstrand–Ryhming nomogram. The age-adjusted relative risk of developing type 2 diabetes was 0.25 (75% lower) in men in the highest quartile for estimated maximum oxygen uptake (mean: 51 mL·kg^{-1}·min^{-1}) compared with men in the lowest quartile (mean: 32 mL·kg^{-1}·min^{-1}). After adjustment for BMI, systolic blood pressure, family history of diabetes, smoking status and alcohol intake, the association between type 2 diabetes risk and cardiorespiratory fitness was attenuated but remained significant (Fig. 2.3). These findings are consistent with those of the Aerobics Centre Longitudinal Study, which also demonstrated an association between low cardiorespiratory fitness and subsequent risk of type 2 diabetes (Wei et al 1999).

Although the findings of observational studies are consistent in indicating a protective effect of physical activity and physical fitness for risk of type 2 diabetes they are not proof of cause and effect. It is possible, for example, that some of the participants in these studies were in the early (undetected) stage of developing type 2 diabetes and that it was this which led to their lower activity levels compared with those who did not go on to develop diabetes. Therefore, to provide more compelling evidence for the role of physical activity in preventing type 2 diabetes intervention studies are required.

Four intervention studies have been conducted to assess the role of physical activity in preventing type 2 diabetes. These are the Malmö Feasibility Study

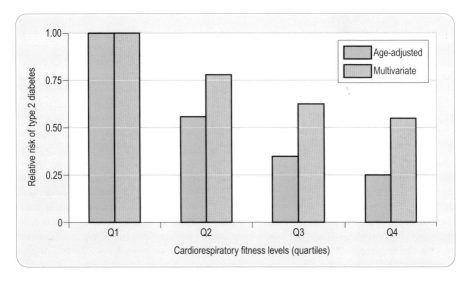

Figure 2.3 Relative risk of type 2 diabetes according to cardiorespiratory fitness levels in 4747 Japanese men followed for 14 years. Multivariate relative risk adjusted for age, BMI, systolic blood pressure, family history of diabetes, smoking status and alcohol intake. Figure drawn from data in Sawada et al (2003).

(Eriksson & Lindgärde 1991), the Da Qing Impaired Glucose Tolerance and Diabetes Study (Pan et al 1997), the Finnish Diabetes Prevention Study (Tuomilehto et al 2001) and the US Diabetes Prevention Program (Knowler et al 2002). All of these studies provide support for the notion that physical activity protects against the development of type 2 diabetes. Further details of these studies can be found in Hardman & Stensel (2003). Below is a brief summary of the findings of the Finnish Diabetes Prevention Study and the US Diabetes Prevention Program.

In the Finnish Diabetes Prevention Study 522 middle-aged, overweight men and women with impaired glucose tolerance were randomly assigned to either an intervention group or a control group. The intervention group received individualized counselling to help them achieve five goals as follows: (1) a reduction in weight of 5% or more, (2) a reduction in total fat intake to less than 30% of energy consumed, (3) a reduction in saturated fat intake to less than 10% of energy consumed, (4) an increase in fibre intake to at least 15 g per 1000 kcal and (5) moderate-intensity exercise for at least 30 minutes each day.

At the end of 4 years the cumulative incidence of type 2 diabetes (diagnosed by an oral glucose tolerance test) was 11% in the intervention group and 23% in the control group, indicating that lifestyle intervention more than halved the risk of diabetes. This lowering of risk occurred despite the fact that weight loss was modest in the intervention group (4.2 kg). Moreover, there were no cases of diabetes in participants who achieved four or five of the intervention programme goals. Also, among the subjects in the intervention group who did not reach the goal of losing 5% of their bodyweight but who achieved the goal of exercising for more than 4 hours per week the odds ratio for diabetes was 0.2 (80% lower risk) compared with those in the intervention group who remained sedentary (Tuomilehto et al 2001). This suggests that even in the absence of major weight loss exercise is effective in preventing type 2 diabetes.

The findings of the Finnish Diabetes Prevention Study were confirmed a year later by those of the Diabetes Prevention Program in the USA. This was a multicentre trial involving 3234 men and women with impaired fasting glucose and impaired glucose tolerance. Participants were randomized to one of three groups: placebo, lifestyle intervention or metformin (a drug used to reduce hepatic glucose production and increase insulin sensitivity). Participants on the lifestyle intervention programme were given the goals of achieving at least a 7% weight loss and 150 minutes of physical activity per week. The average follow-up was 2.8 years, during which time the incidence of diabetes was 11.0, 7.8 and 4.8 cases per 100 person-years in the placebo, metformin and lifestyle intervention groups, respectively. The lifestyle intervention reduced the incidence of diabetes by 58% and metformin by 31% in comparison with the placebo. The lifestyle intervention also reduced the incidence of diabetes by 39% in comparison with the metformin trial. These results held across all age groups and were similar in men and women regardless of ethnic group (Knowler et al 2002).

Collectively large-scale epidemiological and intervention studies provide strong evidence that physical activity is effective in preventing, or at least delaying, the development of type 2 diabetes. In addition, many laboratory-based studies have demonstrated that exercise improves insulin sensitivity and glucose tolerance. Such improvements have been noted in both healthy subjects and in insulin-resistant offspring of diabetic parents (Perseghin et al 1996). Studies have also shown that muscle contraction activates glucose transport by mechanisms which are independent of insulin (Jessen & Goodyear 2005). Readers who want more information on the mechanisms by which physical activity might prevent type 2 diabetes are referred to the following reviews: Gill & Malkova (2006), Hawley (2004), Holloszy (2005).

ROLE OF PHYSICAL ACTIVITY IN MANAGING OBESITY AND DIABETES

Obesity

Some studies have demonstrated large weight/fat losses in obese individuals after relatively short programmes in which exercise is the sole or main form of intervention. One example is a study of 197 obese men undergoing basic military training in the Singapore army. In this study recruits were divided into three categories based on their percentage body fat at baseline, i.e. 24 to <30%, 30 to <35% and ≥35%. After 5 months of training the mean weight loss for each of these groups was 10.7 kg, 13.1 kg and 16.1 kg, respectively (Lee et al 1994). Similarly a study involving obese Bulgarian women resident in a sanatorium has reported a 12.4 kg weight loss after a 45-day programme involving 10 hours of exercise per day (Hadjiolova et al 1982).

Unfortunately such findings are not the norm. A recent review of lifestyle intervention studies concluded that the average weight loss from combined diet and exercise programmes is 3 to 5 kg compared with no treatment or usual care. Moreover, in most studies with long-term follow-up, the initial weight loss is followed by weight regain (Jain 2005). How are these findings reconciled with the findings from studies demonstrating large exercise-induced weight losses? Firstly, most individuals do not have the time and support required to perform large volumes of exercise. Secondly, according to Haslam & James (2005), most obese individuals (80% or more) are insufficiently motivated to maintain long-term lifestyle change.

For those who do have the motivation to maintain a habit of regular exercise over the long term and to adhere to healthy eating guidelines there is evidence that weight loss can be achieved without going to the extremes of military training or residence in a sanatorium. The researcher John Jakicic has conducted extensive research in this area. In one of his studies combined diet and exercise intervention resulted in a 13 kg weight loss in participants who performed an average of 285 minutes of exercise every week (approximately 40 minutes per day) over an 18-month period (Jakicic et al 1999). Moreover, high physical activity levels (11 830 kJ/week) have been identified (along with low energy and fat intakes) as a common feature of individuals who are successful at long-term maintenance of substantial weight loss (Klem et al 1997, Wing & Phelan 2005).

There is some evidence that genetic factors play a role in the extent to which weight loss occurs with exercise. Bouchard and colleagues (1994) studied seven pairs of monozygotic twins over a period of 93 days while they were kept on a constant daily energy intake. Subjects cycled for close to an hour twice a day for 9 out of 10 days. This led to an estimated energy deficit of 244 MJ by the end of the training period. Although the average weight loss was 5 kg, weight loss varied between individuals from 1 to 8 kg. However, the variance between twin pairs was much greater than the variance within twin pairs. These findings suggest that exercise will be more effective as a means of weight loss in some individuals compared with others and that this is due in part to genetic factors. There is evidence to support this conclusion from animal studies (Levin & Dunn-Meynell 2006).

What is the role of exercise in the management of obesity in children? The conclusion of a recent review is that very few randomized controlled trials have investigated this issue and that the trials which have been conducted have been poorly controlled and have not specifically isolated the effects of exercise from those of dietary intervention (Watts et al 2005). At best the data appear inconsistent and when reductions in body fat or BMI have been found they have usually been small. This has not deterred investigators from pursuing this field of research with vigour and a variety of studies have been conducted in an effort to increase the physical activity levels of obese children. In one study, for example, television viewing was contingent on the pedalling of a stationary cycle ergometer. Beneficial changes in body composition were found in this study but as in other studies the changes were small (Faith et al 2001).

Diabetes

Many studies have indicated that physical activity and physical fitness have an important role to play in the treatment of type 2 diabetes. This evidence is pertinent for individuals with type 1 diabetes also, since these individuals suffer from similar complications to those with type 2 diabetes. However, there is only limited evidence available to support a benefit of physical activity for individuals with type 1 diabetes (Wadén et al 2005). Some of the evidence concerning physical activity in the treatment of type 2 diabetes is discussed below. Those wanting a more detailed coverage of this topic are referred to the American College of Sports Medicine Position Stand on exercise and type 2 diabetes (Albright et al 2000).

Fitness appears to provide some protection from the co-morbidities associated with elevations in blood glucose concentration. Kohl and colleagues (1992) examined the relationship between cardiorespiratory fitness (assessed using a maximal-exercise treadmill test), fasting blood glucose concentration and mortality risk in 8715 men followed for an average of 8.2 years. Men were categorized into one of three groups based on their fasting blood glucose concentrations as follows: <6.4 mmol/L, 6.4–7.8 mmol/L and ≥7.8 mmol/L. Low cardiorespiratory fitness was associated with a higher age-adjusted relative risk of death due to all causes in each of these groups. Other prospective cohort studies have demonstrated that low cardiorespiratory fitness and low levels of physical activity are independent predictors of cardiovascular and all-cause mortality in men with type 2 diabetes (Tanasescu et al 2003, Wei et al 2000).

Prospective cohort studies involving women have produced similar findings. One example is a study involving 5125 female nurses with type 2 diabetes. Physical activity was assessed via questionnaire on five occasions over a 14-year period of follow-up. The duration of moderate to vigorous physical activity performed each week was inversely related to the risk of cardiovascular disease (Fig. 2.4). This relationship remained significant after adjustment for smoking, BMI, and other cardiovascular disease risk factors. Moreover, among women who reported no vigorous exercise (i.e. no exercise $\geq$6 METs), walking volume (MET-hours per week) was also inversely related to cardiovascular disease risk (Hu et al 2001b).

In recent years the findings of observational studies concerning physical activity and type 2 diabetes have been supplemented by findings from randomized controlled trials. One example is a multifactorial intervention trial which was conducted in Denmark (Gaede et al 2003). Subjects were randomized to receive conventional treatment or intensive treatment which included both behaviour modification and pharmacological therapy. The intensive treatment group experienced significant decreases in glycosylated haemoglobin values (a marker for blood glucose concentration over the previous 6 to 8 weeks), systolic and diastolic blood pressure, serum cholesterol and serum triglycerides in comparison to the conventional-therapy group. The relative risk of cardiovascular disease was also halved in this group, as was the risk of other diabetic complications such as nephropathy, retinopathy and neuropathy. In this study the exercise prescription for the intensive treatment group involved light-to-moderate exercise for at least 30 minutes three to five times weekly. Unfortunately, the design of the study did not allow the investigators to identify

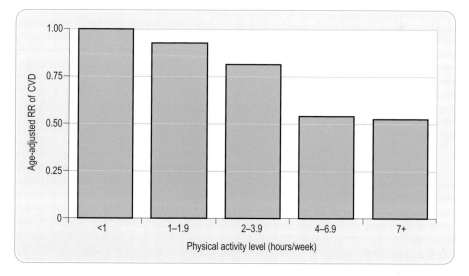

Figure 2.4   The age-adjusted relative risk of cardiovascular disease (CVD; non-fatal myocardial infarction, fatal coronary heart disease and stroke) in 5125 female nurses with type 2 diabetes according to the volume of moderate to vigorous physical activity performed each week. The follow-up duration was 14 years. Figure drawn from data in Hu et al (2001b).

which aspects of the intensive intervention were most effective. This is an area for future research.

The goal of treatment in diabetes is to achieve and maintain near-normal blood glucose and blood lipid concentrations thereby preventing or delaying complications such as cardiovascular disease. Many studies indicate that exercise is beneficial in controlling blood glucose in individuals with type 2 diabetes. A meta-analysis of controlled clinical trials concluded that exercise training significantly reduces glycosylated haemoglobin (HbA_{1c}) concentrations in individuals with type 2 diabetes by an amount that should decrease the risk of diabetic complications (Boulé et al 2001). Most of the studies included in this meta-analysis employed aerobic exercise such as walking and cycling. However, strength training has also been shown to increase insulin-mediated glucose uptake in skeletal muscle in patients with type 2 diabetes (Holten et al 2004). Furthermore, there is evidence that exercise training can enhance β-cell function in patients with type 2 diabetes (Dela et al 2004) in addition to improving insulin sensitivity (Hawley 2004).

EXERCISE PRESCRIPTION FOR THE PREVENTION AND MANAGEMENT OF OBESITY AND DIABETES

Obesity

Guidelines are available regarding the prescription of exercise for preventing and managing obesity (Hill & Wyatt 2005, Jakicic & Otto 2005, Jakicic et al 2001). There is recognition within these guidelines that further research is required to fine-tune the guidance given. It will also be apparent to the reader that there will be individual differences in the response to exercise and therefore some individuals may require more exercise than others to prevent weight gain or to lose weight. Dietary intake will also influence the extent to which exercise is effective in preventing and managing obesity.

Hill & Wyatt (2005) believe that energy expenditure has dropped so low in modern environments that it is very difficult for humans to balance energy intake and energy expenditure. Elsewhere, using data from national surveys, Hill and colleagues (2003) estimate that affecting energy balance by 100 kilocalories (420 kJ) per day could prevent weight gain in most people. They go on to hypothesize that this could be achieved by 15 minutes per day of walking (this is in addition to existing activity). Presumably this habit would need to be maintained throughout life and there is the assumption that energy intake would not increase to compensate for the additional activity.

Other experts give a higher recommendation regarding the amount of exercise required to prevent weight gain. Jakicic & Otto (2005) give an initial target of 150 minutes of exercise per week (20 plus minutes each day). This is based on exercise guidelines for health (US Department of Health and Human Services 1996), which recommend 30 minutes of moderate-intensity physical activity on most, if not all, days of the week. Even this may not be enough, however. In the UK a recent Department of Health (2004) report concluded that for many people 45–60 minutes of moderate-intensity physical activity per day would be required to prevent obesity. In the USA, the Institute of Medicine (2002) has also recommended 60 minutes of exercise per day (420 minutes per week) for weight control.

The American College of Sports Medicine Position Stand on appropriate intervention strategies for weight loss and the prevention of weight regain for adults (Jakicic et al 2001) provides clear and comprehensive guidance for those wishing to lose weight through exercise. Their recommendation is that overweight and obese individuals initially perform a minimum of 150 minutes per week of moderate-intensity physical activity and that for long-term weight loss 200–300 minutes per week are required or ≥2000 kilocalories (8400 kJ). These are not dissimilar to the guidelines for preventing obesity – in fact they are lower than the Institute of Medicine (2002) guidelines. However, the guidelines for weight loss assume that energy intake is reduced by 500 to 1000 kilocalories (2100 to 4200 kJ) per day concurrently with increases in energy expenditure.

Although exercise can be effective in reducing weight without concurrent dietary intervention (Ross et al 2000), exercise is most likely to be effective when it is combined with diet. This is true in reverse also, i.e. dietary intervention is most likely to be effective if it is supplemented by exercise. This is demonstrated by the findings of a recent systematic review that examined the influence of diet alone compared with diet and exercise for managing overweight and obesity. Studies employing both diet and exercise produced 20% greater initial weight loss than studies employing diet alone (13 kg versus 9.9 kg) and 20% greater sustained weight loss after 1 year (6.7 kg versus 4.5 kg). For both forms of intervention, however, almost half of the initial weight loss was regained after 1 year (Curioni & Lourenço 2005).

Overall energy expenditure is probably the most important factor for weight loss through exercise (Jeffery et al 2003). Moreover, there is some evidence that exercise duration is more important for weight loss than exercise intensity (Jakicic et al 2003). It should be recognized, however, that higher physical activity levels are also associated with higher injury rates (Jeffery et al 2003).

Provided that the energy expenditure of exercise is sufficient, the mode of exercise used should not matter. However, the most effective mode of exercise for expending energy is aerobic exercise and walking is one of the most popular activities for individuals wishing to lose weight. Exercise does not need to be performed in a structured setting because at least one study has demonstrated that diet and lifestyle activity (walking instead of driving, taking the stairs instead of the lift, etc.) are as effective for weight loss as diet plus structured aerobic exercise (Andersen et al 1999).

Diabetes

How much physical activity is required to prevent type 2 diabetes? The four intervention studies conducted so far provide some guidance here. In the Finnish Diabetes Prevention Study the recommendation was 30 minutes per day of moderate-intensity activity. In the US Diabetes Prevention Program just over 20 minutes of exercise per day (150 minutes per week) was recommended. In the Da Qing study the recommendation varied from 5–10 minutes of very strenuous exercise to between 30 and 60 minutes of mild exercise. A variety of activities were employed in these studies including walking, running, swimming, cycling, circuit training, volleyball, basketball, dancing, skipping and household tasks. However, none of these studies were able to identify clearly the contribution of physical activity to diabetes prevention.

Recent evidence suggests that although obesity and physical inactivity are both independent predictors of type 2 diabetes risk, the strength of this association is much greater for obesity than for physical inactivity (Weinstein & Sesso 2006). In view of this the optimum exercise prescription for reducing the risk of type 2 diabetes risk may be identical to the prescription for preventing obesity, i.e. 150 minutes per week of moderate-intensity physical activity initially building up to 200 to 300 minutes per week later on. Such doses of exercise have been shown to be effective in improving insulin sensitivity and should therefore assist in preventing type 2 diabetes (Houmard et al 2004, McAuley et al 2002).

The American College of Sports Medicine Position Stand on exercise and type 2 diabetes (Albright et al 2000) gives clear guidelines for the prescription of exercise in type 2 diabetics. These recommend that exercise be performed on at least three non-consecutive days each week at low to moderate intensity (40–70% of maximum oxygen uptake). The recommended duration of each exercise session is 10 to 15 minutes initially building up to 60 minutes per session over time. The exercise mode depends on personal preference and may include a variety of activities including resistance training. Walking is one of the most popular activities for those with type 2 diabetes but for those with complications (see below) non-weight-bearing activities such as cycling and swimming may be preferable.

High levels of leisure time physical activity have been shown to be associated with improved glycaemic control in women with type 1 diabetes (Wadén et al 2005). However, trial and error is required to adjust the insulin dose to prevent either hyperglycaemia or hypoglycaemia. One recent study has shown that overnight hypoglycaemia after exercise is common in children with type 1 diabetes (Tsalikian et al 2005). This indicates the importance of modifying diabetes management after afternoon exercise in those with type 1 diabetes.

CO-MORBIDITIES

Obesity

Aside from type 2 diabetes, obesity is associated with several other co-morbidities including coronary heart disease, hypertension, stroke, several forms of cancer, and arthritis (Haslam & James 2005). The extent to which obesity increases the risk of these co-morbidities is a matter of debate and probably depends on factors such as the severity of obesity and genetic differences between individuals. The extent to which obesity reduces life expectancy is also a matter of controversy. Some writers have concluded that the youth of today may not live as long as their parents (Olshansky et al 2005). However, recent evidence indicates that cardiovascular disease risk factors (excluding diabetes) are less prevalent in obese individuals now than was the case 40 years ago – at least for those living in the USA (Gregg et al 2005). There is also evidence that the impact of obesity on mortality may have decreased over time in developed countries, possibly due to improved public health and medical care (Flegal et al 2005, Mark 2005).

Diabetes

Life expectancy is reduced by 5 to 10 years in individuals with type 2 diabetes if they are diagnosed in middle age, i.e. between 40 and 60 years. In developed countries the age-adjusted relative risk of mortality is approximately twofold higher in type 2 diabetics compared with non-diabetic individuals. The main cause of premature death with type 2 diabetes is cardiovascular disease including coronary heart disease and stroke (Krentz & Bailey 2001). This is due to microvascular disease (affecting the capillaries) and macrovascular disease (affecting larger vessels) and can affect the arteries of the limbs as well as the coronary arteries. Other common problems include hypertension, kidney problems (nephropathy), nerve damage (neuropathy), and eye problems (retinopathy and cataract). These problems are linked to chronically elevted blood glucose concentrations. Diabetics who maintain good control over their blood glucose and blood lipid concentrations have a reduced risk of these complications (Frayn 2003).

Another complication of type 2 diabetes is acute glycaemic reactions and the risk of these may be increased during exercise, particularly in diabetics being treated with insulin or other medications. Therefore, such individuals must take precautions when exercising (for further guidance see Albright et al 2000, McKnight-Menci et al 2005).

GAPS IN THE EVIDENCE AND PRACTICAL ISSUES

Obesity

Further research is required regarding the method used to define obesity. A simple method is needed which will predict body fatness more accurately than BMI. There is also a need for a better indicator of the disease risks associated with obesity. The waist circumference is being used more frequently for such purposes and appears to be promising in this respect. Another need is for further research into the BMI and waist circumference cut-off points related to disease risk in ethnically diverse populations (Haslam & James 2005, Misra et al 2006).

With regard to exercise, randomized controlled trials are required to clarify the role of physical inactivity for future weight gain. Although long-term trials of this nature are not feasible, short-term (up to a year) trials could help to identify more clearly the role of physical inactivity in weight gain. Research is also required to identify the best methods to motivate individuals to become active and to remain active. The influence of the surrounding environment (e.g. urbanization, litter, graffiti, greenery, etc.) on physical activity levels and obesity prevalence also warrants consideration in future (Ellaway et al 2005).

Diabetes

Although several intervention studies have demonstrated that lifestyle intervention is effective in delaying or preventing the development of type 2 diabetes, it is not clear from these trials how important physical activity is in comparison to dietary change. This is a major question for future research. Further research is also required to determine how best to facilitate efficient programmes for the primary prevention of diabetes (Sherwin et al 2002). The role of exercise in preventing type 2 diabetes in ethnic groups known to be at high risk for developing diabetes (e.g. South Asians) is also worthy of consideration in future, as is the role of exercise in preventing type 2 diabetes in children.

Regarding the use of physical activity in the management of diabetes, future research should address the relative contribution of physical activity versus diet in preventing cardiovascular disease and other co-morbidities associated with type 1 and type 2 diabetes. Further information regarding the optimum frequency, mode, intensity and duration of exercise required to prevent and manage diabetes would also be useful.

KEY POINTS

1. Obesity develops when energy intake exceeds energy expenditure over a prolonged period of time. Genetic predisposition increases the risk of obesity.

2. The most commonly accepted definition for obesity in adults is a BMI $\geq$30 kg/m^2. In children and adolescents, one method of defining obesity is the BMI for a given age and sex which predicts a BMI $\geq$30 kg/m^2 in adulthood.

3. Although there are limitations to the accuracy of the BMI for predicting body fatness, it is useful for identifying trends within populations over time. Waist circumference is also a useful marker for obesity and disease risk.

4. Diabetes is a disease characterized by chronic hyperglycaemia. In type 1 diabetes this is caused by a deficient insulin secretion from the pancreas; in type 2 diabetes the main characteristic is resistance to the effects of insulin, although insulin secretion may also be deficient.

5. Obesity causes insulin resistance in some individuals and is associated with an increased risk of type 2 diabetes.

6. The prevalence of obesity and type 2 diabetes is increasing in both children and adults in many countries.

7. There is a large body of observational evidence linking physical inactivity with the development of obesity but the associations are often weak and it is difficult to prove that inactivity precedes the development of obesity.

8. There is strong evidence that physical activity (in combination with dietary intervention) can prevent the development of type 2 diabetes in those at high risk of the disease.

9. Exercise is an effective method for losing weight, particularly if it is combined with dietary intervention. However, a large percentage of people regain the weight they have lost through diet and exercise due to a relapse in eating and exercise behaviours.

10. There is strong evidence that physical activity and physical fitness help to prevent or reduce the severity of cardiovascular disease and other co-morbidities associated with type 2 diabetes.

11. As a general guide, health benefits will accrue if 30 minutes of moderate-intensity exercise is performed on most days of the week. Higher volumes of exercise are probably more beneficial in preventing and managing both obesity and type 2 diabetes.

12. Several health risks are associated with obesity, most notably type 2 diabetes. Type 2 diabetes in turn increases the risk of coronary heart disease, stroke and hypertension, as well as nerve, kidney and eye damage.

13. Further research is required to optimize the role of exercise in the prevention and management of obesity and diabetes.

References

Abate N, Chandalia M 2003 The impact of ethnicity on type 2 diabetes. Journal of Diabetes and Its Complications 17:39–58

Albright A, Franz M, Hornsby G et al 2000 Exercise and type 2 diabetes. Medicine and Science in Sports and Exercise 32:1345–1360

Andersen R E, Wadden T A, Bartlett S J et al 1999 Effects of lifestyle activity vs structured aerobic exercise in obese women. Journal of the American Medical Association 281:335–340

Aylin P, Williams S, Bottle A 2005 Dr Foster's case notes. Obesity and type 2 diabetes in children, 1996–7 to 2003–4. British Medical Journal 331:1167

Baird J, Fisher D, Lucas P et al 2005 Being big or growing fast: systematic review of size and growth in infancy and later obesity. British Medical Journal 331:929–931

Bassuk S S, Manson J E 2005 Epidemiological evidence for the role of physical activity in reducing risk of type 2 diabetes and cardiovascular disease. Journal of Applied Physiology 99:1193–1204

Batterham R L, Cohen M A, Ellis S M et al 2003 Inhibition of food intake in obese subjects by peptide YY_{3-36}. New England Journal of Medicine 349:941–948

Berggren J R, Hulver M W, Houmard J A 2005 Fat as an endocrine organ: influence of exercise. Journal of Applied Physiology 99:757–764

Bouchard C, Tremblay A, Després J P et al 1990 The response to long-term overfeeding in identical twins. New England Journal of Medicine 322:1477–1482

Bouchard C, Tremblay A, Després J P et al 1994 The response to exercise with constant energy intake in identical twins. Obesity Research 2:400–410

Boulé N G, Haddad E, Kenny G P et al 2001 Effects of exercise on glycemic control and body mass in type 2 diabetes mellitus. A meta analysis of controlled clinical trials. Journal of the American Medical Association 286:1218–1227

British Heart Foundation 2005 Coronary heart disease statistics. British Heart Foundation, London

Bullen B A, Reed R B, Mayer J 1964 Physical activity of obese and non-obese adolescent girls appraised by motion picture sampling. American Journal of Clinical Nutrition 14:211–233

Bundred P, Kitchiner D, Buchan I 2001 Prevalence of overweight and obese children between 1989 and 1998: population based series of cross sectional studies. British Medical Journal 322:326–328

Chinn S, Rona R J 2001 Prevalence and trends in overweight and obesity in three cross sectional studies of British children, 1974–94. British Medical Journal 322:24–26

Colditz G A, Willett W C, Stampfer M J et al 1990 Weight as a risk factor for clinical diabetes in women. American Journal of Epidemiology 132:501–513

Cole T J, Bellizzi M C, Flegal K M et al 2000 Establishing a standard definition for child overweight and obesity worldwide: international survey. British Medical Journal 320:1240–1243

Considine R V, Sinha M K, Heiman M L et al 1996 Serum immunoreactive-leptin concentrations in normal-weight and obese humans. New England Journal of Medicine 334:292–295

Cummings D E, Weigle D S, Frayo R S et al 2002 Plasma ghrelin levels after diet-induced weight loss or gastric bypass surgery. New England Journal of Medicine 346:1623–1630

Curioni C C, Lourenço P M 2005 Long-term weight loss after diet and exercise: a systematic review. International Journal of Obesity 29:1168–1174

Dela F, Von Linstow M E, Mikines K J et al 2004 Physical training may enhance β-cell function in type 2 diabetes. American Journal of Physiology Endocrinology and Metabolism 287:E1024–E1031

Department of Health 2004 Physical activity, health improvement and prevention. At least five a week. Department of Health, London

Drake A J, Smith A, Betts P R et al 2002 Type 2 diabetes in obese white children. Archives of Disease in Childhood 86:207–208

Ehtisham S, Barrett T G, Shaw N J 2000 Type 2 diabetes mellitus in UK children – an emerging problem. Diabetic Medicine 17:867–871

Ekelund U, Åman J, Yngve A et al 2002 Physical activity but not energy expenditure is reduced in obese adolescents: a case-control study. American Journal of Clinical Nutrition 76:935–941

Ekelund U, Neovius M, Linné Y et al 2005 Associations between physical activity and fat mass in adolescents: the Stockholm Weight Development Study. American Journal of Clinical Nutrition 81:355–360

Ellaway A, Macintyre S, Bonnefoy X 2005 Graffiti, greenery, and obesity in adults: secondary analysis of European cross sectional survey. British Medical Journal 331:611–612

Eriksson E F, Lindgärde F 1991 Prevention of type 2 (non-insulin-dependent) diabetes mellitus by diet and physical exercise. The 6-year Malmö feasibility study. Diabetologia 34:891–898

Esparza J, Fox C, Harper I T et al 2000 Daily energy expenditure in Mexican and USA Pima Indians: low physical activity as a possible cause of obesity. International Journal of Obesity 24:55–59

Faith M S, Berman N, Heo M 2001 Effects of contingent television on physical activity and television viewing in obese children. Pediatrics 107:1043–1048

Farooqi I S, O'Rahilly S 2005 New advances in the genetics of early onset obesity. International Journal of Obesity 29:1149–1152

Farooqi S, Jebb S A, Langmack G et al 1999 Effects of recombinant leptin therapy in a child with congenital leptin deficiency. New England Journal of Medicine 341:879–884

Flegal K M, Graubard B I, Williamson D F et al 2005 Excess deaths associated with underweight, overweight, and obesity. Journal of the American Medical Association 293:1861–1867

Frayn K N 2003 Metabolic regulation: a human perspective. Blackwell Science, Oxford

Gaede P, Vedel P, Larsen N et al 2003 Multifactorial intervention and cardiovascular disease in patients with type 2 diabetes. New England Journal of Medicine 348:383–393

Gard M, Wright J 2005 The obesity epidemic: science, morality and ideology. Routledge Taylor and Francis, London

Gill J M R, Malkova D 2006 Physical activity, fitness and cardiovascular disease risk in adults: interactions with insulin resistance and obesity. Clinical Science 110:409–425

Gregg E W, Cheng Y J, Cadwell B L et al 2005 Secular trends in cardiovascular disease risk factors according to body mass index in US adults. Journal of the American Medical Association 293:1868–1874

Haapanen N, Miilunpalo S, Pasanen M et al 1997 Association between leisure time physical activity and 10-yr body mass change among working-aged men and women. International Journal of Obesity and Related Metabolic Disorders 21:288–296

Hadjiolova I, Mintcheva L, Dunev S et al 1982 Physical working capacity in obese women after an exercise programme for body weight reduction. International Journal of Obesity 6:405–410

Hancox R J, Milne B J, Poulton R 2004 Association between child and adolescent television viewing and adult health: a longitudinal birth cohort study. Lancet 364:257–262

Hardman A E, Stensel D J 2003 Physical activity and health: the evidence explained. Routledge, London

Haslam D W, James W P 2005 Obesity. Lancet 366:1197–1209

Hawley J A 2004 Exercise as a therapeutic intervention for the prevention and treatment of insulin resistance. Diabetes Metabolism Research Reviews 20:383–393

Hill J O, Wyatt H R 2005 Role of physical activity in preventing and treating obesity. Journal of Applied Physiology 99:765–770

Hill J O, Wyatt H R, Reed G W et al 2003 Obesity and the environment: where do we go from here? Science 299:853–855

Holloszy J O 2005 Exercise-induced increase in muscle insulin sensitivity. Journal of Applied Physiology 99:338–343

Holten M K, Zacho M, Gaster M et al 2004 Strength training increases insulin-mediated glucose uptake, GLUT4 content, and insulin signalling in skeletal muscle in patients with type 2 diabetes. Diabetes 53:294–305

Houmard J A, Tanner C J, Slentz C A et al 2004 Effect of volume and intensity of exercise training on insulin sensitivity. Journal of Applied Physiology 96:101–106

Hu F B, Manson J E, Stampfer M J et al 2001a Diet, lifestyle, and the risk of type 2 diabetes mellitus in women. New England Journal of Medicine 345:790–797

Hu F B, Stampfer M J, Solomon C et al 2001b Physical activity and risk for cardiovascular events in diabetic women. Annals of Internal Medicine 134:96–105

Institute of Medicine 2002 Dietary reference intakes for energy, carbohydrate, fibre, fat, protein, and amino acids. National Academy Press, Washington, DC

International Diabetes Federation 2003 Diabetes atlas, 2nd edn. International Diabetes Federation. Online. Available: www.idf.org/e-atlas. Accessed 31 March 2006

Jacobsen R, Lorenzen J K, Toubro S et al 2005 Effect of short-term high dietary calcium intake on 24-h energy expenditure, fat oxidation, and fecal fat excretion. International Journal of Obesity 29:292–301

Jain A 2005 Treating obesity in individuals and populations. British Medical Journal 331:1387–1390

Jakicic J M, Otto A D 2005 Physical activity considerations for the treatment and prevention of obesity. American Journal of Clinical Nutrition 82(Suppl):S226–S229

Jakicic J M, Winters C, Lang W et al 1999 Effects of intermittent exercise and use of home exercise equipment on adherence, weight loss, and fitness in overweight women. A randomized trial. Journal of the American Medical Association 282:1554–1560

Jakicic J M, Clark K, Coleman E et al 2001 Appropriate intervention strategies for weight loss and prevention of weight regain for adults. Medicine and Science in Sports and Exercise 33:2145–2156

Jakicic J M, Marcus B H, Gallagher K I et al 2003 Effect of exercise duration and intensity on weight loss in overweight, sedentary women. A randomized controlled trial. Journal of the American Medical Association 290:1323–1330

Jeffery R W, Wing R R, Sherwood N E et al 2003 Physical activity and weight loss: does prescribing higher physical activity goals improve outcome? American Journal of Clinical Nutrition 78:684–689

Jessen N, Goodyear L J 2005 Contraction signalling to glucose transport in skeletal muscle. Journal of Applied Physiology 99:330–337

Kahn H S, Tatham L M, Rodriguez C et al 1997 Stable behaviours associated with adults' 10-year change in body mass index and likelihood of weight gain at the waist. American Journal of Public Health 87:747–754

Kimm S Y S, Glynn N W, Obarzanek E et al 2005 Relation between the changes in physical activity and body-mass index during adolescence: a multicentre longitudinal study. Lancet 366:301–307

Klem M L, Wing R R, McGuire M T et al 1997 A descriptive study of individuals successful at long-term maintenance of substantial weight loss. American Journal of Clinical Nutrition 66:239–246

Knowler W C, Barrett-Connor E, Fowler S E et al 2002 Reduction in the incidence of type 2 diabetes with lifestyle intervention or metformin. New England Journal of Medicine 346:393–403

Kohl H W, Gordon N F, Villegas J A et al 1992 Cardiorespiratory fitness, glycaemic status, and mortality risk in men. Diabetes Care 15:184–192

Kragelund C, Omland T 2005 A farewell to the body mass index? Lancet 366:1589–1591

Krentz A J, Bailey C J 2001 Type 2 diabetes in practice. Royal Society of Medicine Press, London

Lahti-Koski M, Pietinen P, Heliövaara M et al 2002 Associations of body mass index and obesity with physical activity, food choices, alcohol intake, and smoking in the 1982–1997 FINRISK Studies. American Journal of Clinical Nutrition 75:809–817

LaMonte M J, Blair S N, Church T S 2005 Physical activity and diabetes prevention. Journal of Applied Physiology 99:1205–1213

Lazar M A 2005 How obesity causes diabetes: not a tall tale. Science 307:373–375

Lee L, Kumar S, Chin Leong L 1994 The impact of five-month basic military training on the body weight and body fat of 197 moderately to severely obese Singaporean males aged 17 to 19 years. International Journal of Obesity 18:105–109

Levin B B, Dunn-Meynell A A 2006 Differential effects of exercise on body weight gain and adiposity in obesity-prone and -resistant rats. International Journal of Obesity 30:722–727

Levine J A, Schleusner S J, Jensen M D 2000 Energy expenditure of nonexercise activity. American Journal of Clinical Nutrition 72:1451–1454

Levine J A, Lanningham-Foster L M, McCrady S K et al 2005 Interindividual variation in posture allocation: possible role in human obesity. Science 307:584–586

Levine J A, Vander Weg M W, Hill J O et al 2006 Non-exercise activity thermogenesis. The crouching tiger hidden dragon of societal weight gain. Arteriosclerosis, Thrombosis, and Vascular Biology 26:729–736

Licinio J, Caglayan S, Ozata M et al 2004 Phenotypic effects of leptin replacement on morbid obesity, diabetes mellitus, hypogonadism, and behaviour in leptin-deficient adults. Proceedings of the National Academy of Sciences 101:4531–4536

Lindsay R S, Funahashi T, Hanson R L et al 2002 Adiponectin and development of type 2 diabetes in the Pima Indian population. Lancet 360:57–58

Littman A J, Kristal A R, White E 2005 Effects of physical activity intensity, frequency, and activity type on 10-y weight change in middle-aged men and women. International Journal of Obesity 29:524–533

Ludwig D S, Gortmaker S L 2004 Programming obesity in childhood. Lancet 364:226–227

McAuley K A, Williams S M, Mann J I et al 2002 Intensive lifestyle changes are necessary to improve insulin sensitivity. Diabetes Care 25:445–452

McCarthy H D, Ellis S M, Cole T J 2003 Central overweight and obesity in British youth aged 11–16 years: cross sectional surveys of waist circumference. British Medical Journal 326:624–626

McCarthy H D, Cole T J, Fry T et al 2006 Body fat reference curves for children. International Journal of Obesity 30:598–602

McKnight-Menci H, Sababu S, Kelly S D 2005 The care of children and adolescents with type 2 diabetes. Journal of Pediatric Nursing 20:96–106

Manson J E, Nathan D M, Krolewski A S et al 1992 A prospective study of exercise and incidence of diabetes among US male physicians. Journal of the American Medical Association 268:63–67

Mark D H 2005 Deaths attributable to obesity. Journal of the American Medical Association 293:1918–1919

Mendez M A, Monteiro C A, Popkin B M 2005 Overweight exceeds underweight among women in most developing countries. American Journal of Clinical Nutrition 81:714–721

Misra A, Vikram N K, Gupta R et al 2006 Waist circumference cut-off points and action levels for Asian Indians for identification of abdominal obesity. International Journal of Obesity 30:106–111

Mokdad A H, Bowman B A, Ford E S et al 2001 The continuing epidemics of obesity and diabetes in the United States. Journal of the American Medical Association 286:1195–1200

Must A, Anderson S E 2006 Body mass index in children and adolescents: considerations for population-based applications. International Journal of Obesity 30:590–594

Ogden C L, Carroll M D, Curtin L R et al 2006 Prevalence of overweight and obesity in the United States, 1999–2004. Journal of the American Medical Association 295:1549–1555

Olshansky S J, Passaro D J, Hershow R C et al 2005 A potential decline in life expectancy in the United States in the 21st century. New England Journal of Medicine 352:1138–1145

Pan X R, Li G W, Hu Y H et al 1997 Effects of diet and exercise in preventing NIDDM in people with impaired glucose tolerance. Diabetes Care 20:537–544

Perseghin G, Price T B, Petersen K F et al 1996 Increased glucose transport-phosphorylation and muscle glycogen synthesis after exercise training in insulin-resistant subjects. New England Journal of Medicine 335:1357–1362

Pinhas-Hamiel O, Zeitler P 2005 The global spread of type 2 diabetes mellitus in children and adolescents. Journal of Pediatrics 146:693–700

Prentice A M, Jebb S A 1995 Obesity in Britain: gluttony or sloth? British Medical Journal 311:437–439

Reilly J J 2006 Diagnostic accuracy of the BMI for age in paediatrics. International Journal of Obesity 30: 595–597

Reilly J J, Armstrong J, Dorosty A R et al 2005 Early life risk factors for obesity in childhood: cohort study. British Medical Journal 330:1357–1359

Rennie K L, Livingstone M B E, Wells J C K et al 2005 Association of physical activity with body composition indexes in children aged 6–8 y at varied risk of obesity. American Journal of Clinical Nutrition 82:13–20

Ross R, Freeman J A, Janssen I 2000 Exercise alone is an effective strategy for reducing obesity and related comorbidities. Exercise and Sport Sciences Reviews 28:165–170

Roth C L, Enriori P J, Harz K et al 2005 Peptide YY is a regulator of energy homeostasis in obese children before and after weight loss. Journal of Endocrinology and Metabolism 90:6386–6391

Sawada S S, Lee I M, Muto T et al 2003 Cardiorespiratory fitness and the incidence of type 2 diabetes: prospective study of Japanese men. Diabetes Care 26:2918–2922

Sherwin R R, Anderson R M, Buse J B et al 2002 The prevention or delay of type 2 diabetes. Diabetes Care 25:742–749

Speiser P W, Rudolf M C J, Anhalt H et al 2005 Consensus Statement: Childhood obesity. Journal of Clinical Endocrinology and Metabolism 90:1871–1887

Stamatakis E, Primatesta P, Chinn S et al 2005 Overweight and obesity trends from 1974 to 2003 in English children: what is the role of socio-economic factors? Archives of Disease in Childhood 90:999–1004

Steinberger J, Jacobs D R, Raatz S et al 2005 Comparison of body fatness measurements by BMI and skinfolds vs dual energy X-ray absorptiometry and their relation to cardiovascular risk factors in adolescents. International Journal of Obesity 29:1346–1352

Steppan C M, Bailey S T, Bhat S et al 2001 The hormone resistin links obesity to diabetes. Nature 409:307–312

Stewart W K, Fleming L W 1973 Features of a successful therapeutic fast of 382 days' duration. Postgraduate Medical Journal 49:203–209

Strauss R S, Pollack H A 2001 Epidemic increase in childhood overweight, 1986–1998. Journal of the American Medical Association 286:2845–2848

Stunkard A J, Sørensen T I A, Hanis C et al 1986 An adoption study of human obesity. The New England Journal of Medicine 314:193–198

Styne D M 2005 Obesity in childhood: what's activity got to do with it? American Journal of Clinical Nutrition 81:337–338

Tanasescu M, Leitzmann M F, Rimm E B et al 2003 Physical activity in relation to cardiovascular disease and total mortality among men with type 2 diabetes. Circulation 107:2435–2439

Tremblay M S, Barnes J D, Copeland J L et al 2005 Conquering childhood inactivity: is the answer in the past? Medicine and Science in Sports and Exercise 37:1187–1194

Tsalikian E, Mauras N, Beck R W et al 2005 Impact of exercise on overnight glycemic control in children with type 1 diabetes mellitus. Journal of Pediatrics 147:528–534

Tuomilehto J, Lindström J, Eriksson J G et al 2001 Prevention of type 2 diabetes mellitus by changes in lifestyle among subjects with impaired glucose tolerance. New England Journal of Medicine 344:1343–1350

US Department of Health and Human Services 1996 Physical activity and health: A report of the Surgeon General. US Department of Health and Human Services, Centers for Disease Control and Prevention, National Center for Chronic Disease Prevention and Health Promotion, Atlanta, GA

Wadén J, Tikkanen H, Forsblom C et al 2005 Leisure time physical activity is associated with poor glycemic control in type 1 diabetic women. Diabetes Care 28:777–782

Wang Y, Rimm E B, Stampfer M J et al 2005 Comparison of abdominal adiposity and overall obesity in predicting risk of type 2 diabetes among men. American Journal of Clinical Nutrition 81:555–563

Wareham N J, Van Sluijs E M F, Ekelund U 2005 Physical activity and obesity prevention: a review of the current evidence. Proceedings of the Nutrition Society 64:229–247

Watts K, Jones T W, Davis E A et al 2005 Exercise training in obese children and adolescents: current concepts. Sports Medicine 35:375–392

Wei M, Gibbons L W, Mitchel T L et al 1999 The association between cardiorespiratory fitness and impaired fasting glucose and type 2 diabetes mellitus in men. Annals of Internal Medicine 130:89–96

Wei M, Gibbons L W, Kampert J B et al 2000 Low cardiorespiratory fitness and physical inactivity as predictors of mortality in men with type 2 diabetes. Annals of Internal Medicine 132:605–611

Weinsier R L, Hunter G R, Desmond R A et al 2002 Free-living activity energy expenditure in women successful and unsuccessful at maintaining normal body weight. American Journal of Clinical Nutrition 75:499–504

Weinstein A R, Sesso H D 2006 Joint effects of physical activity and body weight on diabetes and cardiovascular disease. Exercise and Sport Sciences Reviews 34:10–15

Weyer C, Bodgardus C, Mott D M et al 1999 The natural history of insulin secretory dysfunction and insulin resistance in the pathogenesis of type 2 diabetes mellitus. Journal of Clinical Investigation 104:787–794

Weyer C, Funahashi T, Tanaka S et al 2001 Hypoadiponectinemia in obesity and type 2 diabetes: close association with insulin resistance and hyperinsulinemia. Journal of Clinical Endocrinology and Metabolism 86:1930–1935

Whitaker R C, Wright J A, Pepe M S et al 1997 Predicting obesity in young adulthood from childhood and parental obesity. New England Journal of Medicine 337:869–873

Willett W C, Dietz W H, Colditz G A 1999 Guidelines for a healthy weight. New England Journal of Medicine 341:427–434

Williams P T, Pate R R 2005 Cross-sectional relationships of exercise and age to adiposity in 60,617 male runners. Medicine and Science in Sports and Exercise 37:1329–1337

Williams P T, Wood P D 2006 The effects of changing exercise levels on weight and age-related weight gain. International Journal of Obesity 30:543–551

Williamson D F, Madans J, Anda R F et al 1993 Recreational physical activity and ten-year weight change in a US national cohort. International Journal of Obesity and Related Metabolic Disorders 17:279–286

Wing R R, Phelan S 2005 Long-term weight loss maintenance. American Journal of Clinical Nutrition 82(Suppl):222S–SS5S

Wynne K, Park A J, Small C J et al 2006 Oxyntomodulin increases energy expenditure in addition to decreasing energy intake in overweight and obese humans: a randomised controlled trial. International Journal of Obesity 30:1729–1736

Yusuf S, Hawken S, Ôunpuu S et al 2005 Obesity and the risk of myocardial infarction in 27 000 participants from 52 countries: a case-control study. Lancet 366:1640–1649

Zhang J V, Ren P G, Avsian-Kretchmer O et al 2005 Obestatin, a peptide encoded by the ghrelin gene, opposes ghrelin's effects on food intake. Science 310:996–999

Further reading

Albright A, Franz M, Hornsby G et al 2000 Exercise and type 2 diabetes. Medicine and Science in Sports and Exercise 32:1345–1360

Bassuk S S, Manson J E 2005 Epidemiological evidence for the role of physical activity in reducing risk of type 2 diabetes and cardiovascular disease. Journal of Applied Physiology 99:1193–1204

Frayn K N 2003 Metabolic regulation: a human perspective. Blackwell Science, Oxford. Chapter 10: Diabetes mellitus (pp 281–299), Chapter 11: Energy balance and body weight regulation (pp 300–319)

Haslam D W, James W P 2005 Obesity. Lancet 366:1197–1209

Hawley J A 2004 Exercise as a therapeutic intervention for the prevention and treatment of insulin resistance. Diabetes Metabolism Research Reviews 20:383–393

Hill J O, Wyatt H R 2005 Role of physical activity in preventing and treating obesity. Journal of Applied Physiology 99:765–770

Jakicic J M, Clark K, Coleman E et al 2001 Appropriate intervention strategies for weight loss and prevention of weight regain for adults. Medicine and Science in Sports and Exercise 33:2145–2156

LaMonte M J, Blair S N, Church T S 2005 Physical activity and diabetes prevention. Journal of Applied Physiology 99:1205–1213

Speiser P W, Rudolf M C J, Anhalt H et al 2005 Consensus statement: childhood obesity. Journal of Endocrinology and Metabolism 90:1871–1887

Chapter 3

Cardiac disease and dysfunction

John P Buckley and Patrick J Doherty

CHAPTER CONTENTS

Learning objectives   52
Introduction   52
General epidemiology of cardiovascular
   disease   53
Pathophysiology of coronary heart
   disease   53
Historical overview of physical activity
   and CHD   54
Exertion–related cardiac events   55
Physical activity and exercise in primary
   prevention of CHD   56
   Aerobic endurance exercise for
      preventing CHD   59
   Muscular strength and endurance
      exercise in prevention of CHD   61
   Balance and proprioceptive/coordination
      exercise in prevention of CHD   61
   Summary of preventative exercise
      prescription in CHD   62
Exercise in rehabilitation and secondary
   prevention of CHD   62
   Aerobic endurance exercise for patients
      with CHD   63
   Muscular strength and endurance
      exercise for patients with CHD   64
   Balance and proprioceptive/
      coordination exercise for patients
      with CHD   65
   Summary of rehabilitative and
      secondary preventative exercise
      prescription for CHD   65
Myocardial pumping dysfunction/heart
   failure   66
   Epidemiology of heart failure   66

Exercise in primary prevention of
   heart failure/myocardial
   pumping dysfunction   68
Exercise in rehabilitation and
   secondary prevention of heart
   failure/myocardial pumping
   dysfunction   68
Considerations for patients with
   arrhythmia and/or implantable
   cardioverter defibrillator   74
   Arrhythmia and exercise   74
   Implantable cardioverter
      defibrillators   74
   Summary for arrhythmia and ICD   76
Considerations for exercise and
   cardiac medications   77
   Exercise capacity and medication   78
Practical considerations for exercise
   and rehabilitation of cardiac
   patients   79
   Warm-up and cool-down   79
   Posture and movement   80
   Exertion in activities of daily life   81
Considerations for exercise testing   81
Functional assessment
   considerations   84
   Performance changes   84
   Physiological and perceptual
      response changes   85
Using protocols for assessment   87
Key points   87
References   88
Further reading   96

LEARNING OBJECTIVES

After studying this chapter, you should be able to:

1. Give an account of the epidemiology and pathophysiology of the various types of cardiac disease and dysfunction, with a focus primarily on coronary heart disease and secondarily on other cardiac conditions.
2. Understand the association between pathophysiology and restricted exercise capacity.
3. Describe how physical activity, exercise and physical fitness contribute to the primary prevention of cardiac morbidity and mortality.
4. Consider how physical activity, exercise and physical fitness, with emphasis on their differences, can contribute to the rehabilitation and secondary prevention of cardiac morbidity and mortality.
5. Appreciate the challenges in improving and maintaining exercise behaviour and physical fitness in cardiac patients.
6. Describe the different approaches to exercise prescription and the benefits associated with using relative exercise intensities.
7. Discuss evidence-based physical activity and exercise interventions.
8. Describe exercise testing and exercise prescription procedures that ensure patients' participation is both safe and effective.

Advisory note   Reading and understanding this chapter does not qualify one to embark upon practice as a specialist exercise professional who can work with cardiac populations. Specialist skills training and experience are required and this chapter simply aims to provide an overview or map of the key knowledge, skills and experience required for working with cardiac patients.

INTRODUCTION

For the purposes of this text, the term 'cardiac disease' includes a number of conditions that affect the healthy functioning of the heart, including: coronary artery disease, myocardial pumping dysfunction, electrical conduction abnormalities, and valve disease (Fig. 3.1). Further descriptions of these conditions will be provided in the relevant sections of this chapter. Numerous modifiable and non-modifiable risk factors are associated with the development of cardiac disease (Wood et al 2005). The key modifiable risk factors include: high levels of blood-borne low-density lipoproteins and triglycerides, hypertension, smoking, obesity, type 2 diabetes and of specific importance to this chapter, physical inactivity and low cardiorespiratory fitness (Paffenbarger et al 2001). Physical inactivity (habitual low levels of energy expenditure) and low levels of cardiorespiratory fitness (poor aerobic capacity), which are linked, have each been shown to be independent risk factors. The key non-modifiable risk factors include: age, gender, ethnicity and genetic family history. More recently poor fetal health and low birthweight have been identified as strong predictors of cardiac disease (Henriksen 1999).

The governments of highly urbanized countries have realized that the financial burden associated with poor public health has to be tackled firmly and in the United Kingdom this involves encouraging the nation to eat well, avoid obesity, increase physically activity, and if possible become physically fitter (Department of Health 2004b).

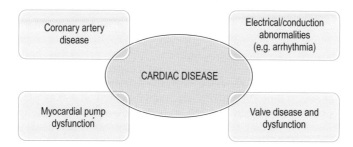

Figure 3.1   Cardiac disease.

GENERAL EPIDEMIOLOGY OF CARDIOVASCULAR DISEASE

The World Health Organization's global estimate of deaths by cardiovascular disease (including cardiac disease, strokes and vascular diseases) stands at 16.7 million (based on 2002 data) with 7.2 million attributed to heart disease and 5.5 million attributed to stroke (WHO 2002). In the UK anyone dying before age 75 years is considered a premature death (Petersen et al 2005; see also www. heartstats.org). Over the past 30 years premature deaths from overall cardiovascular disease (CVD) and specifically coronary (artery) heart disease (CHD) have fallen by 37% and 44%, respectively. Nonetheless, this ongoing collection of statistics continues to show that CVD in the UK and Europe remains a leading cause of mortality. In the UK almost 40% of all deaths are attributable to CVD, of which half are attributable to CHD. Similar rates are found in the USA as in the UK but in Western Europe, Australia and Japan the rates are up to 50% lower than in the UK and USA. In Eastern Europe, however, these are greater by three to four times compared with the UK. More men than women die from CHD (22% of men and 12% of women). The other forms of cardiac disease noted in Figure 3.1 account for about 4% of all deaths (Petersen et al 2005).

A more difficult set of statistics to collect is the prevalence of cardiac disease morbidity (Petersen et al 2005). These data have been collected from people surviving from myocardial infarction, and those living with angina, heart failure, valve disease and arrhythmias. It is individuals with these conditions that form the groups of people eligible for exercise-based rehabilitation (Department of Health 2000). Secondary prevention, including risk factor modification and improved medical and surgical interventions, has been responsible for the large decline in cardiac disease mortality over the past three decades (Tunstall-Pedoe et al 2000). However, up to 60% of this decline can still be attributed to risk factor modification (Unal et al 2004). It will be interesting to see how future trends in cardiac disease change in light of the accelerated prevalence of obesity and type 2 diabetes in younger people since 1990 (see Chapter 2).

PATHOPHYSIOLOGY OF CORONARY HEART DISEASE

Coronary heart disease involves a progressive narrowing of the coronary arterial lumen due to the creation, over many years, of atherosclerotic plaque. This plaque, which makes itself an integral part of the inner lining (endothelium) of the arterial wall, is formed by an outer fibrous cap and filled with either calcified or lipid plaque (Li et al 2003). Depending on how much of the lumen is narrowed by the atherosclerotic plaque (atheroma), it may or may not cause ischaemic symptoms of angina pectoris (pain or tightness in the chest, arm or neck area) when the demand for coronary blood flow is greater than its supply. Diagnosis of ischaemia can only truly be confirmed by either angiography or ECG or preferably both. Typically, lumen occlusions of less than 50% do not cause symptoms of angina but the size of the blockage does not always correlate with the risk of a myocardial infarction (MI) or unstable angina (Libby 2001). This report highlighted that it is plaque stability and not necessarily plaque size which is related to the risk of provoking a coronary event (MI or unstable angina). Ultimately if this fibrous cap is ruptured, from various causes, the lipid-based plaque will leak into the coronary arterial bloodstream, mix with the blood, and form a clot that can cause an acute MI. In a younger adult (<50 years), who has less than a 50% narrowing and no symptoms of angina, an acute MI can occur without warning from an unstable plaque being ruptured (Valika et al 2007). Even with stable plaque, such disease leads to a reduced exercise capacity with early breathlessness. Furthermore the risk of MI, and to lesser extent cardiac arrest, are greatly increased if risk factor reduction is not pursued either by lifestyle changes or by medical management (Fletcher et al 2001, Pashkow et al 1997, Pina et al 2003, Wasserman 1997). The extent of the narrowing of the coronary arteries is only moderately predictive of the cardiorespiratory fitness (and vice versa) in the early stages of the disease, in that some patients, as stated above, may have up to 50% narrowing with minimal awareness during activities of daily living (Fletcher et al 2001, Pina et al 2003, Wasserman 1997).

Libby (2001) has summarized numerous biological factors which increase plaque stability and prevent further growth of atheroma, including reductions of low-density lipoprotein (LDL) cholesterol, increased high-density lipoprotein (HDL) cholesterol, increased nitric oxide release and decreased hypertension and shear stress on the endothelium. These factors decrease the potential of inflammation local to the coronary plaque, all of which are influenced by lifestyle factors of smoking, diet, physical activity and exercise. With regard to physical activity, because it has been engineered out of modern life (Paffenbarger et al 2001), the net effect has been that 60% of people are not sufficiently active to maintain health (WHO 2006). The beneficial dose responses of physical activity and exercise volume (frequency, intensity and duration) will be discussed later in this chapter.

HISTORICAL OVERVIEW OF PHYSICAL ACTIVITY AND CHD

Since the 1950s, it has been established that there is a causal link between levels of human physical activity (caloric expenditure per week) and chronic morbidity, specifically CHD and generally all-cause mortality (Blair et al 1989, Morris et al 1953, Paffenbarger et al 2001). It has also been established that in both primary and secondary (rehabilitation) prevention, there is a decline of 8–17% in premature mortality from CHD with every one metabolic equivalent (MET) increase in aerobic fitness (Franklin & Gordon 2005, Myers et al 2002, 2004). One MET is the amount of oxygen used each minute, per kilogram of body mass, while sitting at rest. The average aerobic capacity of a 50-year-old North American or European adult is 8 to 10 METs (28 to 35 mL $\cdot$ kg^{-1} $\cdot$ min^{-1}) and this declines by approximately 2 METs or 10% per decade (Åstrand et al 2003, Hollenberg et al 2006).

Physical inactivity (expending less than a total of 27 kilocalories per kilogram body mass per day) poses a greater risk to CHD mortality than obesity, high blood pressure and smoking (McPherson et al 2002, Paffenbarger & Lee 1996). In these reports, only a high cholesterol has been shown to be a more potent risk factor. Additionally, low physical fitness (equivalent to not being able to walk 1 mile in under 20 minutes) is as strong a predictor of cardiovascular disease as smoking, high cholesterol, obesity, hypertension and a family history of CHD (Blair et al 1989, 1996, Farrell et al 1998, Laughlin 2004). It is this type of evidence which created the significant momentum for publication of the US Surgeon General's report (Pate et al 1995) and the UK's Chief Medical Officer's report (Department of Health 2004a) on physical activity and public health.

EXERTION–RELATED CARDIAC EVENTS

The American Heart Association (AHA) Committee on exercise, rehabilitation and prevention estimate that 4–20% of MIs occur during or soon after exercise and the risk increases in persons who do not regularly exercise (Pina et al 2003). A similar pattern arises with the triggering of ventricular arrhythmias that can lead to a cardiac arrest during exertion, especially from infrequent bouts of vigorous activity (Mittleman et al 1993, Siscovick et al 1984). Figures 3.2A and B show the significant reduction in exertion-related MIs and cardiac arrests with increased frequency of exercise participation. It is important to note, however, that the exercise risk of triggering an event makes it something of a 'double-edged sword' (Franklin 1999). While exercising, the risk of a cardiac event is significantly heightened in CHD patients, being anywhere between 6 and 164 times greater than the risk for such patients at rest (Cobb & Weaver 1986). With regular exercise training, the risk of an 'event' being provoked during exertion is greatly reduced (Albert et al 2000, Mittleman et al 1993, Siscovick et al 1984). Franklin & Gordon (2005) have summarized in detail the risk of exercise triggering an MI or cardiac arrest (Table 3.1). Whilst the above discussion raises concerns about exertion-related cardiac events, it is important to note the proportion of cardiac events that occur at rest or during sleep. Individuals with underlying myocardial pathology (e.g. right ventricular wall myopathy, Brugada syndrome and

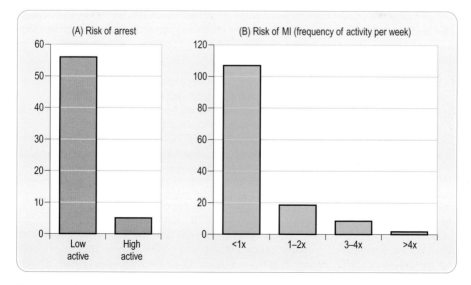

Figure 3.2   Relative risk reduction of cardiac events with regular physical activity. (A) Risk of cardiac arrest (adapted from Siscovick et al 1984). (B) Risk of MI (adapted from Mittleman et al 1993).

Table 3.1 Summary of incidence of cardiac events during exercise

Study authors	Rate of incidence in general population
Malinow et al (1984)	During sports activities: one death per 2 897 057 person-hours
Vander et al (1982)	During physical recreation activities: one non-fatal event per 1 124 200 hours and one fatal event per 887 526 hours
Gibbons et al (1980)	Per 10 000 person-hours: 0.3 to 2.7 events (male) and 0.6 to 6.0 events (female)
Franklin et al (2000)	Fitness centre exercise: one death per 2.57 million 'work-outs' (~50% in non-regular exercisers)
Fletcher et al (2001)	During exercise: one death per 565 000 person-hours
	Rate of incidence in cardiac patient populations
Haskell (1978)	Cardiac rehabilitation exercise: one non-fatal event per 34 673 hours and one fatal event per 116 402 hours
Franklin et al (1998)	Supervised cardiac rehabilitation: One cardiac arrest per 116 906 patient-hours One acute MI per 219 970 patient-hours One fatal event per 752 365 patient-hours One major complication per 81 670 patient-hours

Adapted from Franklin & Gordon (2005, pp. 246–248).

disorders that cause sleep apnoea) have a propensity to die from non-exercise-related cardiac arrest (Nademanee et al 1997, Rodrigeuez et al 1990, Shepard 1992).

PHYSICAL ACTIVITY AND EXERCISE IN PRIMARY PREVENTION OF CHD

This section will review key aspects of how increased physical activity, regular exercise and increased fitness act to prevent CHD or problems associated with it. The three main areas of benefit are:

1. the prevention of cardiac events during physical exertion within the general population, which has been covered in the previous section of this chapter
2. the prevention of coronary artherosclerotic lesions becoming either large, unstable or vulnerable and leading to cardiac-related morbidity and mortality, and
3. the prevention of the accumulation of other CHD risk factors, including increased levels of LDL cholesterol, raised blood pressure, obesity and diabetes, much of which is covered in more detail in Chapter 2 on obesity and diabetes.

Points 1 and 2 above relate to how physical activity, exercise and fitness act as independent risk factors, whereas in point 3 the benefit is achieved indirectly by the influence of physical activity on other key CHD risk factors.

Early evidence for the association between activity and cardiac health came from the 'London Transport Company' study (Morris et al 1953), where they considered the incidence of CHD among 31 000 men aged 35 to 64 who were either drivers (a seated occupation) or conductors (requires standing, walking and climbing stairs). Average mortality was 20% greater in drivers and the first CHD episode in conductors occurred later and was less severe than in drivers. Morris et al hypothesized that a lack of activity in drivers was more than a simple association and possibly causal. Although hotly debated by the medical fraternity (Paffenbarger et al 2001), the work of Morris and co-workers acted as a catalyst for the eventual medical acceptance and promotion of physical activity as a means of decreasing the severity and delaying the onset of CHD. More recently the importance and continued contribution of Morris and his colleagues to science has been acknowledged by leading exercise and public health experts (Paffenbarger et al 2001).

Figure 3.3 illustrates the relationship between physical activity, as measured by weekly energy expenditure, and the risk of developing CHD and death from CHD. There appears to be a threshold energy expenditure of ~1000 kilocalories per week that needs to be attained in order to confer a benefit (Sesso et al 2000). This amount of activity equates to the recommendations for accumulating 30 minutes of activity most days of the week, as highlighted by the US Surgeon General (Pate et al 1995) and the Chief Medical Officer for England and Wales (Department of Health 2004a). When physical activity attains energy expenditures greater than 2000 kilocalories per week, cardiovascular disease risk is reduced by up to 30%. It is important to note that to achieve an energy expenditure of >2000 kilocalories within an average individual's week (equivalent to walking 20 to 25 miles per week), they would probably need to engage in more vigorous activity (e.g. jogging or running). As will be discussed in the next section, more vigorous activity that leads to increased cardio-respiratory fitness clearly demonstrates a much greater benefit than simply adding more activity into daily living (Myers et al 2004, Williams 2001).

As noted in the introductory chapter, physical activity represents any bodily movement that utilizes muscle actions and requires a measurable increase in energy

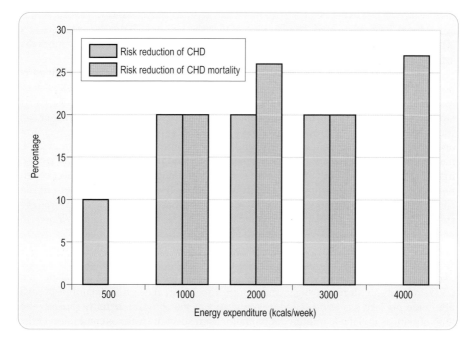

Figure 3.3   Relative risk reduction of acquiring CHD and risk reduction of CHD-related mortality and weekly energy expenditure. Adapted from Sesso et al (2000) and Lee & Paffenbarger (2000).

expenditure, whilst exercise is seen as a subset of physical activity that is structured and targeted at improving physical fitness (ACSM 2006a, Blair et al 1995, 2004, Paffenbarger et al 2001). Within the benefits of increased weekly energy expenditure summarized in Figure 3.3, there still exists some controversy regarding how the dose of the activity is weighted. In this regard it must be acknowledged that energy expenditure is influenced by a combination of factors, including the frequency, intensity and duration of the activity (Kesaniemi et al 2001). The issue of duration now includes the subset of daily fractionalization of bouts that occur throughout a day (Murphy et al 2002). It is known that an increased total dose that specifically includes increased intensity results in a decreased morbidity and lower all-cause mortality (ACSM 2006a, Blair et al 1995, 2004, Lee et al 2003, Paffenbarger et al 2001). This is an important point for health professionals involved with fitness and rehabilitation as the philosophy adopted impacts on programme design, location and resources. In moderately fit individuals, the exercise intensity achieved by increasing physical activity within their occupation and/or lifestyle may be too low to bring about any noticeable benefit. An individual needs to work at levels greater than 50% of peak aerobic capacity to bring about measurable adaptation and reduced risk of CHD and future cardiac events (Blair et al 1995, MacAuley 1999, Pate et al 1995). However, in very unfit individuals whose aerobic capacity is challenged by activities of daily living (probably the overweight, obese and elderly), it could be argued that simply doing more activity within daily life is actually enough to reach the 50% of maximal capacity threshold and thus can be considered fitness training. The American College of Sports Medicine have noted that in some cases working above a threshold of 40% maximal aerobic capacity may be beneficial (ACSM 2006b). Epidemiological findings have more recently emphasized substantive benefits from physical activity and reaffirmed that frequent moderate physical activity and the avoidance of sedentary behaviour substantially improves life expectancy and quality of life (ACSM 2006a, Barengo et al 2004, Blair & LaMonte 2005, Blair et al 2004, Franco et al 2005, Lee et al 2003, Paffenbarger et al 2001). The extent of the sedentary lifestyle (defined as less than one session of moderate activity per week) is estimated at 40% within the UK (Allender et al 2006).

An associated factor noted above is the extent of obesity; this is usually defined by body mass index (BMI) and is described in Chapter 2. The obesity-related risk of death in CHD patients is estimated at 5% for males and 6% for females (Allender et al 2006). Debate continues regarding the relative importance of obesity and inactivity in their contribution to CHD: the 'fatness versus fitness' debate. The work of two research groups, one from Boston (Weinstein et al 2004) and the other from Florida (Wessel et al 2004), has added to the debate by finding in favour of obesity and fitness, respectively. On closer inspection of the data, both studies have some methodological issues in respect of self-report measures of fitness, physical activity and BMI. Notwithstanding this, both studies confirm the importance of obesity and physical inactivity as CHD risk factors. Farrell et al (1998) (Fig. 3.4) and the British Heart Foundation (Allender et al 2006) claim that poor fitness and inactivity, respectively, are much stronger predictors of cardiovascular disease risk than obesity. Furthermore, individuals with higher cardiorespiratory fitness have substantially lower metabolic risk (presence of obesity and/or diabetes) and are less likely to develop the metabolic syndrome (a cluster of factors that lead to diabetes and CVD – obesity, high blood sugar and insulin resistance) (Lee et al 2005). If a population-wide priority has to be stated it would appear that physical activity ranks higher than obesity as it is the 'common denominator' in respect of treatment and intervention in sedentary obese patients (Blair & Church 2004, Hu et al 2004).

The estimated rate of death attributed to physical inactivity in the CHD population is 36% in men and 38% in women (Allender et al 2006, Department of Health 2000, 2004a).

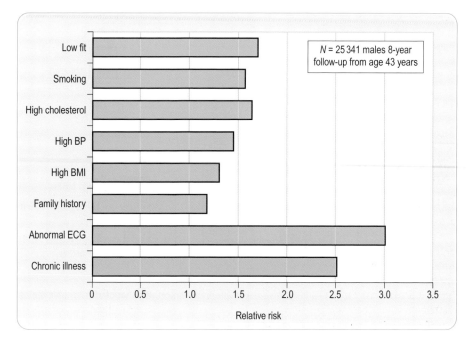

Figure 3.4   Adjusted relative risks of CVD for eight predictors. Adapted from Farrel et al (1998), Blair et al (1996).

This evidence predicts that 9% of deaths could be avoided if people raised their activity status from low to moderate, equating to 30 minutes of aerobic activity on 1–4 days per week. The combined estimated mortality associated with obesity and sedentary life-styles is 41% and 44% for males and females, respectively. UK government policy acknowledges these statistics on obesity and sedentary living and has set obesity and physical activity targets accordingly within National Health Service frameworks and public health initiatives (Department of Health 2000, Department of Health 2001a).

Aerobic endurance exercise for preventing CHD

Cardiorespiratory fitness is mainly increased by aerobic endurance exercise but in some less fit or diseased populations a small benefit can be achieved by muscular strength exercise (ACSM 2006b, Pollock et al 2000). It has been highlighted in the pre-vious section that increased physical activity is beneficial in preventing CHD and CHD-related mortality. However, the debate continues on how much of the benefit is related to increased weekly energy expenditure with or without corresponding increases in cardiorespiratory fitness. The accuracy in measuring daily physical activ-ity and daily energy expenditure is problematic (Tudor-Locke & Myers 2001), whereas measuring cardiorespiratory fitness can be done using a single test and is thus relatively easy. Perhaps it is due in part to the relative ease of accurately measur-ing fitness, compared to measuring physical activity, that increased fitness has been shown to have a statistically stronger and more beneficial association with reductions in CHD morbidity and mortality (Williams 2001). Figure 3.4 (Farrell et al 1998) illus-trates the clear strength of cardiorespiratory fitness as an independent risk factor, compared with other cardiac disease risk factors. Figure 3.5 (Myers et al 2002)

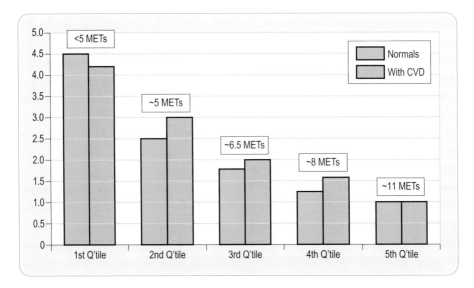

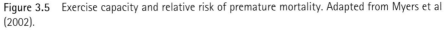

Figure 3.5 Exercise capacity and relative risk of premature mortality. Adapted from Myers et al (2002).

illustrates considerable differences between different levels of cardiorespiratory fitness and specifically CHD mortality. Myers et al (2004) reported up to a 50% reduction in all-cause and cardiovascular disease mortality in those with a higher level of cardiorespiratory fitness.

From the key evidence highlighted, it is apparent that there are two main avenues for preventing CHD through increased physical activity: that which aims to increase weekly energy expenditure within daily life and that which aims to increase cardiorespiratory fitness from more structured vigorous exercise. So far, from a scientific perspective, the latter has demonstrated a greater CHD prevention benefit. However, from a public health perspective, achieving such levels of participation in vigorous structured exercise appears to be an unattainable and/or unsustainable behaviour for large proportions of the population. Hence, public health initiatives have more recently focused on ways in which to reintroduce physical activity into the routine of daily life where experts feel there is a greater chance of successful behaviour change. The main problem is that physical activity has been literally manufactured 'out of life' in the techno-industrialized world through advances in transport and occupational technology and technology-based sedentary leisure pursuits (Paffenbarger et al 2001).

China provides an interesting example of changes in transport modes (Fig. 3.6). In 1986 in Beijing, 58%, 32% and 5% of urban travel was by bicycle, public transport and private car or employer's bus, respectively (Peng 2005). In the year 2000 this had changed to 38%, 27% and 23%, respectively, for these three same modes of urban transport. Bell et al (2002) have been able to show that such changes in transport, as a result of increased prosperity and a shift in the population living in rural to urban locations, are strongly associated with the sharp rises in obesity now prevalent in China (Wang et al 2007). In this vein, it is probably the rise in obesity as a consequence of decreases in active transport that leads to poorer cardiovascular health in such populations, and from this perspective, it is a 'physically active transport' policy and not a nationwide exercise training regimen that is required.

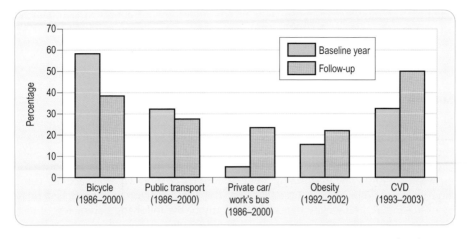

Figure 3.6 Changes in modes of transported, obesity and cardiovascular disease (CVD) in Beijing, China (1986–2003). Adapted from Peng (2005), Wang et al (2007).

The mechanism of increased physical activity and fitness relates to the stability and progression/regression of coronary atherosclerotic plaque. In individuals who fail to expend more than 1000 kilocalories per week (equivalent to walking 1.5 miles per day) coronary disease showed a progression, whereas those who expended 1500 and 2000 kilocalories per week, halted and regressed their atherosclerosis, respectively (Hambrecht et al 1993).

Muscular strength and endurance exercise in prevention of CHD

Unlike cardiorespiratory fitness, there is little evidence of a direct association between muscular strength/muscular endurance and CHD but the enhancing of skeletal musculature does have an indirect influence on various CHD risk factors (McCartney 1998, Pollock et al 2000). These reviews have highlighted the CHD risk factors that benefit, including:

- the prevention or management of diabetes mellitus (glucose control and insulin sensitivity)
- obesity (lean body mass and basal metabolism)
- some more tenuous evidence related to blood pressure and serum lipid management.

The indirect benefit to aerobic fitness is that strength training has been associated with greater submaximal exercise endurance time. Reduced cardiovascular strain has been reported by the attenuation of blood pressure and heart rate responses during acute bouts of heavier lifting activities that involve muscular strength (Lind & McNicol 1967, McCartney 1998, Mitchell et al 1980).

Balance and proprioceptive/coordination exercise in prevention of CHD

There is little evidence that exercise which improves balance and coordination has a direct impact on the prevention of cardiac disease. However, there is an indirect benefit to preventing cardiac disease through the maintenance of joint mobility, stability and movement coordination which underpin the ability to maintain an active life and perform health-benefiting aerobic or muscular endurance exercise. The chapters on exercise and musculoskeletal health (Chapter 5) and exercise in the older person (Chapter 6) will discuss this area in more depth.

Summary of preventative exercise prescription in CHD

From a general physical activity perspective, healthy adults should aim to perform physical activity that equates to expending at least 1000 to 1500 kilocalories per week. For most people this equates to accumulating 30 minutes of activity every day. Greater cardiovascular disease prevention is attained in individuals who increase their aerobic fitness by performing 20 to 60 minutes of more vigorous activity using large muscle groups at least three times per week. More vigorous activity is defined by exercising at an intensity demarcated by any of the following parameters, which aim to reflect either the anaerobic threshold or the threshold of blood lactate accumulation:

- >50–75% $\dot{V}O_2$max or maximal heart rate reserve or
- >65–80% maximal heart rate and/or
- attaining a rating of perceived exertion (RPE) between 12 and 15 of 'somewhat hard' to 'hard' on Borg's RPE scale or 3–5 on Borg's CR-10 scale.

EXERCISE IN REHABILITATION AND SECONDARY PREVENTION OF CHD

In 1772 Dr Heberden reported to the Royal College of Physicians that a patient with chest pain who sawed wood for 30 minutes per day was rid of his symptoms in 6 months (BACR 1995). It would, however, be almost 200 years later (the mid-1950s) that physical activity, as opposed to enforced bed rest, was recognized as the best form of convalescence for individuals with CHD and myocardial infarction (BACR 1995). When trials did begin to emerge in the 1950s, especially in the USA, it was soon clear that those patients who were physically mobilized within days of their event recovered better than those who remained in bed (Froelicher & Myers 2000, May 1950). This not only prevented the deleterious effects of bed rest on their circulation, strength and stamina but such mobilization also prevented the occurrence of a number of other health effects (including psychological well-being) that arise from physical immobilization. Advances in both medical and surgical care in the 1960s contributed to better recovery as exercise started to become accepted. By the 1980s exercise rehabilitation became more prevalent in the UK, with the first randomized controlled trial (RCT) being performed at the North Staffordshire Hospital and demonstrating decreased morbidity and mortality in those who undertook exercise (Carson et al 1982). Overall, exercise has been shown to be an independent significant contributor to the prevention of cardiac and all-cause mortality following myocardial infarction and revascularization interventions (coronary artery bypass surgery and angioplasty) (Jolliffe et al 2001, Oldridge et al 1988). In the studies included in these two meta-analyses, the exercise regimens were of moderate to more vigorous intensity aerobic exercise (50–80% $\dot{V}O_2$max), performed under supervision three times per week with programmes typically lasting for at least 12 weeks. The questions raised by such protocols include: how many participants will continue long term with this volume of activity, are there resources to aid long-term participation, and what might be the benefits of fewer structured sessions but with increased lower-intensity daily physical activities incorporated into day-to-day life?

Aerobic endurance exercise for patients with CHD

Potential mechanisms of increased physical activity and aerobic fitness

In providing a link between the primary and secondary prevention benefits of exercise for CHD, Franklin & Gordon (2005) identified four physiological mechanisms explaining why aerobic exercise has a cardioprotective effect. These mechanisms, which are summarized in Figure 3.7, consist in exercise having an anti-atherosclerotic, anti-thrombotic, anti-ischaemic or anti-arrhythmic effect. Atherosclerosis and thrombosis play a key part in laying down atheromatous plaque (atheroma) that can lead to angina and, worse, a myocardial infarction. Ischaemia is directly related to the extent of the atheroma but as previously noted, it is possible to prevent ischaemia either by: reducing myocardial demand for oxygen through a decreased blood pressure or heart rate; regression of the atheroma (Hambrecht 1993); or improving the vasodilatory mechanism of the coronary arteries as discussed in the next paragraph.

It is only more recently that a potential mechanism has been proposed to explain why regular physical activity and increased aerobic fitness reduce the ischaemic effects and thereby reduce the chances of infarction and/or arrhythmia. Hambrecht et al (2000, 2003) from Germany and Laughlin (Laughlin 2004, Laughlin & Korzick 2001) from the USA have demonstrated that exercise literally 'tones up' the coronary arterial endothelium. The key finding from these reports was that with less than

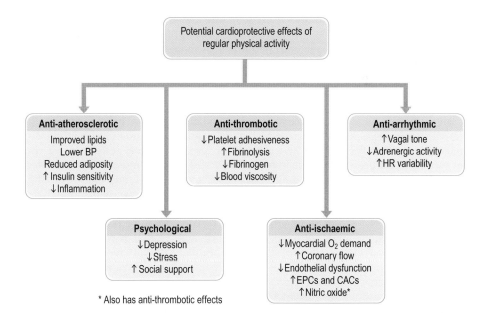

Figure 3.7 Multiple mechanisms by which moderate-to-vigorous exercise training may reduce the risk of non-fatal and fatal cardiovascular events. BP, blood pressure; EPCs, endothelial progenitor cells; CACs, cultured/circulating angiogenic cells; ↑, increased; ↓, decreased; O_2, oxygen. (From Franklin & Gordon 2005, with permission.)

6 weeks of exercise training the coronary arteries improved their ability to dilate more quickly in response to the onset of physical exertion. The mechanism was found to be an increased responsiveness of the arterial endothelium to the presence of exertion-related nitric oxide. Nitric oxide is a key agent in the relaxation of the smooth muscles involved in vasomotor control and hence the benefit is a quicker or more profound vasomotor response that allows for increased myocardial perfusion (reduced ischaemia) and less shear stress on the endothelial wall that could precipitate a rupturing of the atherosclerotic plaque.

Aerobic exercise prescription

Guidelines from the USA and the UK (American Association of Cardiovascular and Pulmonary Rehabilitation (AACVPR), the American College of Sports Medicine (ACSM), the British Association for Cardiac Rehabilitation (BACR) and the Scottish Intercollegiate Guidelines Network (SIGN)) recommend that the exercise dose is similar to that outlined in the previous section for the prevention of CHD in healthy sedentary populations, with some added provisos outlined in Box 3.1. These are, however, general statements and practitioners need to read and apply the specifics in detail following appropriate professional training.

Muscular strength and endurance exercise for patients with CHD

The American Heart Association (Pollock 2000) has provided a position statement from a wide trawl of the evidence, which is freely available from the following website: http://circ.ahajournals.org/cgi/content/full/101/7/828.

The underlying recommendation from this paper is that performing regular strength and muscular endurance exercise is safe and effective for individuals with cardiac disease. This recommendation assumes that appropriate pre-exercise screening and risk stratification have been performed. Although there is no clear evidence that increased muscular strength has a direct effect upon reductions in morbidity and mortality in cardiac disease, the indirect benefits include changes to metabolic risk factor profiles, decreased chances of causing ischaemia during acute muscular exertion, and increased functional movement capacity and quality of life. Metabolic changes include increased fat-free mass, improved blood glucose balance and insulin responsiveness. Decreased occurrences of ischaemia from muscular exertion are related to the fact that for any given weight or force of external resistance, the rise in systolic blood pressure will be less in a larger and stronger muscle. This is related to a reduction in rate pressure product (RPP) for a given level of muscular work. RPP, as described in Box 3.1, is an indirect index of myocardial oxygen demand and is a function of heart rate and systolic blood pressure. Hence, if the rise in systolic blood pressure is less, the rise in peripheral vascular resistance will be less, which in turn will decrease the amount of myocardial work and related myocardial oxygen demand. This provides a good opportunity to highlight the differences in the metabolic systems of cardiac and skeletal muscle. Unlike skeletal muscle, which has an anaerobic metabolic system to provide energy during the acute onset of muscular work, the myocardium relies almost solely on aerobic metabolism; therefore, any impediment to myocardial perfusion will put the myocardium under undue stress, which could lead to an arrhythmia or, worse, a fibrillation (Froelicher & Myers 2002).

The recommended exercise prescription for attaining the above benefits is for patients to perform between 12 and 15 repetitions, of 8 to 10 different major muscle groups, at approximately 60% of a 1-repetition maximum 2 to 3 days per week.

Box 3.1   General provisos for aerobic exercise prescription in CHD

- Appropriate pre-exercise screening and risk stratification has been performed (AACVPR 2004, ACSM 2006a, SIGN 2002).
- The exercise intensity is below the level where the onset of myocardial ischaemia or arrhythmia occurs. This level is best considered in relation to not only a heart rate or rating of perceived exertion but also the rate pressure product. For example, activities involving the upper body at a given heart rate are likely to involve a greater rise in systolic blood pressure compared to lower limb activities (Froelicher & Myers 2000). The rate pressure product is a function of both heart rate and systolic blood pressure that indirectly represents myocardial oxygen demand.
- For higher risk individuals performing activity without appropriate supervision or cardiac monitoring, the intensity of exercise should be at the lower end of the target range.
- Acknowledgement of an individual's functional capacity (the difference between rest and the MET level at which they can no longer sustain aerobic exercise) is of prime consideration. It may be that if activities of daily life pose a challenge, then in some cases the popular public health promotion messages for physical activity may actually be inappropriate and advice about being active at home needs more precise guidance.

Determining an appropriate weight, similar to aerobic exercise, requires careful consideration. In the absence of being able to safely determine a 1-repetition maximum, it is advisable to start at a low resistance and graduate weights until an individual finds the weight that elicits signs of muscular fatigue after the final repetition. The AHA have advised this to be an RPE of 13 to 15 but further research is required on the practical prescription of RPE for strength training in this population.

Balance and proprioceptive/coordination exercise for patients with CHD

It has been reported that cardiac disease is a significant predictor of subsequent falls, especially in women over the age of 60 years (Lawlor et al 2003). Furthermore, because of the risk of osteoporosis and fracture in older women (Bonaiuti et al 2005) together with the increased risk of falling, exercise that enhances bone mineral density and increases strength, balance and coordination is an important feature in cardiac rehabilitation and secondary prevention programmes for older women. Both muscular strength and aerobic endurance exercise have been found to be effective in increasing bone mineral density in the spine and the hip (Bonaiuti et al 2005). Without strength, balance and joint mobility, the ability to perform aerobic activity which directly benefits cardiac health will be diminished. The specifics on prescribing such exercises are detailed in Chapters 6 and 7.

Summary of rehabilitative and secondary preventative exercise prescription for CHD

Both aerobic and muscular strength training are beneficial to patients with CHD. The former has a direct influence on morbidity and mortality, whereas the latter has an influence on risk factors that in turn may influence morbidity and mortality. Aerobic exercise for increasing cardiovascular endurance fitness performed three or more times per week at 50–80% $\dot{V}O_2$max for more than 20 minutes is a common feature reported in the literature. The health promotion message of more moderate activity most days of the week has not yet been widely applied to this population, and hence lacks evidence as a suitable intervention. However, from a behavioural development perspective, this approach may be a good starting point and/or an adjunct to less frequent sessions of more vigorous activity. In all cases, it is important to consider that low, moderate and vigorous intensity are descriptions relative to the individual's own capacity and that on this basis it is individually tailored to each patient/client.

MYOCARDIAL PUMPING DYSFUNCTION/HEART FAILURE

Myocardial pumping dysfunction relates to the loss of the ventricles' ability to create enough blood pressure in order to achieve appropriate circulation to and perfusion of all the organs of the body. This is often referred to as heart failure or left ventricular dysfunction (Hunt et al 2005, Mosterd et al 1999). A significantly overloaded heart, where the amount of blood it can eject (end-systole) is less than the amount that fills the heart (end-diastole), is typically described as congestive heart failure (CHF). In this instance the ejection fraction (the percentage of end-systole to end-diastole) is <50% whereas a normal resting ejection fraction is in the range of 65–70%. During submaximal exercise in healthy individuals this should rise another 10–15% (Brynjolf et al 1984, Stratton et al 1994). Depending on the severity of CHF, the rise in ejection fraction during exercise either is dampened or, worse, decreases (Pokan et al 1998). Failure of the right ventricle, as result of pulmonary disease and/or pulmonary hypertension, can also lead to a poor cardiac output, because of its relation to a decreased Frank–Starling mechanism and its effect on the corresponding ventricular septal wall integrity during contraction (Naeije 2005). Typical symptoms of CHF include shortness of breath, ankle oedema and pulmonary crepitations.

There is no single definitive test for CHF and diagnosis requires a combination of measurements, patient history and symptoms (Hunt et al 2005). A good example of this, as will be discussed later, is that poor left-ventricular ejection fraction is poorly correlated with aerobic exercise capacity (Hanson 1994). The symptomatology includes breathlessness, peripheral oedema, fatigue and poor physical fitness (endurance and muscular strength). The cardiological and physiological measures typically include echocardiography (to assess ejection fraction and wall motion abnormality), exercise tolerance (including ECG and sometimes respiratory responses) and more recently tests for the presence of brain natriuretic peptides (BNP) taken from blood or urine samples (Hunt et al 2005, Ng et al 2003). Changes in BNP are presently being evaluated as a physiological marker specific to individuals with CHF that can be used in evaluating both the extent of heart damage and the benefits of exercise (Bentzen et al 2004). However, the role of BNP testing as a surrogate measure for exercise tolerance and NYHA classification has still to be clearly determined (Abdulla et al 2004).

Within practice and rehabilitation standards (AACVPR 2004, Hunt et al/AHA/ACC 2005, SIGN 2002) the severity of CHF has been classified into four categories based on symptomatology and known as the New York Heart Association (NYHA) classification (Box 3.2).

Epidemiology of heart failure

Since the 1990s, in Western Europe, the UK, the USA and developed nations of Australasia, there has been a wider use and more aggressive medical approach to cardiovascular therapies, including: thrombolytics, antiplatelets, statins, beta-blockade,

Box 3.2   New York Heart Association classifications for heart failure

- *Class I:* patients with no limitation of activities; they suffer no symptoms from ordinary activities.
- *Class II:* patients with slight, mild limitation of activity; they are comfortable with rest or with mild exertion.
- *Class III:* patients with marked limitation of activity; they are comfortable only at rest.
- *Class IV:* patients who should be at complete rest, confined to bed or chair; any physical activity brings on discomfort and symptoms occur at rest.

angiotensin-converting enzyme (ACE) inhibitors, rapid access chest-pain clinics, angiography and revascularization therapies (Tunstall-Pedoe et al 2000). These interventions have led to an increased survival of individuals with ischaemic heart disease (Tunstall-Pedoe et al 2000). This increased survival has led to a corresponding increase in the prevalence of subsequent CHF (Barker et al 2006). As CHF progresses, typically related to left-ventricular systolic function, so do the risks of ventricular tachycardia and fibrillation, where prognosis is poor and survival is unlikely to exceed 5 years (Kannel 2000). As illustrated in Figure 3.8, CHF is one and a half to two times more prevalent in men than in women and this prevalence accelerates after the age of 65 years (Cowie et al 1999).

Data from the Framingham Study reported that the incidence of CHF was related to one or a combination of three main factors: previous myocardial infarction, chronic hypertension and heart-valve disease (Kannel 2000). Other causes of heart failure or valve disease include chronic obstructive pulmonary disease (COPD), congenital cardiomyopathies, viral infections and the toxic side effects from non-cardiac medication (e.g. chemotherapy) or drug abuse. Chronic hypertension showed the greatest

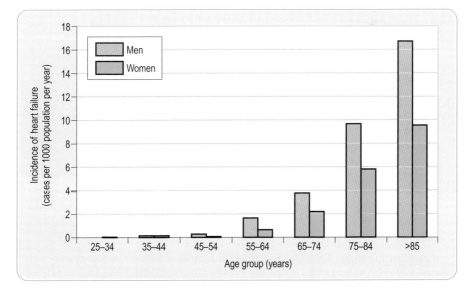

Figure 3.8   UK incidence of heart failure (per 1000 population), by sex and age. From Cowie et al (1999) with permission.

contributor to CHF, accounting for 39% of CHF events in men and 59% in women; MI accounted for CHF in 34% of men and 13% in women; heart-valve disease accounted for 7–8% of CHF. COPD and especially that which leads to pulmonary hypertension is a cause of right-sided heart failure (Naeije 2005). With the prognosis for CHF being relatively poor, as noted earlier, the focus of exercise rehabilitation needs to be on sustaining quality of life through the maintenance or optimization of functional capacity and symptom relief.

Exercise in primary prevention of heart failure/myocardial pumping dysfunction

As discussed in the previous section, heart failure is a condition which mainly develops from chronic hypertension, myocardial infarction or valve disease. Other risk factors that also predict heart failure are similar to those for CHD, including diabetes and hyperlipidaemia (Kannel 2000). With CHF being mainly a condition secondary to other cardiovascular pathologies or risk factors, the prevention of CHF as a result of increased physical activity and aerobic fitness would be a function of the effect of exercise on these same pathologies or primary risk factors. Thus, unlike coronary heart disease, neither lack of physical activity nor low aerobic fitness has been identified as a primary/direct risk factor in heart failure. The guidance for exercise to prevent CHF is outlined either in previous sections in this chapter for preventing CHD, or in Chapter 2 on exercise in obesity and diabetes. From a symptom-limited and functional capacity perspective, the guidance on exercise for pulmonary patients, as detailed in Chapter 4, has many transferable applications to CHF.

Exercise in rehabilitation and secondary prevention of heart failure/myocardial pumping dysfunction

The Cochrane Library systematic review summarizes the benefits of exercise-based rehabilitation for heart failure (Rees et al 2004), as follows:

> *Exercise training improves exercise tolerance and quality of life in people with mild to moderate heart failure.*
>
> *People with heart failure experience breathlessness and restricted activities of daily living because of their restricted heart capacity. This can reduce their amount of exercise, which can further reduce fitness, making their symptoms worse. The review found short-term trials of exercise training in people with mild to moderate heart failure only, which do not represent most of the people who have heart failure. The kinds of exercise programs varied greatly, but most included aerobic exercise rather than resistance training (such as working with weights). Exercise improved people's fitness and quality of life, without causing harm.*

In spite of the many benefits of exercise, this review found limited evidence that exercise training prolongs life, unlike the benefits for those who have had an MI, have chronic ischaemic heart disease or have had coronary bypass surgery. Furthermore, the populations studied were not fully representative of the population of individuals with CHF, especially older individuals (>65 years of age). Nonetheless, in respect of attaining the identified benefits, a number of key physiological elements need to be considered when providing exercise for individuals with CHF:

- the prevention of exercise-induced arrhythmia
- secondary skeletal muscle dysfunction (metabolism and histology)
- age – the exercise needs to be adapted for older people with CHF (see Chapter 6)
- balancing the benefits of aerobic versus strength training
- impact of hydration on exercise capacity.

Exercise-induced arrhythmia

The potential causes of arrhythmia are summarized in Figure 3.9A. These include: myocardial irritation through a rapid rise in heart rate and high levels of adrenaline or noradrenaline (catecholamines) and ischaemia brought about by myocardial oxygen supply (poor coronary perfusion) not meeting myocardial oxygen demand (dictated by heart rate and increased myocardial contractility). Poor coronary perfusion can be a function of three factors: coronary atheroma impeding blood flow, poor vasodilatory response or decreased coronary flow from a drop in aortic pressure. Four main precautions for preventing these factors (Doherty 2006, Foster & Porcari 2002, Franklin & Gordon 2005) are:

1. There is gradual pre-conditioning warm-up.
2. The activities do not involve any sudden increases in exercise intensity during the conditioning stage.
3. The target exercise intensity is mild to moderate.
4. Exercise is followed by a gradual decremented cool-down.

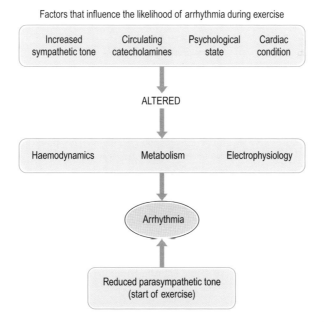

Figure that influence the likelihood of arrhythmia during exercise

Figure 3.9A   Factors that influence the likelihood of arrhythmia during exercise. (Developed from Beckerman et al 2005, Kelly 1996, Pashkow et al 1997.)

(Continued)

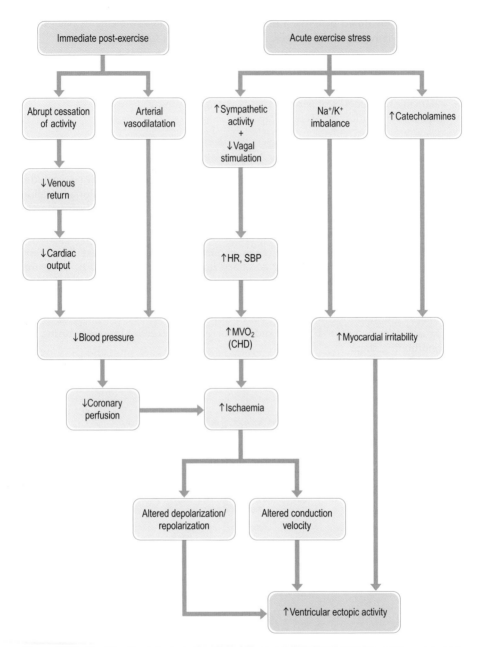

Figure 3.9B—Cont'd Physiological alterations accompanying acute exercise and recovery and their possible sequelae. HR, heart rate; SBP, systolic blood pressure; MVO_2, myocardial oxygen uptake; CHD, coronary heart disease. (From Franklin & Gordon 2005, with permission.)

Further rationale for these precautions is covered later in the section 'Practical considerations for exercise and rehabilitation of cardiac patients'.

The nature of CHF, typically in individuals with a history of CHD and left-ventricular dysfunction, greatly increases the risk of arrhythmia especially during physical exertion (Hunt et al 2005). In this population such arrhythmias (ventricular tachycardia, ventricular fibrillation) are the primary cause of sudden cardiac death (Hunt et al 2005). In more advanced stages of CHF, the anti-arrhythmic therapy may include the use of implantable cardioverter defibrillators (ICDs). Specific recommendations for exercising patients with ICDs are covered in a subsequent section of this chapter. Beyond this patients may be considered for either heart transplant or ventricular assist devices (VADs). Heart transplant and VAD are to be covered in this book but the reader is recommended to review the literature on these two fascinating areas.

Secondary muscle dysfunction and reduced functional capacity

A very important aspect for the exercise scientist and practitioner to note are the related pathological consequences that CHF imposes upon pulmonary and skeletal muscle function. Poor functional capacity stems well beyond the influence of a poor cardiac output (Pina et al 2003). Similar to individuals with pulmonary disease (highlighted in Chapter 4), CHF leads to a cascade of impairments to skeletal and pulmonary (intercostal and diaphragm) muscle histology and biochemistry (Gosker et al 2000). Such impairments include a reduced vasodilatory capacity of muscle capillaries, a change from type I oxidative to type II glycolytic muscle fibres in skeletal muscle and the opposite in diaphragm muscle. Reduced vasodilatation response to exertion in individuals with CHF is believed to be linked to arterial endothelial function and its loss of ability to react to the presence of nitric oxide (Gosker et al 2000, Pina et al 2003). It would appear that there is some internal signalling to preserve central circulation, where in healthy individuals it has been demonstrated at maximal exercise that 76% of blood volume is distributed to the exercising muscle as compared to 51% in individuals with CHF (Pina et al 2003, Sullivan et al 1989, Wada et al 1997). The biochemical changes that correspond to muscle fibre type changes in skeletal muscle, making them less fatigue resistant, include decreases in creatine phosphate (PCr) and ATP stores, decreases in stored glycogen and corresponding increases in lactate and pyruvate. Mitochondrial density is impaired and related muscle and mitochondrial enzyme activity is decreased, which decreases the provision of muscle metabolism through fatty acid oxidation and other aerobic processes. These impairments caused by CHF are due to disuse, chronic tissue hypoxia, oxidative stress, nutritional depletion and systemic inflammation (Gosker et al 2000, Pina et al 2003).

Originally it was thought that these changes were due to decreased muscle activation through enforced inactivity, which resulted from poor nutritive blood flow relative to a decreased cardiac output. However, more recently, evidence has pointed towards a neuro-hormonal signalling linked to responses of reduced vasomotor sensitivity (noted above in relation to nitric oxide), hypoxia, inflammation and oxidative stress within the body that also affects such changes within skeletal muscle (Khan & Sinoway 2000, Onder et al 2006, Troosters et al 2004). One of the catalysts to this thinking has been the independent effects of ACE inhibitor (angiotensin-converting-enzyme inhibitor) medication on skeletal muscle function (Onder et al 2006). ACE inhibitors are standard therapy for CHF (Wood et al 2005) and not only bring about a relative increase in stroke volume via reduced cardiac 'afterload' (decreased peripheral arterial resistance), but also have a number of effects on skeletal muscle, including mechanical, metabolic, anti-inflammatory, nutritional, neurological and angiogenic actions. One might think that ACE inhibitors are a 'magic bullet' that can replace exercise training but individuals with CHF will still continue to have significant metabolic and enzymatic changes in their skeletal muscles and a loss of muscle mass (Gosker et al 2000, Pina et al 2003).

It is now fairly well established that regular exercise cannot directly improve myocardial function in CHF, and that increases in $\dot{V}O_2max/\dot{V}O_2$ peak and endurance time from aerobic and strength training are attained through reversing the deleterious effects that CHF imposes on skeletal muscle (Hanson 1994, Pina et al 2003). The muscle myopathy described above predicts nearly 50% of the variance in functional capacity in CHF and provides a clear rationale as to why resting ejection fraction poorly predicts functional capacity (Hanson 1994, Pina et al 2003).

Aerobic endurance exercise in heart failure

As noted in the Cochrane Library Systematic Review (Rees et al 2004), most of the trials on the benefits of exercise in CHF used aerobic endurance type activity. In addition to the NYHA classification, Hanson (1994) specifically summarized classifications for functional aerobic capacity in CHF into four fitness categories:

- normal ≥ 7 METs ($\dot{V}O_2max \geq 24.5$ mL $\cdot$ kg^{-1} $\cdot$ min^{-1})
- mild 5–7 METs ($\dot{V}O_2max$ 17.5–24.5 mL $\cdot$ kg^{-1} $\cdot$ min^{-1})
- moderate 3–5 METs ($\dot{V}O_2max$ 10.5–17.5 mL $\cdot$ kg^{-1} $\cdot$ min^{-1})
- severe <3 METs ($\dot{V}O_2max$ <10.5–24.5 mL $\cdot$ kg^{-1} $\cdot$ min^{-1}).

These values suggest that individuals who have mild or moderate CHF classifications may find that many activities in daily life (typically 2–5 METs; Ainsworth et al 1993) are equivalent to intensities associated with exercise training thresholds (>50% $\dot{V}O_2max$). In the absence of performing an aerobic fitness test it is likely that individuals who find activities of 2–5 METs hard or extremely hard will probably have a $\dot{V}O_2max$ less than 10–15 mL $\cdot$ kg^{-1} $\cdot$ min^{-1}. It is also important to appreciate that the relationship between resting left-ventricular ejection fraction and the above four categories is weak (Hanson 1994). This phenomenon highlights, as stated earlier, the importance of peripheral skeletal muscle factors as being key contributors to aerobic exercise capacity in CHF. As with exercise recommended in other cardiac populations, the benefits have been shown to occur in those who have performed exercise three or more times per week (Rees et al 2004). The guidelines of the AHA (Pina et al 2003) have, however, highlighted that there has been no setting of a standardized formula with regard to intensity and duration. They recommend setting exercise on an individualized basis, which relates to the patient's ability to utilize either a continuous or more typically an interval approach to aerobic endurance training that lasts >20 minutes. The important aspect to remember is that in individuals with less than 6 METs of maximal capacity ($\dot{V}O_2max$ <20 mL $\cdot$ kg^{-1} $\cdot$ min^{-1}), when their exercise intensity is progressed, what may feel like a small increment in exercise intensity (e.g. increase of walking speed by 1 km $\cdot$ h^{-1}) to a healthy individual (who has a $\dot{V}O_2max$ >35 mL $\cdot$ kg^{-1} $\cdot$ min^{-1} or 10 METs) represents a much larger relative increase for the CHF individual. For the low fit CHF individual walking at a speed of 3.5 km $\cdot$ h^{-1}, which for example represents a recommended intensity of 60–70% $\dot{V}O_2max$ (70–80% HRmax or ventilatory threshold), an increase in walking speed of 1 km $\cdot$ h^{-1} would represent an increase of 15–20% of the $\dot{V}O_2max$ being required.

If the person is already exercising at 70% $\dot{V}O_2$max this would most certainly have increased the intensity above the ventilatory threshold and because such intensities are poorly tolerated, potentially lead to ischaemic responses previously described. Hence the interval approach, with bouts of active rest, can help prevent sustained periods of activity at too high an intensity (Meyer 2001, Meyer et al 1997). The use of smaller muscle group aerobic endurance or strength training exercises, which have a high local metabolic demand but a low central cardiorespiratory demand, may provide a useful alternative to whole-body exercise (Tyni-Lenne et al 2001, Volaklis & Tokmakidis 2005). Strength training could be used as a means of active recovery during the interval between whole-body aerobic exercises. In very low fit individuals, muscular strength and endurance exercises of smaller muscle groups may be an appropriate starting point before attempting to engage in longer-duration large muscle group or whole-body aerobic exercise.

An area that is developing further credence is the use of inspiratory muscle training in CHF, which has been shown to improve exercise endurance and peak $\dot{V}O_2$ and is an aid in coping with breathlessness brought on by exercise in CHF (Mancini et al 1995).

Muscular strength and endurance exercise in heart failure

The onset of physiological disability (exercise intolerance) imposed by heart failure has been described as occurring in parallel to the ageing process but in an accelerated manner (Geilen et al 2005). Muscle atrophy, along with the numerous histochemical and biochemical problems highlighted above, is a key aspect of decreased physical functioning (Opasich et al 1999). It has been argued that a baseline of muscular strength underpins all activity (Latham et al 2004), especially those activities of a short duration but vital to independent living (walking a short distance, getting in and out of bed or a chair, climbing a short flight of stairs). Only when skeletal joints can be supported and stabilized is it possible to perform more enduring, repeated aerobic activity (e.g. walking, stepping, cycling). These features are also associated with reductions in quality of life related to the ageing process in individuals older than 70 years (Latham et al 2004). With the largest proportion of individuals with CHF being older than 70 years (Fig. 3.8), and considering all the above factors, it is obvious why strength training should form an important component of exercise. Furthermore, age, cardiorespiratory disease, inactivity, poor strength and coordination are all independent and collective risk factors for falling, osteoporosis and fractures (Lawlor et al 2003). These aspects and the guidance for exercise prescription of resistance strength training were covered in the section on muscular strength and endurance training in CHD. The same principles can be applied safely and effectively in CHF (Levinger et al 2005, Volaklis & Tokmakidis 2005). The only precaution is that individuals with CHF may be somewhat weaker than those who have CHD or are younger, and the mode of resistance apparatus may have to be lighter hand/leg weights or the use of elasticated 'dyna-bands'. In summary, strength training exercise in CHF:

- helps in reversing the effects of muscle myopathy associated with CHF, without causing large demands on central cardiorespiratory function
- can contribute to increases in $\dot{V}O_2$ peak and submaximal aerobic endurance
- is most beneficial if it can either be a starting point in aiding progression towards more whole-body aerobic exercise or is combined with an aerobic exercise programme.

Balance and proprioceptive/coordination exercise in heart failure

As covered in Chapter 6 and noted above, in concert with muscle strength losses and atrophy resulting from CHF and/or ageing, balance and coordination are important factors in being active to prevent falls and fractures and maintaining quality of life. Tai chi exercise that involves the development of local muscular strength, proprioception and balance has been reported to enhance quality of life, increase 6-minute walking distance and decrease B-type natriuretic peptide levels in CHF (Yeh et al 2004).

CONSIDERATIONS FOR PATIENTS WITH ARRHYTHMIA AND/OR IMPLANTABLE CARDIOVERTER DEFIBRILLATOR

Arrhythmia and exercise

As noted earlier, exercise-induced arrhythmia continues to be a distinct possibility at the start of exercise, during and at the end of exercise, and is influenced by decreased vagal tone, latency of the sympathetic nervous system and circulating catecholamines (Beckerman et al 2005, Belardinelli 2003, Braith and Edwards 2003, Kelly 1996, Malfatto et al 1996, Mayordomo & Batalla 2002, Pashkow et al 1997). Generally there is a mixed message as to the likelihood of arrhythmia. For instance, exercise testing and exercise is effective at provoking arrhythmias (Beckerman et al 2005) and others have stated that exercise testing and training is safe and effective in patients with arrhythmia (Allen et al 1988). Vigorous exercise training is not associated with an increased incidence of ventricular arrhythmias in elderly athletes (Pigozzi et al 2004). Exercise can induce or prevent arrhythmias and exercise training lessens the likelihood of arrhythmia (Belardinelli 2003, Malfatto et al 1996). Approximately 5–10% of myocardial infarctions are associated with vigorous physical activity (Thompson et al 2003). As illustrated in Figure 3.2, the relative risk of both exercise-related myocardial infarction and sudden death is greatest in individuals who are the least physically active and still performing unaccustomed vigorous physical activity. A summary of the factors contributing to arrhythmia during exercise is shown in Figure 3.9A.

Regular exercise over an 8-week period in post-MI patients has been shown to improve parasympathetic tone, increase heart rate variability, reduce the incidence of arrhythmia and improve prognosis (Malfatto et al 1996). Assuming appropriate precautions are taken, as discussed at the end of this chapter, aerobic endurance training and strength training can be performed safely and effectively in patients with arrhythmias (Fitchet et al 2003, Vanhees et al 2001).

Implantable cardioverter defibrillators

The first prospective randomized control trial in ICD patients with low capacity (ejection fraction <35%) demonstrated that exercise-based rehabilitation (including aerobic circuit training) has significant and beneficial outcomes in terms of aerobic fitness and psychological well-being (Fitchet et al 2003). Similar findings have been found in larger retrospective studies with a 20% mean improvement in aerobic fitness following regular aerobic exercise training (Vanhees et al 2001). Most importantly the intensity and variety of physical activity, as seen in daily life, needs to be reflected in the exercise phase of the cardiac rehabilitation programme so that patients can gain the greatest benefit. Aerobic and skilled flowing movement, muscular endurance and flexibility should dominate the exercise and physical activity sessions. Such activities are very well tolerated, effective and lead to optimal carryover (Belardinelli 2003, Fitchet et al 2003, Fletcher et al 2001, Pina et al 2003). A note of caution is required for those few patients who are at risk of ICD electrical-lead failure. This situation is rare, but often known immediately postoperatively and exists because the only viable route to the ventricle required the ICD wire to bend slightly more than normal. During exercise it is important to avoid excessive shoulder range of movement and/or highly repetitive vigorous shoulder movements (Fitchet et al 2003, Lampman & Knight 2000, Pashkow et al 1997, Pina et al 2003). Light to moderate resistance activities performed within a normal range of movement that closely match functional activities have been used successfully in patients with an ICD (Fitchet et al 2003).

Exercise prescription should utilize one of the standard best-practice approaches of monitoring, e.g. rating of perceived exertion or target heart rate (ACSM 2006a, Fletcher et al 2001). However, a note of caution is required when prescribing exercise intensity based on standard heart rate approaches. The use of standard 75% target heart rate in patients with slow ventricular tachycardia will often mean that the target exercise heart rate is above the detection threshold of the ICD (Fitchet et al 2003). Sinus tachycardia is a normal response to exercise and although most modern ICDs have algorithms designed to differentiate sinus from ventricular tachyarrhythmias, there are still occasions when uncomfortable, inappropriate therapy is administered (Begley et al 2003, Luthje et al 2005). Every effort should be made to reduce patient anxiety, in regard to perceived physical activity and exercise risks, in order to achieve the best outcome post implant (Lewin et al 2001, Sears et al 2001).

The important points that need consideration prior to prescribing exercise or giving advice on physical activity are: (1) the ICD detection threshold setting in beats per minute; (2) whether the device is set for ventricular tachycardia (VT) or ventricular fibrillation (VF); (3) rapid onset setting; (4) sustained ventricular tachycardia settings; (5) ICD therapy, e.g. anti-tachycardia pacing or shocks; (6) use and dose of beta-blockade (Doherty 2006). Figure 3.10 shows conceptually how points 1 to 4 are considered by the ICD in terms of exercise heart rate. Knowledge of all these factors and their interrelationship can reduce the anxiety of patients and clinicians involved in setting physical activity and exercise targets. For example, a patient who is taking beta-blockade and has an ICD VF setting of 180 beats per minute with a rapid onset setting of 30 beats and set for shock therapy (defibrillation) is very unlikely to experience inappropriate shocks or arrhythmia with moderate-intensity exercise.

All exercise sessions should start with a warm-up and finish with a cool-down period, both of which should last for 10 to 15 minutes, so that the cardiovascular system has time to adjust to the alteration in circulatory and respiratory demand (Fletcher et al 2001, Pina et al 2003). The sequence of exercise should vary from arm work to trunk and leg work, with flexibility and coordination exercises following the more strenuous exercises. The main part of the training programme should consist of graded aerobic circuit training exercises lasting 30 to 40 minutes and incorporating multijoint movements with part bodyweight and moderate resistance (ACSM 2006a, Fitchet et al 2003, Fletcher et al 2001, Lampman & Knight 2000, Pashkow et al 1997).

In general, most exercises should be performed standing, with horizontal and seated arm exercises kept to a minimum. Seated arm exercise, especially at or above shoulder height, is associated with reduced venous return, reduced end-diastolic volume, a concomitant decrease in cardiac output and increased likelihood of arrhythmia (Fitchet et al 2003, Lampman & Knight 2000, Pashkow et al 1997). If seated exercise is to be performed then the intensity of exercise should be lowered and the emphasis placed on muscular endurance. Mild leg exercise, for example alternate

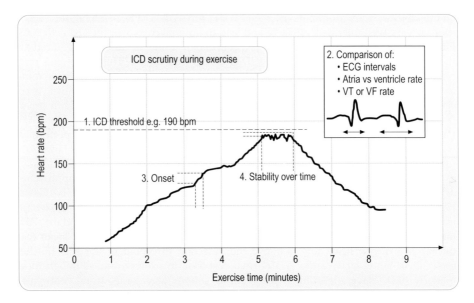

Figure 3.10   Implantable cardioverter defibrillator (ICD) monitoring during exercise.

heel raises, when combined with arm exercise, reduces the haemodynamic response compared with strict arm work (Toner et al 1990).

Physical fitness is soon lost if training is not continued at a level sufficient to maintain the effect (ACSM 2006a, Fitchet et al 2003, Fletcher et al 2001, Pina et al 2003, Rees et al 2004). The terms reversibility, deconditioning and detraining all describe the rapid loss of fitness that follows a relatively permanent cessation of training. Moderate physical activity as well as leisure and sport are known to benefit health and where possible these should be pursued most days of the week. Continuous physical activity of 30 minutes or more is considered most effective, although multiple activity sessions of 10 to 15 minutes, on the same day, have also demonstrated significant health improvement (ACSM 2006a, Blair et al 2004, Fitchet et al 2003).

Summary for arrhythmia and ICD

Physical activity and exercise has a substantial role in enabling patients with an ICD to take control of their condition. Exercise can be performed safely without increasing the risk of cardiac complications so long as the exercise is prescribed at the appropriate intensity and the exercise session incorporates an effective warm-up and cool-down period. The initial assessment of patients with an ICD and the pre-exercise review requires that certain information be obtained to inform the physical activity prescription. This includes ICD heart rate settings, ICD therapy settings and medication used to control the rate and rhythm of the heart. The mode of exercise needs to be similar to daily activity in order to gain the most from exercise sessions and maintain the effect over years. A long-term, preferably lifestyle, approach to physical activity and exercise is essential if patients are to achieve the greatest benefits.

CONSIDERATIONS FOR EXERCISE AND CARDIAC MEDICATIONS

Numerous medications are used to manage cardiac disease, each of which has a specific physiological task with related side effects and factors that can positively and negatively interact with exercise. This area could fill a whole chapter and/or a book but not to make any mention of it would be negligent. Further information may be found in Reents (2000).

This section aims to be a very brief overview from which the reader can at least develop an appreciation of key underlying factors. There are six general areas of cardiac medications, namely those that:

- increase coronary blood flow, which preserves or increases myocardial oxygen supply, e.g. nitrates
- reduce myocardial oxygen demand, e.g. beta-blockers
- stabilize or maintain electrical control of the myocardium (prevent dysrhythmia), e.g. anti-arrhythmics
- prevent atherosclerosis, e.g. statins
- decrease blood viscosity, e.g. antiplatelets
- control fluid levels, e.g. diuretics.

The typical medications prescribed to individuals with cardiac disease to achieve the above list of benefits include: beta-blockers, nitrates, calcium channel blocker, digitalis, diuretics, vasodilators, anti arrhythmic agents, anti thrombotics and lipid management agents. Many of these medications have multiple effects, for example the beta-adrenergic receptor antagonist (beta-blocker), which is one of the most widely prescribed medications in cardiac disease (Beanlands et al 2000, Department of Health 2000). Beta-blockers reduce the sympathomimetic effects of adrenaline and noradrenaline. The main consequence is that they decrease both the heart rate (chronotropic effect) and the force of myocardial contraction (inotropic effect). In doing this not only is myocardial oxygen demand decreased, but the oxygen supply to the myocardium is preserved; the period of diastole is preserved, allowing greater time for coronary arteries to fill and perfuse the myocardium (Beanlands et al 2000). Eighty per cent of myocardial perfusion occurs during diastole and the period of diastole is shortened with any increase in heart rate (Myers et al 2002). By decreasing heart rate and myocardial work, the risk of provoking ischaemia and arrhythmia is decreased.

Along with beta-blockers, most individuals with cardiac disease (unless contra-indicated) will also be taking:

- aspirin as an antiplatelet in the event that an atheroma ruptures, which could prevent a clot forming within a coronary artery or cerebral artery, leading to a myocardial or cerebral infarction (stroke), respectively
- ACE inhibitor, a powerful peripheral vasodilator which, as mentioned in the section on heart failure, reduces 'afterload' and thereby brings about a relative increase in stroke volume
- statin for lowering cholesterol.

Patients who need further treatment to bring about enhanced myocardial perfusion and/or reduced myocardial workload through vasodilatation and decreased peripheral resistance, respectively, may also be given a long-acting nitrate or a calcium channel blocker (e.g. amlodipine). Other calcium channel blockers include diltiazem and verapamil, which not only act as vasodilators but also act upon both the electrical conduction and contractility of the myocardium, decreasing myocardial

Table 3.2   Main cardiac medication groups and the heart conditions for which they are used (with permission from BACR Phase IV Training, Farnham, Surrey, UK)

	Ischaemic heart disease and angina	Hypertension	Heart failure and poor left ventricular function	Arrhythmias
Nitrates	✓		✓	
Beta-blockers	✓	✓	✓	✓
Calcium channel blockers	✓	✓		✓
Antiplatelets/ anticoagulants	✓	✓	✓	✓
Diuretics		✓	✓	
ACE inhibitors		✓	✓	
Digoxin			✓	✓
Amiodarone				✓

oxygen demand and preventing arrhythmia. When arrhythmias are more serious, patients may be treated with amiodarone. A summary of typical cardiac drug groups is provided in Table 3.2. From a practical perspective, individuals who require medications to augment coronary perfusion or manage myocardial dysrhythmias beyond the effects of beta-blockade and ACE inhibitors are likely to be individuals at 'higher risk' of an exertion-related event.

In the event that an individual has had coronary artery bypass surgery, coronary angiography and stenting, or a valve replacement, or has arrhythmias, it is likely he or she will be prescribed clopidogrel or warfarin in addition to aspirin, to prevent the formation of a secondary thrombosis (Wood et al 2005). Such a thrombosis could cause a myocardial infarction, pulmonary embolism or a cerebral infarction that precipitates a stroke.

Exercise capacity and medication

Generally in patients who are stable and have no angina or heart failure, cardiac medications will not increase exercise capacity and in some cases (beta-blockers) exercise capacity will decrease (Franklin & Gordon 2005, pp. 176–183). In individuals with good ventricular function and no residual ischaemia, beta-blockers reduce relative exercise performance as a result of the following: a reduced maximal heart rate (by 20–40 beats per minute) and maximal contractility and thus reduced $\dot{V}O_2$max, vasoconstriction to peripheral tissues including skeletal muscle, prevention of bronchodilatation in the pulmonary system (contraindicated for asthmatics and those with COPD), slowed oxygen kinetics and a reduced ability to mobilize and utilize free fatty acids for muscle metabolism (Lamont et al 1997). However, for individuals with compromised left ventricular function and myocardial ischaemia on exertion, beta-blockers have been demonstrated to enhance submaximal physical performance and increase ventilatory efficiency (Wolk et al 2005, Abraham 2000). Some individuals on beta-blockade may complain of lethargy and cold extremities and some may feel depressed, all of which could affect motivation to be physically active.

For individuals with angina, arrhythmias and heart failure, the increase in functional exercise capacity can be related to a raised threshold before arrhythmias or ischaemia occur. Sensibly patients will not be tested or exercised at intensities above such a threshold and hence determining a true maximal capacity, where all three systems (cardiac, pulmonary and skeletal muscle) can be taken to maximum level, is not possible. The increased exercise capacity due to the use of medications is therefore not necessarily a true or absolute physiological maximum that will meet the criteria for 'maximum' (Winter et al 2006). This is why in clinical populations the term $\dot{V}O_2$ peak is often used as opposed to $\dot{V}O_2$max.

PRACTICAL CONSIDERATIONS FOR EXERCISE AND REHABILITATION OF CARDIAC PATIENTS

Exercise is only part of the rehabilitation process along with advice, counselling and lifestyle management education (AACVPR 2004, BACR 1995). The considerations discussed in this section are applicable to any form of exertion whether it is performed in the early inpatient phase (phase I), early discharge phase (phase II) or the mid-to-latter phases (phases III and IV) of cardiac rehabilitation, or long term in supervised exercise sessions or within activities of daily living. Individuals with cardiac disease will typically have other co-morbidities including obesity, diabetes, hypertension, pulmonary disease, mental health conditions or neuro-musculoskeletal disorders linked with the ageing process (Beswick et al 2004). Therefore adaptations for exercise sessions and the psychosocial milieu in which they take place also need considering so that patients attain amounts of physical activity that will be beneficial.

The most obvious practical consideration for exercise, supervised or unsupervised, is to prevent physical exertion from triggering a cardiac event. Events include the provocation of dizziness, angina, arrhythmia, myocardial infarction, ventricular fibrillation and cardiac arrest. The risks of provoking more severe events were summarized in Table 3.1 and Figure 3.2. In general, exercise movements, posture and changes in intensity must be performed so as not to cause sudden drops in myocardial perfusion or sudden changes in electrical stimulation that augment areas of myocardial irritability (Figs 3.9A and B).

Warm-up and cool-down

During structured moderate to vigorous exercise it is recommended to precede or follow the main exercise session with a 10- to 15-minute period of lighter activity (AACVPR 2004, Foster & Porcari 2002, SIGN 2002). The warm-up should graduate the intensity from rest up to 40–50% $\dot{V}O_2$max (heart rate reserve maximum) or 50–60% HRmax and/or 9 to 11 on Borg's RPE scale (AACVPR 2004, Borg 1998, Foster & Porcari 2002, SIGN 2002). The rationale behind this from a safety perspective is that it takes this amount of time for coronary arteries to fully dilate (Edwards et al 2004, Kelion et al 2001) and correspondingly prevent acute rises in circulating catecholamines (sympathetic stimulation) that could irritate the myocardium (Fig. 3.9B). From an exercise performance perspective, it allows enough time for the shunting of blood from the viscera to the skeletal muscles, the lungs, the heart and the skin. Ensuring the skeletal muscle is adequately perfused is important so as to meet the needs of aerobic metabolism and overcome muscle performance limitations caused by the oxygen deficit. As noted earlier, this also takes into consideration the time needed to reach a 'steady-state' level of submaximal activity (oxygen kinetics). In individuals on beta-blockade or with poor left-ventricular function the time it takes to reach steady state is 3 to 4 minutes longer than in healthy individuals (Hughson & Kowalchuk 1991). A final and important matter to appreciate is that in individuals with low levels of aerobic fitness, there is a much narrower difference between light and moderate-to-vigorous activity, and the potential to over-exert during the warm-up is greater than in healthy, fitter individuals. Those with low levels of aerobic fitness may have to begin their warm-up performing mobility exercises in a chair. See Chapter 6 for such recommendations.

The key factors in an active cool-down are aiding the clearance of sympathetic stimulants including metabolites (e.g. blood lactate) and catecholamines (e.g. adrenaline) from the blood, while maintaining venous return and thus myocardial perfusion. The latter is aimed at preventing acute postural hypotension and correspondingly returning heart rate back to near resting levels. As highlighted in Figures 3.9A and B, the failure to achieve any one or a combination of any of the above factors can precipitate ischaemia and arrhythmia. It has long been known that an active recovery with low-intensity exercise, following moderate to vigorous exercise, helps return blood lactic acid to resting levels more quickly compared with immediate rest (Newman et al 1937). More recently it has been demonstrated that an active recovery also helps to return heart rate sooner to resting levels but with better maintenance of venous return as compared with immediate rest (Takahashi & Miyamoto 1998). These studies linked such a phenomenon with an increase in cardiac vagal tone as a result of the active recovery. Wolk et al (2005) reported that in heart failure patients, the time-course to heart rate recovery was related to the prevalence of poorer echocardiographic, neurohormonal and/or haemodynamic prognostic indexes. This not only highlights the importance of a proper cool-down but suggests that monitoring heart rate recovery may provide clinically relevant prognostic information. The BACR (2006) recommend that patients are observed up to 30 minutes post exercise, especially where they may have a shower (a warm humid environment, in an upright somewhat static posture) that is conducive to postural hypotension. The use of a post-exercise social or education session provides a natural opportunity for this observation period to occur.

Posture and movement

During submaximal exercise, for a given oxygen uptake, cardiac output is greater in supine than in upright positions (Leyk et al 1994). The implication of this for cardiac patients is that the greater the cardiac output, the greater the myocardial oxygen demand, which increases the likelihood of ischaemia and ischaemic-related events. Hence it is not advisable to get patients to perform activities in a lying position or give them supine activities after a dynamic upright activity. Quick changes in posture that increase blood flow into the thoracic cavity are known to trigger angina in patients with CHD (Klein et al 1993). Changes in posture which cause blood pooling in the lower limbs (e.g. when an individual goes from a lying or seated position to an upright position) can induce postural hypotension (Bradley & Davis 2003). In this situation there is a sudden decrease in both systolic and diastolic pressure which could lead to a sudden decrease in venous return, reduced aortic pressure and a consequent reduction in myocardial perfusion that may invoke ischaemia. In older individuals or those on vasodilating (e.g. ACE inhibitors, nitrates) and sympathetic blocking agents (beta-blockers, calcium channel blockers), where autonomic responses to such a challenge are blunted, hypotension can be augmented (Shi et al 2000, 2003). Therefore in all cases of exercise or within activities of daily living, sudden changes in posture either from upright to supine or from a sitting/supine to upright should be avoided.

In many exercise situations, exercise equipment may be used, including ergometers (treadmills, cycle or rowing ergometer, circuit equipment, steps, free weights, machine weights, etc.). Repetitive movements from these may exacerbate the effects of medications, including dizziness (e.g. treadmill) or postural hypotension following seated exercise (e.g. rowing and cycling). Furthermore, movement in and around equipment can create physical hazards. Care needs to be taken, especially for patients on clopidogrel or warfarin, where there is an increased risk of bruising or even bleeding/haemorrhaging from accidental impact (Fitzmaurice et al 2002).

Exertion in activities of daily life

Within the confines of a carefully designed and managed exercise session, which includes attention to warm-up, cool-down and posture, associated cardiac events can be avoided. It is, however, in activities of daily life that individuals may unconsciously perform acute bouts of activity that trigger exertion-related ischaemia (Freedman & Wong 1998). Therefore, individuals with cardiac disease need to be informed of how to prevent, in both domestic and/or occupational settings, the triggering of hypotensive events, sudden increases in venous return or acute rises in heart rate, blood pressure and catecholamines. Freedman & Wong (1998) reported that mental stress was an uncommon trigger of either silent or symptomatic ischaemia. Preventative recommendations should include performing heavier activity (e.g. gardening) only when preceded and followed by lighter activity (e.g. light housework), avoiding acute changes in posture (either from lying or sitting to upright or vice versa) by performing light mobility exercises and deeper breathing for a minute or two prior to getting up out of a chair, and walking on the level for a minute before climbing a set of stairs.

CONSIDERATIONS FOR EXERCISE TESTING

There are numerous guidelines and protocols on the clinical exercise testing of patients with cardiac disease and it is not considered necessary to go into the details of protocols and diagnostic assessment techniques here. Organizations such as the American College of Sports Medicine (2006a, 2006b) and the British Association of Sport and Exercise Sciences (Winter et al 2006) provide in-depth information. This section highlights the reasons or rationale for choosing a particular test.

Tests are performed for one of three reasons:

1. clinical diagnosis, prognosis, treatment decisions, and risk stratification
2. assessment of functional capacity to monitor changes related to exercise training
3. applying results to exercise prescription or physical activity guidance.

Clinical testing for diagnosis and prognosis typically involves symptom-limited or clinical end-point testing which takes the patient to the highest possible intensity. A typical end-point for protocols within the UK, other than symptoms or clinical changes, is to stop the test when the patient attains 100% age-adjusted maximal heart rate (AAMHR) calculated as 220 minus age. A major problem with the AAMHR method, and even those with updated algorithms, is that it represents a gross expression of heart rate change that fails to take account of how much above rest the heart rate has risen. This variability is illustrated in Figure 3.11, where even patients without symptoms or signs of ischaemia attained a maximal heart rate that was on

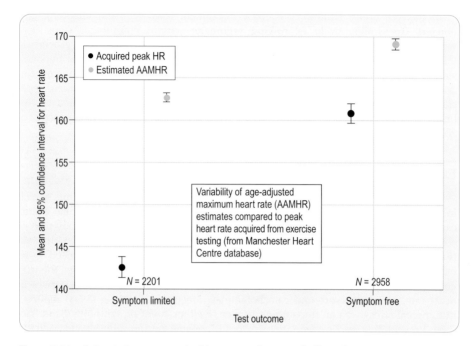

Figure 3.11   Estimated versus acquired heart rate from treadmill testing.

average more than 10 beats per minute below their AAMHR. The other factor here that also needs to be considered is why the patient decided to stop. Hence three factors need to be considered when the heart rate response data are either used to stop the test or used in subsequent exercise prescription: what was the resting heart rate so that a Karvonen range (Karvonen 1959) can be determined; was the patient on any chronotropic medication (e.g. beta-blocker); and did the patient achieve a true maximum or did they stop for reasons of poor motivation, fear, lack of motor control or orthopaedic limitation? Considering these factors increases in importance when managing patients with lower functional capacities (<7 METs) or those of a higher risk who have symptoms or clinical changes at intensities lower than 7 METs (ACSM 2006b). Why 7 METs? The physiological demands for being able to cope with activities of daily living are typically in the range of 3.5 to 5.0 METs (Ainsworth et al 1993), which represents 50–70% of 7 METs. This means that such individuals may be at clinical and relatively high intensity thresholds that could easily provoke ischaemia or arrhythmia just performing activities of daily life. Furthermore, as discussed earlier and to follow, there is a strong correlation between a poor prognosis, morbidity and mortality in individuals with exercise capacities of less than 7 METs.

From a medical practitioner's perspective, the aim of an exercise test is to determine a point where ischaemia or arrhythmias/dysrhythmia can be provoked or ventricular function fails to increase with increased work rates. If problems arise at intensities less than 10 METs then further investigations or aggressive medical or surgical therapy are typically pursued. Myers et al (2002) have demonstrated that individuals with cardiovascular disease who attain greater than 10 METs will have a reduced future risk of cardiac events and early mortality.

In the UK routine clinical measurements include 12-lead ECG and blood pressure responses as recommended by the British Cardiovascular Society (www.bcs.org.uk). Systolic blood pressure measurement is used not only for determining whether cardiac output rises with increases in exercise intensity but also for calculating an additional measure of haemodynamics known as the rate pressure product (RPP). RPP has been quoted since 1974 (Nelson et al 1974) in the literature but is only recently finding acceptance. It is a composite measure of the product of heart rate and systolic blood pressure (HR × systolic BP × 0.01) that is strongly associated with myocardial oxygen consumption (ACSM 2006b, Fletcher 1998, Gibbons et al 2002, Nelson et al 1974, Thompson et al 2003, Wasserman et al 1999). High RPP values are strongly associated with clinical symptoms in patients with angina. From a physical activity advice perspective it is the RPP at the clinical threshold (ischaemia, arrhythmia, pump failure) that is important and not just heart rate. Upper-body activity is known to have a higher RPP and thus greater myocardial oxygen demand than lower-body exercise for a given heart rate (Toner et al 1990). Thus RPP caters for independent variations in heart rate or blood pressure and is a more accurate reflection of myocardial demand than heart rate alone. It is, however, known that when exercising at a given heart rate, when leg exercise is added to arm exercise (e.g. in rowing ergometry), systolic blood pressure decreases, and rate pressure and whole body oxygen uptake will be similar to exercising with legs only (e.g. walking) (Toner et al 1990, Buckley et al 1999b). Aerobic exercise training has been found to increase the RPP threshold for clinical changes and reducing symptoms (Nelson et al 1974, Thompson et al 2003). RPP values (expressed in hundreds × 10²) from the Manchester Heart Centre database, as illustrated in Figure 3.12, tend to be in the range of 230 and

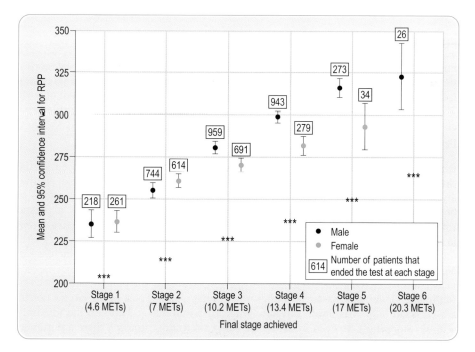

Figure 3.12 Rate pressure product (RPP) for referred cardiac patients during treadmill testing (from the Manchester Heart Centre database; Bruce protocol: 4840 referred cardiac patients). *** 75% RPP exercise training threshold based on mean test results from each stage.

325 during treadmill testing in referred cardiac patients. As with most exercise-related physiological responses, there is a gender bias in favour of males demonstrating a higher threshold for RPP as the intensity of exercise increases (Doherty 2003). This reiterates the need for relative (as a proportion of the individual's own maximum or peak capacity) and not absolute expressions of exercise intensity when advising patients and producing guidelines. On average RPP training thresholds in cardiac rehabilitation exercise programmes are much lower than peak exercise testing RPP values (Fig. 3.12). The data in Figure 3.12 agree with other reports, where values of between 250 and 280 are well tolerated during exercise training (Nelson et al 1974, Thompson et al 2003).

In the USA, pulmonary responses and sometimes echocardiographs are measured during exercise ECG testing in cardiopulmonary patients. Such integration of testing parameters has been described as part of the assessment of cardiac conditions in athletic populations (Winter et al 2006). In the UK, the National Health Service resources are typically limited and only a few specialist centres linked to research will include pulmonary function assessments. The addition of pulmonary function testing allows for a greater assessment of the integration between cardiac function, pulmonary function and skeletal muscle performance (McConnell et al 1995). Such tests can more specifically determine which system (cardiac, pulmonary, muscle) is the limiting factor in overall functional capacity. From this, subsequent exercise and drug therapy can be better tailored to the individual. Take for example an individual with heart failure. With the addition of pulmonary function testing it can be determined if and when the breathlessness is being affected by cardiac or pulmonary dysfunction and how much of the exercise capacity is limited by skeletal muscle dysfunction. The addition of blood lactate responses, from a simple capillary sample, adds further information to skeletal muscle performance limitations.

FUNCTIONAL ASSESSMENT CONSIDERATIONS

Functional physiological outcomes during exercise come under two broad categories: performance changes or physiological response changes to a given exercise work rate (submaximal or maximal). Many testing protocols allow for the measurement of both. These field-based assessments can also be used for exercise prescription guidance.

Performance changes

Performance changes are those that will demonstrate a clear increase in either the duration or intensity of exercise a patient can achieve. Peak or maximal levels that an individual can attain have been highly correlated with longer-term prognosis in both healthy and CVD populations (Myers et al 2002). In general terms, a person unable to attain a peak level equivalent to 6 METs has a risk of premature death that is almost twice that of an individual with a peak capacity of 10 METs. Myers et al (2002) showed that once an individual can attain 10 METs, any further increase in aerobic fitness has only a small impact on further reducing risk.

Performance changes are typically those recognizable by the patient, either perceptually (e.g. 'I can walk faster or longer now on the walking part of the circuit') or by the clinician (e.g. 'Mrs Smith can now walk for 5 minutes at 3 kph on the treadmill without stopping'). So even in the absence of a set testing protocol, there are numerous opportunities within an exercise circuit to objectively note changes in exercise performance. The least that is required in order to make an objective measure is that it is reliable (e.g. the stepping height or the treadmill speed can be accurately repeated from one occasion to the next).

To gain further objectivity within outcome measures, a standardized protocol is typically used (treadmill test, cycle ergometer, step test, shuttle walk, etc.).

If a testing protocol is designed to take an individual to a peak level then their 'peak performance level' achieved can be used as an objective outcome. This is unwise in many cases unless it is being done with appropriate ECG monitoring and advanced life support (ALS) trained personnel available. It is therefore important to check what type of protocol is being used to know whether the patient is required to attain a specified submaximal or maximal level. Typically if a patient is required to work to greater than 65–70% $\dot{V}O_2$max or 80% HRmax, as the recommended upper limit for standardized exercise rehabilitation sessions, then caution is necessary. If submaximal protocols are being used, then it is important to have physiological (HR, blood pressure) and perceptual responses (RPE or breathlessness scales) that correspond to a given level of performance (speed, work rate, duration).

Physiological and perceptual response changes

As described earlier, the gold standard for exercise testing responses of cardiac patients is the use of both cardio (ECG) and respiratory (expired gas analysis) measures during an incremental peak/maximal test, e.g. the Bruce protocol (Bruce et al 1973). The use of expired gas analysis is rare in the UK except in specialist centres of research.

The four measures available, typically taken and recommended in the UK during early discharge or outpatient cardiology clinics, are the ECG (heart rate and ECG changes), blood pressure, estimated METs and RPE. With modern technology of wireless chest-strap telemetry heart rate monitors, it is very practicable to measure heart rate within a cardiac rehabilitation setting along with RPE. Therefore if the rehabilitation gym has a treadmill, then submaximal components of the Bruce or modified Bruce protocol can be repeated as a means of measuring improvement against initial clinical testing results taken previously for purposes of diagnosis and prognosis.

Example 1

For patients who have attained two stages of the Bruce protocol, and no problems occurred during stage 1, it would be possible to reassess a patient's heart rate and RPE during stage 1 on the treadmill in the gym and compare this to the original stress test. This requires the biomedical engineering department to ensure that the cardiology treadmill and the gym treadmill have been calibrated with each other.

But what about if the patient is on beta-blockers? As long as the dosage has not been changed and it is at a similar time of day on each testing occasion then the heart rate measurement will be valid.

Example 1 uses the very same principle as implementing protocol-specific shuttle walk tests, cycle ergometer or step tests. The important point is that the exact same speed or work rate needs to be set for the initial and final assessment. The outcome variable becomes the heart rate and RPE at a given speed or work rate. If heart rate has decreased by more than 5 beats per minute or RPE by 1.5 points or more at the same work rate then this can be stated as a significant improvement in aerobic fitness (Buckley et al 2004).

If it is not practical to carry out such standardized tests, then a station within the circuit can be designated as an assessment station where heart rate and RPE are measured as a suitable (not equal) alternative.

Example 2

A circuit of exercise contains a station with 2 or more minutes of shuttle walking. If the shuttle distance markers are accurately set for each session then all that needs to be done is to count the number of shuttles performed in that period. As required, the patient is expected to work to a given target heart rate and RPE. By recording heart rate and RPE for a given walking speed (total number of shuttles multiplied by the distance of each shuttle and divided by the time in minutes) it can easily be seen if the patient's heart rate and RPE are either lower for the same speed or are the same for a faster speed (see Table 3.3).

The conversion of the shuttle walking speed into METs, where a walking speed of 50 m per minute is ~2.5 METs and 70 m per minute is 3.6 METs, is derived from the ACSM (2006a). In the example shown in Table 3.3 it can be clearly seen that the patient is walking 20 m per minute faster or 1 MET harder for the same heart rate and RPE.

Example 3

A circuit of exercise contains a cycle ergometer station that is for 2 or more minutes. If the cycle ergometer resistance can be accurately set for each session and the patient pedals at the same speed then all that needs to be done is record heart rate and RPE for a given speed and resistance (if the cycle displays watts, even better). It can then be easily seen if the patient's heart rate and RPE are either lower for the same work rate or are the same for greater cycle work rate.

Example 4

A circuit of exercise contains a station with 2 or more minutes of box-stepping exercise. If the box-step height is kept the same for each session and the number of steps achieved in the 2 minutes is counted, it can then be seen if the patient's heart rate and RPE are either lower for the same stepping rate or are the same for a faster stepping rate.

Table 3.3 Example of response measures taken during an exercise class/circuit that can be used as a means of charting progress and change, in the event there is a limited opportunity to perform a specific test

Measure	Test 1 beginning of rehabilitation programme	Test 2 completion of rehabilitation programme
Walking shuttles completed in 2 minutes	10	14
Shuttle distance	10 metres	10 metres
Shuttle speed	10 shuttles × 10 m × 2 minutes = 50 m per minute	14 shuttles × 10 m × 2 minutes = 70 m per minute
Estimated MET value for walking speed	2.5	3.6
Heart rate	112	112
RPE	14	14

USING PROTOCOLS FOR ASSESSMENT

Various protocols for assessing changes in fitness and physical activity are now widely recommended within exercise for health promotion and rehabilitation (ACSM 2006a, SIGN 2002). Functional/practical fitness tests include timed walks, shuttle walking, treadmill, cycle ergometer and step testing protocols that have been traditionally used to predict $\dot{V}O_2max$. However, the validity of these in cardiac populations is not widely evidenced, often because normal age-estimated heart rate responses are altered either by medication or the presence of dysrhythmias (Buckley et al 1999a). This does not mean that their use for cardiac patients is redundant where, as explained before, these tests have been demonstrated to be reliable and sensitive enough to show changes from baseline in physical performance and changes in key responses (heart rate and RPE) (Buckley et al 2004). Another benefit of such protocols is that they provide an initial introduction for the patient to submaximal exercise to establish or evaluate both physiological and psychological baseline responses to exercise. In this case the exercise professional is provided with important information that relates to the actual exercise intensities at which the patient will be working during an exercise training session. Furthermore it provides an opportunity to gauge how the patient responds in terms of self-efficacy, motivation and motor skill, all of which are helpful in anticipation of the sometimes psychologically or socially challenging environment of a rehabilitation programme (Rejeski 1901).

More recent physical activity initiatives such as the use of pedometers have been employed both as measurement and motivational tools within health promotion (Tudor-Locke 2002). These have not been widely evaluated in cardiac populations and the make and model are very important to their reliability and validity (De Cocker et al 2006). Therefore, advice in using these with cardiac populations needs to be tailored for the individual patient. The standardized message of either 10 000 steps per day or 30 minutes of activity per day (Department of Health 2004a) is a health promotion message targeted at healthy sedentary individuals within the general population. Hence, the use of pedometer or accelerometer for evaluating present levels of activity within appropriate activities of daily living for cardiac patients may seem a potentially good practice but it is the specific advice about target volumes of activity which need to be adjusted; handing out generalized prescription guidelines could easily pose a risk for the older, frailer, higher-risk or less fit patient.

Choosing an appropriate exercise measure, whether within the exercise circuit or from specific protocols, is of paramount importance for practitioners so that objective information can be used to help patients effectively transfer from one phase of rehabilitation to the next.

KEY POINTS

1. Aerobic exercise and, in some reports, muscular strength exercise can contribute significantly to the reduction in future cardiac disease morbidity and mortality in individuals with and without cardiac disease.
2. Aerobic fitness, related to both aerobic power ($\dot{V}O_2max$) and aerobic endurance, is a strong independent risk factor of cardiac morbidity and all-cause mortality.
3. Physical activity, related to an individual's weekly energy expenditure above basal metabolic rate, is inversely related cardiac disease related morbidity and mortality.

4. Aerobic fitness is a stronger independent predictor of morbidity and mortality compared with physical activity. However, it is difficult sometimes to delineate between the individual effects of aerobic fitness versus total weekly caloric energy expenditure (physical activity). Furthermore, measuring total weekly energy expenditure in both free-living and structured exercise is much more difficult than measuring aerobic fitness.
5. Exercise professionals need to assess the risk of adverse cardiac events in patients prior to their participation and in order to determine an exercise intensity which optimizes safety, efficacy and personal needs (physically, psychologically and socially).
6. In planning safe and effective exercise, cardiac function related to overall physical function needs to be considered in light of autonomic-electrical rhythm control, coronary artery and myocardial integrity.

References

AACVPR (American Association of Cardiovascular and Pulmonary Rehabilitation) 2004 Guidelines for cardiac rehabilitation programs, 4th edn. Human Kinetics, Champaign, IL

Abdulla J, Kober L, Torp-Pedersen C 2004 Methods of assessing the functional status of patients with left ventricular systolic dysfunction in interventional studies: can brain natriuretic peptide measurement be used as surrogate for the traditional methods? Cardiovascular Drugs and Therapy 18(3):219–224

Abraham W T 2000 Beta-blockers: the new standard of therapy for mild heart failure. Archives of Internal Medicine 160(9):1237–1247

ACSM 2006a Guidelines for exercise testing and prescription. Lippincott Williams & Wilkins, Baltimore

ACSM 2006b Resource manual for guidelines for exercise testing and prescription. Lippincott Williams & Wilkins, Baltimore

Ainsworth B E, Haskell W L, Leon A S et al 1993 Compendium of physical activities: classification of energy costs of human physical activities. Medicine and Science in Sports and Exercise 25:71–80

Albert C M, Mittleman M A, Chae C U et al 2000 Triggering of sudden death from cardiac causes by vigorous exertion. New England Journal of Medicine 343(19):1355–1361

Allen B J, Casey T P, Brodsky M A et al 1988 Exercise testing in patients with life-threatening ventricular tachyarrhythmias: results and correlation with clinical and arrhythmia factors. American Heart Journal 116:997–1002

Allender S, Peto V, Scarborough P, Rayner M 2006 Coronary heart disease statistics. British Heart Foundation, London

Åstrand P, Rodahl K, Dahl H, Stromme S 2003 Text book of work physiology: physiological bases of exercise. Human Kinetics, Champaign, IL

Barengo N C, Hu G, Lakka T A 2004 Low physical activity as a predictor for total and cardiovascular disease mortality in middle-aged men and women in Finland. European Heart Journal 25:2204–2211

Barker W H, Mullooly J P, Getchell W 2006 Changing incidence and survival for heart failure in a well-defined older population, 1970–1974 and 1990–1994. Circulation 113(6):799–805

Beanlands R S, Nahmias C, Gordon E et al 2000 The effects of beta(1)-blockade on oxidative metabolism and the metabolic cost of ventricular work in patients with left ventricular dysfunction: a double-blind, placebo-controlled, positron-emission tomography study. Circulation 102:2070–2075

Beckerman J, Wu T, Jones S, Froelicher V F 2005 Exercise test-induced arrhythmias. Progress in Cardiovascular Disease 47:285–305

Begley D A, Mohiddin S A, Tripodi D et al 2003 Efficacy of implantable cardioverter defibrillator therapy for primary and secondary prevention of sudden cardiac death in hypertrophic cardiomyopathy. Pacing and Clinical Electrophysiology 26:1887–1896

Belardinelli R 2003 Arrhythmias during acute and chronic exercise in chronic heart failure. International Journal of Cardiology 90:213–218

Bell A C, Ge K, Popkin B M 2002 The road to obesity or the path to prevention: motorized transportation and obesity in China. Obesity Research 10(4):277–283

Bentzen H, Pedersen R S, Nyvad O, Pedersen E B 2004 Effect of exercise on natriuretic peptides in plasma and urine in chronic heart failure. International Journal of Cardiology 93(2–3):121–130

Beswick A D, Rees K, Griebsch I et al 2004 Provision, uptake and cost of cardiac rehabilitation programmes: improving services to under-represented groups. Health Technology Assessment 8:iii–iv, ix–x, 1–152

Blair S N, Church T S 2004 The fitness, obesity, and health equation: is physical activity the common denominator? JAMA 292:1232–1234

Blair N, Lamonte J 2005 How much and what type of physical activity is enough? What physicians should tell their patients. Archives of Internal Medicine 165:2324–2325

Blair S N, Kohl H W 3rd, Paffenbarger R S Jr et al 1989 Physical fitness and all-cause mortality. A prospective study of healthy men and women. JAMA 262:2395–2401

Blair S N, Kohl H W 3rd, Barlow C E et al 1995 Changes in physical fitness and all-cause mortality. A prospective study of healthy and unhealthy men. JAMA 273:1093–1098

Blair S N, Kampert J B, Kohl H W 3rd et al 1996 Influences of cardiorespiratory fitness and other precursors on cardiovascular disease and all-cause mortality in men and women. JAMA 276:205–210

Blair S N, Lamonte M J, Nichaman M Z 2004 The evolution of physical activity recommendations: how much is enough? American Journal of Clinical Nutrition 79:913–920

Bonaiuti D, Arioli G, Diana G et al 2005 SIMFER rehabilitation treatment guidelines in postmenopausal and senile osteoporosis. Europa Medicophysica 41:315–337

Borg G 1998 Borg's perceived exertion and pain scales. Human Kinetics, Champaign, IL

Bradley J G, Davis K A 2003 Orthostatic hypotension. American Family Physician 68:2393–2398

Braith R W, Edwards D G 2003 Neurohormonal abnormalities in heart failure: impact of exercise training. Congestive Heart Failure 9:70–76

British Association for Cardiac Rehabilitation (BACR) 1995 Guidelines for cardiac rehabilitation. Blackwell Science, Oxford

British Association for Cardiac Rehabilitation 2006 Phase IV exercise instructor manual, revised edn. Human Kinetics, Leeds

Bruce R A, Kusumi F, Hosmer D 1973 Maximal oxygen intake and nomographic assessment of functional aerobic impairment in cardiovascular disease. American Heart Journal 85:546–562

Brynjolf I, Kelbaek H, Munck O et al 1984 Right and left ventricular ejection fraction and left ventricular volume changes at rest and during exercise in normal subjects. European Heart Journal 5:756–761

Buckley J, Holmes J, Mapp G 1999a Exercise on prescription; cardiovascular activity for health. Butterworth-Heinemann, Oxford

Buckley J P, Davis J A, Simpson T 1999b Cardio-respiratory responses to rowing ergometry and treadmill exercise soon after myocardial infarction. Medicine and Science in Sports and Exercise 31:1721–1726

Buckley J P, Sim J, Eston R G et al 2004 Reliability and validity of measures taken during the Chester step test to predict aerobic power and to prescribe aerobic exercise. British Journal of Sports Medicine 38:197–205

Carson P, Phillips R, Lloyd M et al 1982 Exercise after myocardial infarction: a controlled trial. Journal of the Royal College of Physicians London 16(3):147–151

Cobb L A, Weaver W D 1986 Exercise: a risk for sudden death in patients with coronary heart disease. Journal of the American College of Cardiology 7(1):215–219

Cowie M R, Wood D A, Coats A J et al 1999 Incidence and aetiology of heart failure; a population-based study. European Heart Journal 20(6):421–428

De Cocker K, Cardon G, de Bourdeaudhuij I 2006 Validity of the inexpensive Stepping Meter in counting steps in free living conditions: a pilot study. British Journal of Sports Medicine 40:714–716

Department of Health 2000 National service framework for coronary heart disease. Department of Health, London

Department of Health 2004a At least five a week: evidence on the impact of physical activity and its relationship to health. Department of Health, London

Department of Health 2004b Choosing health: making healthy choices easier. HMSO, London

Doherty P 2003 Haemodynamics during exercise testing. Cardiology News 6:10–12

Doherty P J 2006 Physical activity and exercise for patients with implantable cardioverter defibrillators. British Journal of Cardiac Nursing 1:327–331

Edwards D G, Schofield R S, Lennon S L et al 2004 Effect of exercise training on endothelial function in men with coronary artery disease. American Journal of Cardiology 93:617–620

Farrell S W, Kampert J B, Kohl H W 3rd et al 1998 Influences of cardiorespiratory fitness levels and other predictors on cardiovascular disease mortality in men. Medicine and Science in Sports and Exercise 30(6):899–905

Fitchet A, Doherty P J, Bundy C et al 2003 Comprehensive cardiac rehabilitation programme for implantable cardioverter-defibrillator patients: a randomised controlled trial. Heart 89:155–160

Fitzmaurice D A, Blann A D, Lip G Y 2002 Bleeding risks of antithrombotic therapy. BMJ 325:828–831

Fletcher G F 1998 Current status of cardiac rehabilitation. American Family Physician 58:1778–1782

Fletcher G F, Balady G J, Amsterdam E A et al 2001 Exercise standards for testing and training: a statement for healthcare professionals from the American Heart Association. Circulation 104:1694–1740

Foster C, Porcari J P 2002 The physiologic basis for the warm-up in therapeutic exercise programs. American Journal of Medicine and Sports 4(2):157–158

Franco O H, de Laet C, Peeters A et al 2005 Effects of physical activity on life expectancy with cardiovascular disease. Archives of Internal Medicine 165:2355–2360

Franklin B 1999 Exercise and cardiovascular events: a double-edged sword? Journal of Sports Science 17(6):437–442

Franklin B, Gordon N 2005 Contemporary diagnosis and management in cardiovascular exercise. Handbooks in Health Care Co., Newtown, PA, p 80

Franklin B A, Bonzheim K, Gordon S, Timmis G C 1998 Safety of medically supervised outpatient cardiac rehabilitation exercise therapy: a 16-year follow-up. Chest 114:902–906

Franklin B A, Conviser J M, Stewart B et al 2000 Sporadic exercise: a trigger for acute cardiovascular events? [abstract]. Circulation 102(Suppl II):II-612

Freedman S B, Wong C K 1998 Triggers of daily life ischaemia. Heart 80:489–492

Froelicher V F, Myers J N 2000 Exercise and the heart. W B Saunders, Pittsburgh

Gibbons L W, Cooper K H, Meyer B M, Ellison R C 1980 The acute cardiac risk of strenuous exercise. JAMA 244:1799–1801

Gibbons R J, Balady G J, Bricker J T et al 2002 ACC/AHA 2002 guideline update for exercise testing: summary article. A report of the American College of Cardiology/American Heart Association Task Force on Practice Guidelines (Committee to Update the 1997 Exercise Testing Guidelines). Journal of the American College of Cardiology 40:1531–1540

Gosker H R, Wouters E F, van der Vusse G J, Schols A M 2000 Skeletal muscle dysfunction in chronic obstructive pulmonary disease and chronic heart failure: underlying mechanisms and therapy perspectives. American Journal of Clinical Nutrition 71(5):1033–1047

Hambrecht R, Niebauer J, Marburger C et al 1993 Various intensities of leisure time physical activity in patients with coronary artery disease: effects on cardiorespiratory fitness and progression of coronary atherosclerotic lesions. Journal of the American College of Cardiology 22(2):468–477

Hambrecht R, Wolf A, Gielen S et al 2000 Effect of exercise on coronary endothelial function in patients with coronary artery disease. New England Journal of Medicine 342(7):454–460

Hambrecht R, Adams V, Erbs S et al 2003 Regular physical activity improves endothelial function in patients with coronary artery disease by increasing phosphorylation of endothelial nitric oxide synthase. Circulation 107(25):3152–3158

Hanson P 1994 Exercise testing and training in patients with chronic heart failure. Medicine and Science in Sports and Exercise 26(5):527–537

Haskell W L 1978 Cardiovascular complications during exercise training of cardiac patients. Circulation 57:920–924

Henriksen T 1999 Foetal nutrition, foetal growth restriction and health later in life. Acta Paediatrica Supplement 88(429):4–8

Hollenberg M, Yang J, Haight T J, Tager I B 2006 Longitudinal changes in aerobic capacity: implications for concepts of aging. Journal of Gerontology. A Biological Sciences and Medical Sciences 61:851–858

Hu G, Tuomilehto J, Silventoinen K et al 2004 Joint effects of physical activity, body mass index, waist circumference and waist-to-hip ratio with the risk of cardiovascular disease among middle-aged Finnish men and women. European Heart Journal 25:2212–2219

Hughson R L, Kowalchuk J M 1991 Beta-blockade and oxygen delivery to muscle during exercise. Canadian Journal of Physiology and Pharmacology 69:285–289

Hunt S A, Abraham W T, Chin M H et al 2005 ACC/AHA 2005 guideline update for the diagnosis and management of chronic heart failure in the adult: a report of the American College of Cardiology/American Heart Association Task Force on Practice Guidelines Circulation 112(12):e154–e235

Jolliffe J A, Rees K, Taylor R S et al 2001 Exercise-based rehabilitation for coronary heart disease. Cochrane Database Systematic Review CD001800

Kannel W B 2000 Vital epidemiologic clues in heart failure. Journal of Clinical Epidemiology 53(3):229–235

Karvonen M 1959 Problems of training of the cardiovascular system. Ergonomics 2:207–215

Kelion A D, Webb T P, Gardner M A et al 2001 The warm-up effect protects against ischemic left ventricular dysfunction in patients with angina. Journal of the American College of Cardiology 37:705–710

Kelly T M 1996 Exercise testing and training of patients with malignant ventricular arrhythmias. Medicine and Science in Sports and Exercise 28:53–61

Kesaniemi Y K, Danforth E Jr, Jensen M D et al 2001 Dose-response issues concerning physical activity and health: an evidence-based symposium. Medicine and Science in Sports and Exercise 33(6 Suppl):S351–S358

Khan M H, Sinoway L I 2000 Muscle reflex control of sympathetic nerve activity in heart failure: the role of exercise conditioning. Heart Failure Reviews 5(1):87–100

Klein H O, Nuriel H, Levi A et al 1993 Pronus angina (angina pectoris induced by stooping or crouching). A proposed mechanism. Chest 104:65–70

Lamont L S, Romito R A, Finkelhor R S, Kalhan S C 1997 Beta 1-adrenoreceptors regulate resting metabolic rate. Medicine and Science in Sports and Exercise 29:769–774

Lampman R M, Knight B P 2000 Prescribing exercise training for patients with defibrillators. American Journal of Physical Medicine and Rehabilitation 79:292–297

Latham N K, Bennett D A, Stretton C M, Anderson C S 2004 Systematic review of progressive resistance strength training in older adults. Journal of Gerontology. A Biological Sciences and Medical Sciences 59(1):48–61

Laughlin M 2004 Joseph B Wolfe Memorial lecture. Physical activity in prevention and treatment of coronary disease: the battle line is in exercise vascular cell biology. Medicine and Science in Sports and Exercise 36(3):352–362

Laughlin M H, Korzick D H 2001 Vascular smooth muscle: integrator of vasoactive signals during exercise hyperemia. Medicine and Science in Sports and Exercise 33(1):81–91

Lawlor D A, Patel R, Ebrahim S 2003 Association between falls in elderly women and chronic diseases and drug use: cross sectional study. BMJ 327:712–717

Lee I M, Paffenbarger R S Jr 2000 Associations of light, moderate, and vigorous intensity physical activity with longevity. The Harvard Alumni Health Study. American Journal of Epidemiology 151(3):293–299

Lee I M, Sesso H D, Oguma Y, Paffenbarger R S Jr 2003 Relative intensity of physical activity and risk of coronary heart disease. Circulation 107:1110–1116

Lee S, Kuk J L, Katzmarzyk P T et al 2005 Cardiorespiratory fitness attenuates metabolic risk independent of abdominal subcutaneous and visceral fat in men. Diabetes Care 28:895–901

Levinger I, Bronks R, Cody D V et al 2005 Resistance training for chronic heart failure patients on beta blocker medications. International Journal of Cardiology 102(3):493–499

Lewin R J, Frizelle D J, Kaye G C 2001 A rehabilitative approach to patients with internal cardioverter-defibrillators. Heart 85:371–372

Leyk D, Essfeld D, Hoffmann U et al 1994 Postural effect on cardiac output, oxygen uptake and lactate during cycle exercise of varying intensity. European Journal of Applied Physiology and Occupational Physiology 68:30–35

Li C, Ebenstein D, Xu C et al 2003 Biochemical characterization of atherosclerotic plaque constituents using FTIR spectroscopy and histology. Journal of Biomedical Materials Research A 64:197–206

Libby P 2001 What have we learned about the biology of atherosclerosis? The role of inflammation. American Journal of Cardiology 88(7B):3J–6J

Lind A R, McNicol G W 1967 Muscular factors which determine the cardiovascular responses to sustained and rhythmic exercise. Canadian Medical Association Journal 96(12):706–715

Luthje L, Vollmann D, Rosenfeld M, Unterberg-Buchwald C 2005 Electrogram configuration and detection of supraventricular tachycardias by a morphology discrimination algorithm in single chamber ICDs. Pacing and Clinical Electrophysiology 28:555–560

McCartney N 1998 Role of resistance training in heart disease. Medicine and Science in Sports and Exercise 30(10 Suppl):S396–S402

Macauley D 1999 Benefits and hazards of exercise, BMJ Publication Group, London

McConnell T R, Laubach C A, Clark B A 1995 Value of gas exchange analysis in heart disease. Journal of Cardiopulmonary Rehabilitation 15:257–261

McPherson K, Britton A, Causer L 2002 Monitoring the progress of the 2010 target for coronary heart disease mortality: Estimated consequences on CHD incidence and mortality from changing prevalence of risk factors. National Heart Forum, London

Malfatto G, Facchini M, Bragato R et al 1996 Short and long term effects of exercise training on the tonic autonomic modulation of heart rate variability after myocardial infarction. European Heart Journal 17:532–538

Malinow M R, McGarry D L, Kuehl K S 1984 Is exercise testing indicated for asymptomatic active people? Journal of Cardiac Rehabilitation 4:376–379

Mancini D M, Henson D, La Manca J et al 1995 Benefit of selective respiratory muscle training on exercise capacity in patients with chronic congestive heart failure. Circulation 91(2):320–329

May S H 1950 A program for active rehabilitation of the cardiac patient. N Y State Journal of Medicine 50:1231–1233

Mayordomo J, Batalla A 2002 Characteristics of patients with ventricular arrhythmias induced with exercise testing. International Journal of Cardiology 83:299–300

Meyer K 2001 Exercise training in heart failure: recommendations based on current research. Medicine and Science in Sports and Exercise 33(4):525–531

Meyer K, Samek L, Schwaibold M et al 1997 Interval training in patients with severe chronic heart failure: analysis and recommendations for exercise procedures. Medicine and Science in Sports and Exercise 29(3):306–312

Mitchell J H, Payne F C, Saltin B, Schibye B 1980 The role of muscle mass in the cardiovascular response to static contractions. Journal of Physiology 309:45–54

Mittleman M A, Maclure M, Tofler G H et al 1993 Triggering of acute myocardial infarction by heavy physical exertion. Protection against triggering by regular exertion. Determinants of Myocardial Infarction Onset Study Investigators. New England Journal of Medicine 329(23):1677–1683

Morris J N, Heady J A, Raffle P A et al 1953 Coronary heart-disease and physical activity of work. Lancet 265:1111–1120

Mosterd A, Hoes A W, de Bruyne M C et al 1999 Prevalence of heart failure and left ventricular dysfunction in the general population. The Rotterdam Study. European Heart Journal 20:447–455

Murphy M, Nevill A, Neville C et al 2002 Accumulating brisk walking for fitness, cardiovascular risk, and psychological health. Medicine and Science in Sports and Exercise 34:1468–1474

Myers J, Prakash M, Froelicher V et al 2002 Exercise capacity and mortality among men referred for exercise testing. New England Journal of Medicine 14:793–801

Myers J, Kaykha A, George S et al 2004 Fitness versus physical activity patterns in predicting mortality in men. American Journal of Medicine 15:912–918

Nademanee K, Veerakul G, Nimmannit S et al 1997 Arrhythmogenic marker for the sudden unexplained death syndrome in Thai men. Circulation 96:2595–2600

Naeije R 2005 Pulmonary hypertension and right heart failure in chronic obstructive pulmonary disease. Proceedings of the American Thoracic Society 2(1):20–22

Nelson R R, Gobel F L, Jorgensen C R et al 1974 Hemodynamic predictors of myocardial oxygen consumption during static and dynamic exercise. Circulation 50:1179–1189

Newman E, Dill D, Edwards T, Webster F 1937 The rate of lactic acid removal in exercise. American Journal of Physiology 118:457–462

Ng L L, Loke I, Davies J E et al 2003 Identification of previously undiagnosed left ventricular systolic dysfunction: community screening using natriuretic peptides and electrocardiography. European Journal of Heart Failure 5(6):775–782

Oldridge N B, Guyatt G H, Fischer M E, Rimm A A 1988 Cardiac rehabilitation after myocardial infarction. Combined experience of randomized clinical trials. JAMA 260(7):945–950

Onder G, Vedova C D, Pahor M 2006 Effects of ACE inhibitors on skeletal muscle. Current Pharmaceutical Design 12(16):2057–2064

Opasich C, Ambrosino N, Felicetti G et al 1999 Heart failure-related myopathy. Clinical and pathophysiological insights. European Heart Journal 20(16):1191–1200

Paffenbarger R, Lee I M 1996 Physical activity and fitness for health and longevity. Research Quarterly for Exercise and Sport 67:11–28

Paffenbarger R S Jr, Blair S N, Lee I M 2001 A history of physical activity, cardiovascular health and longevity: the scientific contributions of Jeremy N Morris, DSc, DPH, FRCP. International Journal of Epidemiology 30:1184–1192

Pashkow F J, Schweikert R A, Wilkoff B L 1997 Exercise testing and training in patients with malignant arrhythmias. Exercise and Sport Science Reviews 25:235–269

Pate R R, Pratt M, Blair S N et al 1995 Physical activity and public health. A recommendation from the Centers for Disease Control and Prevention and the American College of Sports Medicine. JAMA 273:402–407

Peng Z-R 2005 Urban transportation strategies in Chinese cities and their impacts on the urban poor. Presented to the 84th Annual Conference of the Transportation Research Board, Washington DC

Petersen S, Peto V, Scarborough P, Rayer M 2005 Coronary heart disease statistics. British Heart Foundation Health Promotion Research Group. Online. Available: www.heartstats.org

Pigozzi F, Alabiso A, Parisi A et al 2004 Vigorous exercise training is not associated with prevalence of ventricular arrhythmias in elderly athletes. Journal of Sports Medicine and Physical Fitness 44:92–97

Pina I L, Apstein C S, Balady G J et al 2003 Exercise and heart failure: A statement from the American Heart Association Committee on exercise, rehabilitation, and prevention. Circulation 107:1210–1225

Pokan R, Hofmann P, Von Duvillard S P et al 1998 The heart rate performance curve and left ventricular function during exercise in patients after myocardial infarction. Medicine and Science in Sports and Exercise 30:1475–1480

Pollock M L, Franklin B A, Balady G J et al 2000 AHA Science Advisory. Resistance exercise in individuals with and without cardiovascular disease: benefits, rationale, safety, and prescription: An advisory from the Committee on Exercise, Rehabilitation, and Prevention, Council on Clinical Cardiology, AHA; Position paper endorsed by the ACSM

Reents S 2000 Sport and exercise pharmacology. Human Kinetics, London

Rees K, Taylor R S, Singh S et al 2004 Exercise based rehabilitation for heart failure. Cochrane Database Systematic Review CD003331

Rejeski W 1981 The perception of exertion: a social psychophysiological integration. Journal of Sport and Exercise Psychology 3:305–320

Rodriguez L M, Waleffe A, Brugada P et al 1990 Exercise-induced sustained symptomatic ventricular tachycardia: incidence, clinical, angiographic and electrophysiologic characteristics. European Heart Journal 11(3):225–232

Sears S F Jr, Rauch S, Handberg E, Conti J B 2001 Fear of exertion following ICD storm: considering ICD shock and learning history. Journal of Cardiopulmonary Rehabilitation 21:47–49

Sesso H D, Paffenbarger R S Jr, Lee I M 2000 Physical activity and coronary heart disease in men: the Harvard Alumni Health Study. Circulation 102(9):975–980

Shepard J Jr 1992 Hypertension, cardiac arrhythmias, myocardial infarction, and stroke in relation to obstructive sleep, apnea. Clinics in Chest Medicine 13:437–458

Shi X, Wray D W, Formes K J et al 2000 Orthostatic hypotension in aging humans. American Journal of Physiology. Heart and Circulatory Physiology 279:H1548–H1554

Shi X, Huang G, Smith S A et al 2003 Aging and arterial blood pressure variability during orthostatic challenge. Gerontology 49:279–286

SIGN (Scottish Intercollegiate Guidelines Network) 2002 Publication Number 57, Cardiac Rehabilitation

Siscovick D S, Weiss N S, Fletcher R H, Lasky T 1984 The incidence of primary cardiac arrest during vigorous exercise. New England Journal of Medicine 311(14):874–877

Stratton J R, Levy W C, Cerqueira M D et al 1994 Cardiovascular responses to exercise. Effects of aging and exercise training in healthy men. Circulation 89(4):1648–1655

Sullivan M J, Knight J D, Higginbotham M B, Cobb F R 1989 Relation between central and peripheral haemodynamics during exercise in patients with chronic heart failure. Muscle blood flow is reduced with maintenance of arterial perfusion pressure. Circulation 80(4):769–781

Takahashi T, Miyamoto Y 1998 Influence of light physical activity on cardiac responses during recovery from exercise in humans. European Journal of Applied Physiology and Occupational Physiology 77(4):305–311

Thompson P D, Buchner D, Pina I L et al 2003 Exercise and physical activity in the prevention and treatment of atherosclerotic cardiovascular disease: a statement from the Council on Clinical Cardiology (Subcommittee on Exercise, and Prevention) and the Council on Nutrition, Physical Activity, and Metabolism (Subcommittee on Physical Activity). Circulation 107:3109–3116

Toner M M, Glickman E L, McArdle W D 1990 Cardiovascular adjustments to exercise distributed between the upper and lower body. Medicine and Science in Sports and Exercise 22:773–778

Troosters T, Gosselink R, Decramer M 2004 Chronic obstructive pulmonary disease and chronic heart failure: two muscle diseases? Journal of Cardiopulmonary Rehabilitation 24(3):137–145

Tudor-Locke C 2002 Taking steps toward increased physical activity: using pedometers to measure and motivate. Research Digest: President's Council on Physical Fitness and Sports, Series 3

Tudor-Locke C E, Myers A M 2001 Challenges and opportunities for measuring physical activity in sedentary adults. Sports Medicine 31(2):91–100

Tunstall-Pedoe H, Vanuzzo D, Hobbs M et al 2000 Estimation of contribution of changes in coronary care to improving survival, event rates, and coronary heart disease mortality across the WHO MONICA Project populations. Lancet 355:688–700

Tyni-Lenne R, Dencker K, Gordon A et al 2001 Comprehensive local muscle training increases aerobic working capacity and quality of life and decreases neurohormonal activation in patients with chronic heart failure. European Journal of Heart Failure 3(1):47–52

Unal B, Critchley J A, Capewell S 2004 Explaining the decline in coronary heart disease mortality in England and Wales between 1981 and 2000. Circulation 109:1101–1107

Valika A A, Pica M, Goldstein J 2007 Normal coronary arteries are rare in young patients with acute myocardial infarction. Catheterization and Cardiovascular Intervention 70(5):683–690

Vander L, Franklin B, Rubenfire M 1982 Cardiovascular complications of recreational physical activity. Physician and Sports Medicine 10:89–96

Vanhees L, Schepers D, Heidbuchel H et al 2001 Exercise performance and training in patients with implantable cardioverter-defibrillators and coronary heart disease. American Journal of Cardiology 87:712–715

Volaklis K A, Tokmakidis S P 2005 Resistance exercise training in patients with heart failure. Sports Medicine 35:1085–1103

Wada A, Tsutamoto T, Fukai D et al 1997 Comparison of the effects of selective endothelin ETA and ETB receptor antagonists in congestive heart failure. Journal of the American College of Cardiology 30(5):1385–1392

Wang Y, Mi J, Shan X Y et al 2007 Is China facing an obesity epidemic and the consequences? The trends in obesity and chronic disease in China. International Journal of Obesity (London) 31(1):177–188

Wasserman K 1997 Diagnosing cardiovascular and lung pathophysiology from exercise gas exchange. Chest 112:1091–1101

Wasserman K, Hansen J, Sue D et al 1999 Principles of exercise testing and interpretation, Lippincott Williams & Wilkins, Baltimore

Weinstein A R, Sesso H D, Lee I M et al 2004 Relationship of physical activity vs body mass index with type 2 diabetes in women. JAMA 292:1188–1194

Wessel T R, Arant C B, Olson M B et al 2004 Relationship of physical fitness vs body mass index with coronary artery disease and cardiovascular events in women. JAMA 292:1179–1187

WHO 2002 The world health report 2002 – reducing risks, promoting healthy life. World Health Organization, Geneva

WHO 2006 Cardiovascular disease. World Health Organization, Geneva

Williams P T 2001 Physical fitness and activity as separate heart disease risk factors: a meta-analysis. Medicine and Science in Sports and Exercise 33:754–761

Winter E, Jones A, Davison R et al 2006 Sport and exercise physiology testing guidelines. Volume II: Exercise and clinical testing. The British Association of Sport and Exercise Sciences Guide. Routledge, London

Wolk R, Johnson B D, Somers V K et al 2005 Effects of beta-blocker therapy on ventilatory responses to exercise in patients with heart failure. Journal of Cardiac Failure 11: 333–339

Wood D, Wray R, Poulter N et al 2005 JBS 2: Joint British Societies' guidelines on prevention of cardiovascular disease in clinical practice. Heart 91(Suppl 5):v1–v52

Yeh G Y, Wood M J, Lorell B H et al 2004 Effects of tai chi mind-body movement therapy on functional status and exercise capacity in patients with chronic heart failure: a randomized controlled trial. American Journal of Medicine 117(8):541–548

Further reading

Brubaker P H, Kaminsky L A, Whaley M H 2002 Coronary artery disease: essentials of prevention and rehabilitation programs. Human Kinetics, Champaign, IL

Fardy P, Franklin B A, Porcari J, Verrill D E 1998 Training techniques in cardiac rehabilitation. Human Kinetics, Champaign, IL

Froelicher V F, Myers J N 2006 Exercise and the heart, 5th edn. Saunders, Philadelphia, PA

Chapter 4

Lung disease and dysfunction

Alison McConnell

CHAPTER CONTENTS

Learning objectives   97
Introduction   98
The pathophysiology of COPD   99
The pathophysiology of asthma   103
Evidence for a therapeutic effect of
    exercise in respiratory disease   104
Exercise training in COPD   104
Exercise training in asthma   107
Evidence-based guidance on exercise
    training in COPD   109
Overload (intensity)   110

Specificity   111
Reversibility   112
Evidence-based guidance on exercise
    training in asthma   112
Summary   113
Key points   113
References   114
Further reading   118

LEARNING OBJECTIVES

After studying this chapter, you should be able to:

1. Appreciate the personal, social and financial burdens imposed by respiratory illness.
2. Gain an insight into the pathophysiology of the two major respiratory illnesses (asthma and COPD).
3. Understand the factors limiting exercise tolerance in respiratory illness.
4. Understand the interplay of expiratory flow limitation, hyperinflation, inspiratory muscle work and dyspnoea.
5. Understand and be able to distinguish roles of deconditioning and disease-specific pathology in exercise limitation.
6. Understand the role of exercise in managing exercise limitation in patients with respiratory illness.
7. Gain an insight into the appropriate prescription of exercise for patients with respiratory illness, including type and modality.
8. Understand how to assess outcome efficacy following the implementation of exercise training in patients with COPD.
9. Gain an appreciation of the current knowledge gaps with respect to exercise training in patients with respiratory illness.

INTRODUCTION

There is now ample evidence that programmes of physical exercise are beneficial to the health and quality of life of people with lung disease. Indeed, the question is no longer 'does physical exercise benefit respiratory patients?', but rather 'how can exercise be structured to optimize benefits?'.

The British Lung Foundation (BLF) estimates that around 14% of the UK's population live with some kind of respiratory illness. This encompasses diseases as wide-ranging as tuberculosis, lung cancer, asthma and bronchitis. However, the two most prevalent respiratory diseases are asthma and chronic obstructive lung disease (COPD); the latter is an umbrella term principally for chronic bronchitis and emphysema. This chapter will focus on the most prevalent respiratory illnesses of asthma and COPD, but the principles espoused are applicable to individuals with a wider range of respiratory illnesses.

According to Asthma UK, 5.2 million people in the UK are currently receiving treatment for asthma (~8%). Unlike COPD, which is primarily a condition of middle age (see below), asthma afflicts both children and adults, with children forming the fastest growing section of the population affected by the disease (1.1 million children (10%) and 4.1 million adults (8%)). Estimates by the BLF for the prevalence of COPD are that around 3 million people in the UK are affected by COPD (~4.5%), but only 900 000 are currently diagnosed (British Thoracic Society (BTS) 2000). Bearing these numbers in mind, it is perhaps no surprise that respiratory disease is the most common reason for an emergency admission to hospital (BTS 2000).

Whilst the underlying causes of asthma remain unknown, the aetiology of COPD is well understood. COPD is primarily a disease associated with exposure to tobacco smoke, although there are occupational factors, such as coal dust, and some inherited disorders that can also cause COPD. Generally, the symptoms of COPD manifest themselves in middle age, whilst asthma can strike at any time of life. The dissimilarities continue in respect of the pathophysiology and its consequences for exercise tolerance. COPD is a progressively worsening, physically devastating disease with systemic, as well as respiratory, repercussions (Celli 1995). Whilst COPD patients' exercise tolerance is primarily limited by dyspnoea (breathlessness), there is a widespread muscle dysfunction that contributes to functional compromise (Orozco-Levi 2003). Because COPD is primarily a smoking-related illness, patients have co-morbidities that necessitate cautious implementation of certain forms of physical exercise. In contrast, people with asthma are limited only by the efficacy of their disease management; indeed there are many examples of people with asthma becoming world and Olympic champions. Unfortunately, these individuals are the exception, and not the rule, since many people with asthma are afraid to take exercise either because it makes them feel dyspnoeic, and/or because they fear it will trigger an 'attack' that may result in death (Emtner et al 1998). Accordingly, levels of physical activity and aerobic fitness in people with asthma are low (Satta 2000), which is of particular concern in children, who represent the fastest growing section of the asthmatic population. However, recent observations in elite athletes indicate that exercise is not universally beneficial from a respiratory perspective. Firstly, it has been shown that prevalence of asthma in elite athletes is more than twice that occurring in the general population (Dickinson et al 2005); secondly, certain sports are associated with particularly high prevalence rates (Dickinson et al 2005). This has been linked to environmental factors such as air pollution, and/or airway remodelling due to the damaging effects of high levels of respiratory moisture loss (Rundell & Jenkinson 2002).

THE PATHOPHYSIOLOGY OF COPD

COPD is a disorder characterized primarily by destruction of the lung parenchyma/ vasculature and dysfunction of the small and large airways. The disease shows great heterogeneity between individuals and its diagnosis is made primarily on the basis of spirometry and symptoms. However, the diagnostic criteria differ between different national and international societies, which may have led to underdiagnosis of COPD (Lindberg et al 2005). Diagnosis is beyond the scope of this chapter, which will focus upon the role of exercise in patients with an existing diagnosis of their respiratory illness. However, it is important to be aware that not all COPD patients will present for exercise training with the same pattern of disability. Furthermore, over the past decade, it has become increasingly recognized that the pathophysiological repercussions of COPD are not confined to the lungs. The systemic manifestations of COPD include weight loss (cachexia) and muscle dysfunction (Decramer et al 2005). It has been suggested that cachexia and peripheral (limb) muscle dysfunction may be secondary to the presence of chronic inflammatory processes in the muscles of patients with COPD (Montes de Oca et al 2005).

Breathlessness and exercise intolerance are the cardinal symptoms of COPD, and show a progressive worsening with disease progression. Patients with COPD have lower spontaneous activity levels than age-matched controls (Sandland et al 2005), and deconditioning undoubtedly plays a part in the deterioration of muscle quality and exercise intolerance. The mechanisms underlying the development and progression of muscle dysfunction in patients with COPD remain poorly understood, but are currently the subject of intense interest. Notwithstanding this current lack of mechanistic insight, the characteristics and functional repercussions of muscle dysfunction in COPD are well described. In both the respiratory and peripheral muscles, there are alterations in muscle mass, fibre type distribution and metabolic capacity, but these differ between muscle groups (Table 4.1).

The changes depicted in Table 4.1 are due to the combined influences of reduced whole-body activity levels, systemic inflammation, nutritional imbalance, electrolyte disturbances and (iatrogenic) steroid-induced myopathy. The fact that the diaphragm appears to show adaptations that are consistent with the development of a fatigue-resistant phenotype, i.e., to be partially protected, is thought to be due to the differing

Table 4.1 Morphological and metabolic changes in the quadriceps and diaphragm of patients with COPD (ATS/ERS 1999, Decramer et al 1996, Maltais et al 2000, Orozco-Levi 2003)

Peripheral muscles		Respiratory muscles
↓	Proportion of type I fibres	↑
↑	Proportion of type II fibres	↓
↓	Size of type I fibres	↓
↓	Size of type II fibres	↓
↓	Capillarization	↑
↓	Intramuscular pH	?
↓	ATP concentration	?
↓	Mitochondria	↑
↓	Aerobic enzyme activities	→
↑	Anaerobic enzyme activities	→

activity profiles of the respiratory and peripheral muscles (see below) (Orozco-Levi 2003). In addition, there is evidence that the lower limbs are impaired to a greater extent than the upper limbs, and this is also thought to be due to different patterns of use of the upper and lower limbs (Franssen et al 2005).

The reduction in muscle mass that accompanies COPD is proportionately greater than the loss of total body mass (Bernard et al 1998). Weight loss in COPD is due to a combination of factors that result in an imbalance between energy requirements and dietary intake. Resting and exercise energy expenditure may be elevated due to both metabolic and mechanical inefficiency, whilst systemic inflammation may also contribute via its influence on hypermetabolism at rest and appetite. In addition, the release of pro-inflammatory cytokines by neutrophils and macrophages may contribute to cachexia (Schols et al 1996), resulting in loss of muscle mass. Symptoms such as dyspnoea may also impair appetite and dietary intake. Simply correcting nutritional imbalance does not necessarily lead to a recovery of muscle mass (Schols 2003). However, a combination of nutritional support and exercise has been shown to result in functional improvements (Schols 2003).

The pathophysiological factors that contribute to exercise limitation in COPD are known to include increased inspiratory muscle work (see next paragraph), inspiratory muscle weakness, early lactic acidosis, increased ventilatory demand relative to capacity, gas exchange abnormalities, dynamic airway compression and expiratory flow limitation, cardiovascular factors, and peripheral muscle abnormalities (Ambrosino & Strambi 2004).

Dyspnoea is the main symptom leading to exercise limitation in patients with COPD, but limb muscle abnormalities also lead to limitation due to increased sense of limb effort. Dyspnoea is a complex sensory experience, but one that is influenced strongly by the intensity of inspiratory muscle work; the greater the intensity of this work, the greater the intensity of dyspnoea (McConnell & Romer 2004a).

The expiratory flow limitation observed in COPD is due to pathological changes that result in reduced lung recoil and airway tethering, as well as intrinsic airway narrowing. The mechanical repercussions of expiratory flow limitation are important contributors to dyspnoea, and hence, exercise limitation. Whilst the most obvious mechanical defect is obstruction during expiration, the most important mechanical and sensory consequences are upon inspiration. Incomplete lung emptying in the presence of airways obstruction results in a phenomenon known as 'dynamic lung hyperinflation', which has negative repercussions for the inspiratory muscles. Figure 4.1 illustrates how expiratory flow limitation and premature airway closure stimulate an adaptive response that shifts the tidal flow loop towards total lung capacity (TLC), increasing end-expiratory lung volume (EELV), i.e., dynamic hyperinflation. Hyperinflation impairs both the capacity of the inspiratory muscles to generate pressure (due to their length-tension relationship; see inset of Fig. 4.1), and the demands placed upon them for inspiratory pressure generation (due to an increase in the elastic load). Although dynamic hyperinflation serves to maximize tidal expiratory flow under conditions of expiratory flow limitation (by moving the tidal flow loop away from the maximum envelope), there is a requirement to breathe at higher ranges of the total lung capacity (reducing inspiratory capacity) where the inspiratory muscles are weaker, and the elastic load presented to the inspiratory muscles by the lungs and chest wall is higher. This creates a 'restrictive' ventilatory deficit in which the demand for inspiratory muscle force is increased, whilst their ability to generate force is reduced. Hyperinflation and/ or expiratory flow limitation also exacerbate inspiratory muscle loading in two further ways:

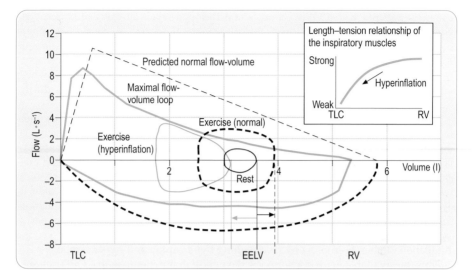

Figure 4.1 Dynamic hyperinflation. Comparison of the response of the exercise tidal flow volume in a person with expiratory flow limitation (EFL) (solid blue lines), compared with that predicted for someone with normal lungs (dashed black lines). Note that in the presence of EFL there is encroachment upon the inspiratory capacity in order to increase minute ventilation (flow volume loop shifts to the left and end-expiratory lung volume (EELV) increases). The person with normal lungs (dashed black lines) is able to increase minute ventilation by utilizing both their inspiratory and expiratory reserve volumes (EELV decreases). The inset illustrates the length–tension relationship of the inspiratory muscles, showing that as lung volume increases (as occurs in hyperinflation), the inspiratory muscles become weaker. TLC, total lung capacity; RV, residual volume.

- by forcing inspiratory time to shorten (to allow more time for expiration, which moves the inspiratory muscles to a weaker portion of their force–velocity relationship (the faster a muscle contracts, the lower its force-generating capacity))
- by generating positive end-expiratory pressure (PEEP – expiration ends before all of the forces acting on the lung are in equilibrium, so inspiration is initiated under a positive expiratory load).

As outlined above, the diaphragms of patients with COPD appear to undergo an endurance training adaptation in response to the chronic inspiratory loading conditions described above (Levine et al 1997). However, there is also seemingly contradictory evidence that patients with COPD exhibit inspiratory muscle weakness and reduced endurance (Orozco-Levi 2003). The healthy diaphragm is composed predominantly of two types of muscles fibres; one with high endurance, but low power (type I, 45%); the other with low endurance, but high power (type II, 55%). Patients with long-standing COPD have an abnormally high proportion of the former (type I, 64%; type II, 36%), which is believed to be an endurance training adaptation to continuous inspiratory muscle loading (Levine et al 1997). Thus, patients with COPD appear to be well adapted to generating low flow rates for long periods of time (such as at rest), but this adaptation robs them of the type II muscle fibres required to generate the high pressures and flow rates required during exercise. In the same way that marathon runners cannot match the pace of sprinters or middle distance runners over short distances, patients with COPD cannot attain the high levels of exercise hyperpnoea required to sustain exercise. Indeed, the adaptations described above do not appear to protect the inspiratory muscles of COPD patients from exercise-induced fatigue (Kyroussis et al 1996). This is probably a function of the lower force-generating capacity of the inspiratory muscles in COPD (Levine et al 2003, Orozco-Levi 2003), which requires the muscle to work at a greater proportion of its maximum capacity during exercise.

The demand for exercise ventilation in patients with COPD is elevated by their deconditioned state, their inefficient breathing pattern, and their gas exchange impairment. Deconditioning and myopathy lead to a premature reliance upon anaerobic metabolism, which evokes an early respiratory compensation for the resulting metabolic acidosis. The tachypnoeic breathing pattern that results from the mechanical defects described above increases the dead space/tidal volume ratio, which reduces alveolar ventilation and results in an increased requirement for minute ventilation. Gas exchange impairments, due to loss of lung diffusing area and ventilation/perfusion abnormalities, also contribute to an increased ventilatory requirement via the stimulation of chemoreceptors by the resulting hypercapnia and hypoxaemia.

Thus, the available evidence supports the notion that patients with COPD not only have relatively weak, fatigue-prone inspiratory muscles, but that they also have an increased demand for ventilatory work during exertion. The latter stems from the direct effects of hyperinflation upon respiratory mechanics, as well as an elevated demand for minute ventilation.

The treatment and management of COPD represents a huge burden on the healthcare system. In the UK it is estimated that the hospitalization of patients with COPD accounts for 54% of direct costs within the secondary care system (Britton 2003). Significantly, the utilization of healthcare resources by patients with COPD is more closely related to their respiratory and peripheral muscle function than to the severity of their airway obstruction (Decramer et al 1997). Furthermore, one-year survival following hospitalization due to an exacerbation is positively related to functional status prior to the exacerbation (Connors et al 1996). In other words, the functional ability of patients with COPD is the most important predictor of both morbidity and mortality, making it an extremely worthwhile therapeutic target.

Finally, it is also relevant to mention that, not unsurprisingly, the physiological changes associated with COPD are also accompanied by psychosocial repercussions including depression and social isolation (Ambrosino & Strambi 2004). All of the negative repercussions of COPD that have been described in the preceding section are amenable to the beneficial effects of exercise, which is why pulmonary rehabilitation has become an increasingly important part of the management of COPD. This is amply illustrated by the inclusion of pulmonary rehabilitation in the most recent NICE guidelines for the management of COPD (NICE 2004), which state that pulmonary rehabilitation 'should be made available to all appropriate patients'. Unfortunately, a British Thoracic Society survey on pulmonary rehabilitation provision in the UK concluded that only 1.7% of the COPD patients who could benefit from pulmonary rehabilitation actually have access to it (BTS/BLF 2003). Furthermore, although pulmonary rehabilitation is strongly recommended for patients with COPD, it is not always practical. Many patients with COPD have co-morbidities that render them unable to walk, including recent myocardial infarction and unstable angina. Accordingly, it is necessary to apply insights into the underlying mechanisms for exercise limitation in COPD in order to identify practical solutions for individual patients. This is addressed in a later section dealing with exercise training ('Evidence-based guidance on exercise training in COPD').

THE PATHOPHYSIOLOGY OF ASTHMA

Surprisingly, there is no internationally agreed definition of asthma, but the International Consensus Report of 1992 described asthma as 'a chronic inflammatory disorder of the airways ... in susceptible individuals, inflammatory symptoms are usually associated with widespread but variable airflow obstruction and an increase in airway response to a variety of stimuli. Obstruction is often reversible, either spontaneously or with treatment' (NHLBI/NIH 1992). Symptoms include wheeze, dyspnoea, chest tightness and cough, which are variable, intermittent, and provoked by triggers that include exercise. However, diagnosis is complicated by the fact that asthma shares some of its symptomatology with a range of other common respiratory diseases. Furthermore, patients can be completely asymptomatic unless an airway response is stimulated by a specific trigger, e.g. exercise. Thus, it is recommended that diagnosis be made on the basis of both symptoms and assessment of lung function. Diagnosis is beyond the scope of this chapter, which focuses upon exercise prescription in patients with a pre-existing diagnosis.

Airflow limitation in asthma is principally due to incursion of the airway lumen due to oedema of the airway mucosa, accumulation of mucus and airway smooth muscle contraction. The resulting narrowing is known as a bronchoconstriction. The mechanical abnormalities associated with bronchoconstriction mimic closely those described in COPD; however, there are important differences. For example, there is less reduction in static lung recoil pressure and more widespread intrathoracic airway narrowing in asthma (Pride & Macklem 1986). In addition, the increased airway collapsibility in patients with COPD is not seen in asthma. Finally, the reversible nature of airways obstruction in asthma results in relatively short-lived periods of resistive loading being applied to the inspiratory muscles. This undoubtedly influences their capacity to express training adaptations, as they appear to in patients with chronic pulmonary disease (Levine et al 1997).

In the presence of bronchoconstriction, exercise limitation in asthma is brought about primarily by dyspnoea. As is the case in COPD, the mechanical changes associated with bronchoconstriction most likely increase the intensity of dyspnoea via their effect upon the requirement for increased inspiratory muscle work. Experimental support for this suggestion has come from Bellofiore et al (1996), who found that the strongest determinant of dyspnoea during methacholine-induced bronchoconstriction was inspiratory motor drive, which explained 82% of the total variance in dyspnoea. Thus, dyspnoea in asthma is primarily a function of an increase in the intensity of inspiratory muscle work.

There is no clear consensus regarding the strength of the inspiratory muscles in patients with asthma compared to healthy people, but it is universally accepted that bronchoconstriction-induced hyperinflation is associated with a functional deficit in inspiratory muscle strength (see inset of Fig. 4.1) (Weiner et al 1990). As is the case in COPD, the major mechanical consequences of airway narrowing are increased flow resistive work, increased elastic work and PEEP (resulting from dynamic lung hyperinflation), as well as reduced dynamic lung compliance (Lougheed et al 1995). Lougheed et al (1993) used methacholine-induced bronchoconstriction to examine the interrelationship between bonchoconstriction, hyperinflation and dyspnoea. Multiple regression analysis indicated that change in inspiratory capacity (an index of dynamic hyperinflation) was the most powerful predictor of dyspnoea during bronchoconstriction, accounting for 74% of the variance in perceptual ratings. These observations are supported by more recent evidence confirming that hyperinflation is a major determinant of dyspnoea in patients with asthma (Martinez-Moragon et al 2003). In common with patients with COPD, the aerobic fitness of patients with asthma is also generally low (Satta et al 1997). It is therefore likely that poor aerobic conditioning also contributes to an increased ventilatory requirement, which will further exacerbate hyperinflation. In combination, the higher ventilation and consequent hyperinflation conspire, individually and in combination, to elevate the overall demands placed upon the inspiratory muscles during exercise.

It is important to appreciate that patients with asthma do not experience bronchoconstriction as a single sensation. Airway narrowing is associated with sensations of both increased respiratory effort (load) and chest tightness, which are distinct from one another (Moy et al 2000). However, the sensation that has been linked to exercise intolerance is respiratory effort, which suggests that this should be the focus of therapeutic interventions. As is the case in patients with COPD, the increased demand for inspiratory muscle work in patients with asthma can be alleviated by non-pharmacological interventions that strengthen the inspiratory muscles and/or reduce the ventilatory requirement.

Finally, it is worth mentioning that it's not uncommon for patients with COPD to also have asthma, but differentiating the two conditions clinically is very difficult.

EVIDENCE FOR A THERAPEUTIC EFFECT OF EXERCISE IN RESPIRATORY DISEASE

It is important to appreciate that exercise is just one component of a structured programme of pulmonary rehabilitation. The other essential components are (AACVPR 2004):

- assessment
- education and training
- promotion of long-term adherence
- psychosocial intervention (including smoking cessation).

The goals of pulmonary rehabilitation programmes are to reduce symptoms, to improve the ability to undertake activities of daily living, and to increase patient independence (ACCP/AACVPR 1997, ATS 1999, BTS 2001). Exercise training is a vital part of pulmonary rehabilitation programmes, with a proven efficacy in terms of exercise capacity (ACCP/AACVPR 1997, Lacasse et al 2002). The current chapter will confine itself to considering the role of exercise within a structured rehabilitation programme.

EXERCISE TRAINING IN COPD

The earliest reports of exercise training interventions in patients with COPD emerged during the early 1970s. Unfortunately, the value of exercise training was underestimated for many years by the results of early studies. These reported that COPD patients appeared to be incapable of achieving a physiological training effect (Belman & Kendregan 1981, Mungall & Hainsworth 1980). These same studies reported improvements in the functional capacity of the patients, but the authors ascribed the changes to 'psychological' factors, or a desensitization to dyspnoea. During the 1970s and 1980s it was argued that patients were too limited by their disease to be capable of exercising at an intensity that was sufficient to elicit classical training responses such as increases in muscle enzyme activities (Belman & Kendregan 1981) or central cardiac adaptations (Mungall & Hainsworth 1980). This misconception led to the view that, because most patients were limited by the ventilatory mechanics, improving their systemic function would yield no benefit.

Thankfully, these views have been overtaken by a plethora of evidence from well-designed randomized controlled trials (RCTs) that attest to the trainability of patients with COPD, and the impressive improvements in physiological function, exercise capacity and health-related quality of life that result (Troosters et al 2005).

Typically, RCTs implementing exercise training programmes for patients with COPD have incorporated three main types of training: (1) lower limb training (endurance and resistance), (2) upper limb training (endurance and resistance), (3) inspiratory muscle training (resistance). Exercise modalities such as cycling, walking and/or stair climbing have been implemented. Limb resistance training has normally involved muscle groups around the shoulder girdle and the leg extensors/flexors. Training has normally been undertaken two to three times per week.

The outcome measures used to assess the efficacy of any intervention need to be both relevant to the context and sensitive to the intervention. For example, assessing the outcome of an aerobic training intervention in COPD patients using a sprint test would be inappropriate in terms of both relevance and sensitivity. Typically, exercise performance has been assessed in COPD patients using incremental tests to the limit of tolerance, fixed intensity tests to the limit of tolerance, and/or timed walk tests. Troosters et al (2005) have calculated the average effect size for various outcome measures of exercise performance from a sample of controlled trials. For incremental tests, the average improvement was between 11% and 18%, depending upon whether the variable measured was peak work rate or peak oxygen uptake ($\dot{V}O_2$), respectively. In constant intensity tests, which are arguably more relevant to everyday life, the time to the limit of tolerance improved by an average 87%. Because of its high external validity, the test of physical capacity that is most often used is the 6-minute walk test. As the name suggests, patients are requested to cover the greatest distance possible in 6 minutes. The minimum clinically important improvement has been estimated to be 54 metres (Redelmeier et al 1997). The pooled effect size calculated from 12 randomized controlled trials of pulmonary rehabilitation by Lacasse and colleagues was just below this at 49 metres (Lacasse et al 2002); however, there was a trend for longer programmes (>6 months), incorporating more sessions, to yield greater improvements. Factors that may influence this outcome are the intensity and duration of the training, as well as its setting (supervised, unsupervised, inpatient, outpatient, domiciliary).

Viewed from a slightly different perspective, Troosters and colleagues calculated the number of patients that needed to be treated in order for one patient to display a clinically significant increase in exercise tolerance (Troosters et al 2005). This was estimated to be three; in other words, meaningful improvements in exercise tolerance can be obtained in ~30% of patients. This might appear a modest success rate, until it is put into context; when the functional improvements gained by adding rehabilitation to a patient's treatment are compared to those of adding a bronchodilator (Oga et al 2000), the relative changes in 6-minute walking distance are 49 metres versus 6 metres, respectively.

The mechanisms underlying improvements in exercise tolerance can be divided broadly into two groups: (1) changes derived from the influence of training per se (ameliorating effects of deconditioning and myopathy); (2) changes derived from disease-specific improvements in ventilatory mechanics. In respect of the former, these include improvements in mechanical efficiency, muscle force (Troosters et al 2000), oxidative capacity and the lactate threshold (Casaburi et al 1991). In the case of the latter, improvements in breathing pattern and the ventilatory demand (which reduces dynamic hyperinflation) have been implicated (Casaburi 1995, Gigliotti et al 2003, Porszasz et al 2005).

Arguably the most important outcome measure of any intervention in patients is health-related quality of life (HRQL). In this context, pulmonary rehabilitation also outperforms pharmacological treatments convincingly. Troosters and colleagues (2005) analysed the outcomes of a number of RCTs of corticosteroids, long-acting bronchodilators and combination therapies. According to their analysis, 15 of the 16 trials failed to generate changes in HRQL that exceeded the minimum clinically important difference (MCID). In contrast, 11 of 13 pulmonary rehabilitation trials generated improvements that exceeded the MCID (Troosters et al 2005).

It is noteworthy that dyspnoea is more closely related to HRQL than to the severity of disease, as determined by the American Thoracic Society (ATS) system for disease staging (Hajiro et al 1999). Since pharmacologically induced improvements in lung function also do not seem to result in clinically meaningful increases in exercise tolerance (Oga et al 2000) or quality of life (Troosters et al 2005), there is a strong argument in favour of interventions that target dyspnoea. Reduction in exertional dyspnoea is an almost ubiquitous finding in well-controlled studies of pulmonary rehabilitation (Gigliotti et al 2003). Not only is there a reduction in the ventilatory requirement for a given intensity of exercise (Casaburi 1995), but there is also a reduction in the intensity of dyspnoea associated with a given level of ventilation (O'Donnell et al 1998). A reduction in the ventilatory requirement of a given task leads to a reduction in the extent of dynamic hyperinflation (Porszasz et al 2005), which is the primary determinant of dyspnoea and exercise limitation (O'Donnell 2001). A reduction in the intensity of dyspnoea at a given level of ventilation is most likely the result of training-induced improvements in inspiratory muscle function (O'Donnell et al 1998), which result in a reduction in the magnitude of the inspiratory motor drive required to generate a given level of ventilation (McConnell & Romer 2004a).

The role of specific inspiratory muscle training (IMT) in patients with COPD has been a hotly debated topic for many years. Interpretation of the literature relating to IMT in patients with COPD has been hampered by studies with inadequate experimental designs. Flaws have included a failure to apply basic training theory, which resulted in a failure to elicit muscle adaptations to training, e.g. strength improvements. The negative outcomes of these studies contributed to early scepticism about the value of IMT. However, the most recent meta-analysis of IMT supports the notion that specific IMT increases inspiratory muscle strength, reduces dyspnoea and improves functional exercise capacity in patients with COPD (Lotters et al 2002). Lotters et al (2002) examined 15 studies, seven of which incorporated measures of dyspnoea. Studies included in the analysis had randomized controlled designs and set training loads $\geq 30\%$ of the maximum strength of the inspiratory muscles in the treatment group. The effect sizes for changes in dyspnoea during exercise and daily activities were statistically significant and the largest of the outcomes assessed. This positive influence of inspiratory muscle strengthening upon dyspnoea is also supported by observations in healthy young people, where pressure threshold IMT has also been associated with a reduced whole-body effort sensation and improved athletic performance (McConnell & Romer 2004b). Collectively, these data support the notion that IMT attenuates respiratory effort sensation, irrespective of the functional status of the inspiratory muscles.

Finally, in the most recent study of IMT in patients with COPD, Beckerman and colleagues examined the influence of IMT over a 1-year period. As well as outcomes such as exercise tolerance and dyspnoea, they also examined use of healthcare resources over the 12-month period of the study (Beckerman et al 2005). Significantly, IMT led to patients spending fewer days in hospital after an exacerbation, and making fewer primary consultations. Given the high absolute costs associated with treatment of respiratory exacerbations in secondary care, these data suggest that the cost/benefit of IMT is extremely favourable.

EXERCISE TRAINING IN ASTHMA

Pulmonary rehabilitation programmes in general, and exercise training in particular, have been much less widely explored or applied in people with asthma, compared to those with COPD. The earliest published reports of exercise interventions in patients with asthma appeared in the late 1960s and early 1970s. These early studies were undertaken on children, who along with adolescents have remained the main focus of research in this area (Welsh et al 2005).

A wide variety of training interventions have been used to assess the efficacy of physical training in asthma. Unfortunately, some studies have failed to achieve minima for intensity and duration, and this may explain their lack of efficacy. Two main modes of aerobic exercise have been employed, namely running or swimming. The rationale for using swimming is that the warm, humid surroundings create a less 'asthmogenic' environment (Rosimini 2003). However, there are clear issues with respect to the accessibility and appropriateness of swimming as a form of habitual exercise, as there is a large skill component to being able to swim at an intensity sufficient to induce an aerobic training effect. In addition, there are concerns that a chlorinated environment may be damaging to the lung (Helenius & Haahtela 2000), and it is noteworthy that asthma prevalence amongst elite swimmers is twice that of elite summer sports athletes (Dickinson et al 2005). Other activities that have been associated with successful outcomes include cycling, circuit training, skipping, gymnastics and competitive team sports. Typically, training responses have been assessed in terms of $\dot{V}O_2$max or peak $\dot{V}O_2$, as well as timed run tests (akin to the 6-minute walk for COPD patients) and heart rate, blood lactate concentrations, and ventilatory responses to identical intensities of exercise.

The authors of a recent Cochrane review (Ram et al 2005) of exercise training in asthma concluded that it improved cardiorespiratory 'fitness' ($\dot{V}O_2$max by 5.4 mL·kg^{-1}·min^{-1}; $n = 7$ randomized controlled trials (RCT), selected from a total of 49). However, there was no evidence of a beneficial effect of exercise training upon lung function ($n = 4$–5 RCTs). Cochrane reviews are well known for the rigorous, but rigid statistical methods that are applied, and it is not unusual for Cochrane reviews to conclude that insufficient evidence exists to support a particular outcome in response to an intervention.

Taking a more pragmatic approach, Welsh et al (2005) came to a slightly more optimistic conclusion. Their review concentrated upon the influence of physical training upon exercise tolerance, severity and incidence of exercise-induced asthma (EIA), and symptoms in children and adolescents. In agreement with Ram and colleagues (2005), they concluded that there was strong evidence for improvements in aerobic capacity ($n = 22$ studies), and that training may restore this to normal levels. The authors also concluded that there was some weak evidence for a reduction in symptoms ($n = 5$ studies), but that there was no support for a reduction in the severity or incidence of exercise-induced asthma (EIA) post training ($n = 13$). With respect to exacerbations and impact on daily life, the authors concluded that the literature provided some support for beneficial effects upon hospitalizations, wheeze frequency, absenteeism from school, doctor consultations and medication use.

The issue of exercise training having a beneficial influence upon EIA symptoms and exacerbations is an important one and has received recent support from a mouse model of atopic (allergic) asthma (Pastva et al 2004). The rationale for a beneficial effect is that atopic asthma is characterized as an inflammatory process that, over time, results in tissue damage and airway remodelling (Pastva et al 2004). Consequently, the immune system has a pivotal role in asthma. Since exercise modulates immune function in healthy human beings it is reasonable to posit that exercise may be capable of exerting a beneficial influence upon airway function in atopic asthma. The evidence within the human literature is difficult to interpret, with studies showing positive effects on some, but not all, aspects of the disease, e.g. symptoms, hospitalizations, medication consumption, and severity of EIA (Welsh et al 2005). However, it is important to bear in mind the large inter- and intra-individual variation that exists in 'free-living' human beings, and that the influence of exercise upon immune function can be negative, as well as positive. There has also been considerable variation in methodologies between studies. Hence, despite its obvious limitations, an animal model in which all aspects of the animal's environment, diet and exercise can be controlled offers a more rigorous test of the hypothesis. In short, Pastva and colleagues (2004) observed a reduction in factors linked to airway inflammation in their mouse model after moderate physical training. Further, the authors argued that moderate exercise may provide a protective effect that attenuates airway remodelling and reduces asthma symptoms. These conclusions suggest that studies designed to address this specific question are warranted in human beings.

On the specific issue of EIA, the weight of evidence appears to be tipped in favour of there being no influence upon the severity of EIA after exercise training (Welsh et al 2005). However, there are two theoretical rationales for the severity of EIA being reduced; firstly through the effects described above upon airway inflammation (Pastva et al 2004), and secondly via a reduction in the ventilatory requirement for exercise that accompanies improvements in aerobic fitness. Since EIA is triggered by airway drying, it follows that a reduction in the quantity of air breathed during exercise may lead to a reduction in airway water loss, and a corresponding reduction in the severity of the resulting bronchoconstriction. An unequivocal answer to this question awaits well-designed and controlled studies in human beings.

Whilst there may be disagreement about the range of benefits that are achievable following physical training in patients with asthma, what is unequivocal is that moderate exercise training does not adversely affect symptoms or severity of EIA. Given the other health benefits associated with greater levels of physical activity, and the lower than normal levels of activity in patients with asthma, there would seem to be no further support required for promoting exercise training in asthma. Furthermore, exposure to exercise in the safe and controlled environment of a rehabilitation programme provides patients with the confidence to exercise, and reduces the fear and anxiety that many associate with the normal exertional dyspnoea (Emtner et al 1998). There is, however, one note of caution to add. There is a growing awareness, and concern, regarding the prevalence of exercise-induced bronchoconstriction in elite athletes, which is more than twice that in the general population (Dickinson et al 2005). It is possible that intense, daily training for endurance-based events may induce airway remodelling that results in the development of exercise-induced bronchoconstriction in athletes without atopy (allergy). Hence, moderation is advised in the therapeutic use of exercise.

Finally, as has been the case in patients with COPD, the role of specific inspiratory muscle training (IMT) has been examined. The rationale for IMT in asthma is similar to that for COPD, as hyperinflation, and the attendant increase in inspiratory muscle work, is a feature of both diseases (see above). However, a recent Cochrane review concluded that there were still insufficient data to recommend IMT routinely, and that more trials were required (Ram et al 2003). Although IMT has been less widely studied in asthma than in COPD, those data that exist are universally supportive of the efficacy of IMT. To date, there have been four RCTs of IMT in patients with asthma, all of which have been in adults, and all emanate from the same laboratory (Weiner et al 1992, 2000, 2002a, 2002b).

An impressive feature of studies of IMT in patients with asthma is the reduction in β_2-agonist (bronchodilator) consumption that accompanies IMT. In the three studies from Weiner's group in which this has been quantified, the reduction has ranged from 38% to 78%, being greatest in those with the highest baseline consumption (Weiner et al 1992, 2000, 2002b). In another study, Weiner and colleagues examined the interrelationship between inspiratory muscle strength, dyspnoea and bronchodilator consumption (Weiner et al 2002a). Although they observed no correlation between baseline measures of inspiratory muscle strength and intensity of dyspnoea in their sample of 30 patients, they observed a highly significant correlation between change in inspiratory muscle strength and change in the intensity of dyspnoea following IMT. Indeed, 93% of the variance in dyspnoea was accounted for by the improvement in inspiratory muscle strength. Thus, IMT appears to be particularly helpful for patients with high levels of dyspnoea and β_2-agonist consumption.

However, a note of caution is also called for at this point, because there is a small group of patients with asthma for whom further reductions in the intensity of dyspnoea sensation may be life-threatening. According to one study, around 26% of patients with asthma have abnormally low perceptions of dyspnoea (Magadle et al 2002); this was associated with low consumption of medication, increased emergency department visits, hospitalizations, near-fatal asthma attacks, and deaths during follow-up (Magadle et al 2002). It would therefore be inappropriate to implement IMT in this subgroup. However, available evidence suggests that patients with normal or high sensation of dyspnoea do not become desensitized to bronchoconstriction following IMT. Weiner et al (2000) noted that IMT did not result in exaggerated ablation of dyspnoea, and concluded that IMT was safe, at least for use in patients with mild asthma. Further research is required to identify those patients with asthma who are likely to derive the greatest benefit from IMT.

Thus, for patients with high perception of dyspnoea, high consumption of medication, low levels of physical activity, and mild asthma, IMT may offer the rare combination of an intervention that improves quality of life, whilst simultaneously reducing consumption of medication.

EVIDENCE-BASED GUIDANCE ON EXERCISE TRAINING IN COPD

It has taken over 30 years for respiratory medicine to reach a point where exercise training is considered to be a routine part of mainstream treatment for COPD (AACVPR 2004). However, the fact that exercise appears to be so much more potent in terms of its efficacy than pharmacotherapy with respect to exercise tolerance and quality of life (Troosters et al 2005) remains less well appreciated. The questions that remain unanswered are concerned primarily with how to optimize the efficacy of exercise training and how to maintain the benefits. Readers who are exercise scientists will appreciate that these questions will take considerable time and resource to answer, since the permutations and combinations of training methods are almost without limit. Optimization of training interventions also represents a particular challenge in a group of patients with such heterogeneity, where one size does not fit all. However, by applying an understanding of the mechanisms underlying exercise intolerance of patients with COPD (see above) it is possible to refine the search and to explore some obvious candidate training methods. Indeed, this has already begun, and data are beginning to emerge.

The principal limitation for patients with COPD is the intolerable dyspnoea that is associated with physical exertion. This is primarily attributable to the elevated inspiratory muscle work that results from dynamic hyperinflation and an exaggerated ventilatory response to exercise. In addition, there is a generalized deconditioning and muscle weakness, especially of the lower limbs. Thus, exercise training should be formulated to address these specific impairments. However, patients with COPD are older adults who are current or ex-smokers, with low levels of physical activity. This means that co-morbidities such as coronary heart disease, chronic heart failure, increased risk of stroke, etc. (Holguin et al 2005, Huiart et al 2005) must be borne in mind before prescribing exercise for these patients. Ischaemic heart disease is a common cause of death in patients with COPD (Huiart et al 2005).

The fundamentals of training theory are as applicable to patients with respiratory illness as they are to the elite athlete.

Overload (intensity)

Pulmonary rehabilitation programmes for patients with COPD have tended to emphasize endurance training at intensities that can be sustained for 20 to 30 minutes. For some patients, this is impossible, because of a progressive acidaemia and associated hyperinflation and dyspnoea that results. However, interval training (30 s intense exercise/30 s active recovery) has been shown to yield similar physiological improvements, but with shorter training sessions (Vogiatzis et al 2002). In addition, because of a slower development of dynamic hyperinflation during interval exercise, patients are able to interval train for three times longer, and to increase the total amount of work done (Vogiatzis et al 2004). Furthermore, research from healthy athletes suggests that interval training is a more effective method of increasing the lactate threshold than moderate, sustained exercise. Accordingly, this approach appears to be worthy of further exploration.

So far as prescribing the training intensity is concerned, RCTs have used various percentages of peak work rate, $\dot{V}O_2max$ or heart rate (normally $\geq 60\%$). A dose-response effect has been observed such that high-intensity exercise (60–80% of the peak work rate achieved during an incremental test) yields greater improvements in exercise tolerance than does lower-intensity exercise (30% of peak work rate) (Casaburi et al 1991). Clearly, the duration of the exercise bout is dependent upon its intensity. Interval training allows higher intensities to be undertaken, but for shorter durations (typically 30 seconds to 3 minutes). Generally, when applying interval training techniques, it is recommended that a 30-minute training session be subdivided into shorter bouts of higher-intensity exercise (70–100% of the peak work rate) (Troosters et al 2005). The use of symptom intensity, specifically dyspnoea, may provide a more pragmatic, and relevant, alternative to the use of peak work rate, $\dot{V}O_2max$ or heart rate. A rating of 4–6 on the Borg CR-10 scale has been recommended for sustained exercise (Horowitz et al 1996). The latter principle should also be applied periodically during the programme in order to maintain the 'overload' stimulus, i.e., intensity can be incremented as function improves, and this should be based upon symptom limitation (Troosters et al 2005).

The duration of the programme is another area in which there is uncertainty, and scant systematic evidence. Although it is possible to elicit physiological changes in just a few weeks, it has been argued that this is too short an intervention to effect the behavioural changes required for a lifestyle shift. There is also evidence to support larger physiological changes with longer programmes (>3 months) (Troosters et al 2005). Accordingly, a minimum duration of 8 weeks has been recommended (Troosters et al 2005).

Specificity

Although many RCTs have utilized cycle ergometry, it may be more appropriate for patients to walk, or stair climb, as these activities mimic more closely activities of daily living. Certainly, walking training has not been shown to be any less effective than cycle ergometry.

Upper body muscles function as accessory muscles of breathing in patients with COPD. Perhaps for this reason, activities of daily living that involve the upper limbs often elicit dyspnoea. Accordingly, the benefits of upper limb training have been assessed. Available evidence supports a beneficial influence of upper limb training upon dyspnoea (Gigliotti et al 2005), but specific adaptations appear to be smaller than for the lower limbs (Franssen et al 2005), most likely because their function is less profoundly impaired than that of the lower limbs.

Strength training in patients with COPD has a rationale based upon the generalized myopathy that is present. However, it has not been as widely applied to limb muscles as whole-body endurance training and its role is correspondingly less clear. What can be concluded from the literature is that lower and upper limb strength can be improved. Interestingly, a handful of studies have directly compared the outcome of strength and endurance training. For quality of life, strength training had a larger effect than endurance training. For exercise performance, the data were less clear, but strength training was no less effective than endurance training (Puhan et al 2005). Somewhat surprisingly, there appear to be no additional benefits to exercise performance, HRQL or symptoms of combining strength training with endurance training (Puhan et al 2005). Despite this, current recommendations are that both should be implemented concurrently (Troosters et al 2005), perhaps because muscle strength is an independent contributor to survival and utilization of healthcare resources.

There is a strong theoretical rationale for strength training of the inspiratory muscles, which is well supported by the literature (Lotters et al 2002, McConnell & Romer 2004a). Inspiratory muscle training (IMT) improves exercise tolerance, dyspnoea and quality of life as a stand-alone intervention, but it is unclear whether it provides any added benefits when implemented concurrently with whole-body endurance training, except in patients with inspiratory muscle weakness (Lotters et al 2002). However, the role of IMT as a precursor to endurance or interval training has yet to be explored, and it is possible that the reduction in dyspnoea that can be achieved with IMT may enable patients to exercise at higher intensities during subsequent endurance/interval training. Furthermore, there are no contraindications to IMT, and it is safe for patients for whom endurance/interval or other forms of strength training are inappropriate due to co-morbidities. Specific guidance on implementation of IMT is available elsewhere (McConnell et al 2005).

An intervention that is related to IMT is the use of 'breathing retraining'. This phase means different things to different people, but one aspect of this treatment that is not recommended is the use of diaphragm breathing, i.e., the conscious expansion of the abdominal wall during diaphragmatic inspiration. In particular, one study showed that diaphragm breathing reduced the mechanical efficiency of breathing and increased the intensity of dyspnoea relative to spontaneous breathing (Gosselink et al 1995).

Reversibility

The time course of the reversibility of training adaptations is pertinent to the question of how best to maintain the benefits derived from initial training. Patients are normally enrolled in either inpatient or outpatient programmes that run for several weeks, or even months. After this, they are encouraged to undertake home-based activities in order to sustain the benefits. To date, the evidence suggests that this does not result in a maintenance of function, which returns to pre-training levels over a 24-month period, even if the patients return for outpatient training once per month, and are given weekly telephone support (Ries et al 2003). A strategy that has yet to be evaluated in an RCT is to provide short blocks of structured training in an effort to retard the decline in function once the initial training period is completed. Fundamentally, if patients are to maintain the benefits derived from rehabilitation, they need to make a lifestyle change that incorporates daily physical activity, or at least structured activity two to three times per week. This is a public health challenge that is not confined to patients with COPD, and an important selection criterion must surely be the patient's commitment to such a lifestyle change.

EVIDENCE–BASED GUIDANCE ON EXERCISE TRAINING IN ASTHMA

Unlike COPD, there are no specific guidelines issued by national or international societies for exercise training in patients with asthma; there is also a much smaller evidence base. Most studies have been conducted on children and adolescents, who are likely to have less systemic impairment, and different exercise preferences than middle-aged and elderly COPD patients. Notwithstanding this, the same general principles can be applied in terms of the duration and intensity of physical activity, and the rationale and evidence favouring adjuncts such as inspiratory muscle training are sound. Prescription should therefore be made on the basis of guidelines for COPD for adults, and using best practice guidance for promoting physical activity in children and adolescents.

Since exercise induces bronchoconstriction, it needs to be administered carefully, and airway function needs to be monitored. Basic precautions include administration of short-acting bronchodilators prior to exercise (at least 10 minutes), and their availability throughout. Patients should also be encouraged to monitor their symptoms, and to respond appropriately to any deterioration in these. In addition, patients should also monitor their peak expiratory flow rate pre- and post-exercise to ensure that their asthma is properly controlled. This latter measure is only necessary during periods of change (e.g. initiating a programme of exercise; change to medication; after an upper respiratory tract infection, etc.), or if the patient is concerned by their symptoms.

The environment in which exercise is undertaken must also be borne in mind. In atopic asthmatics, avoiding specific allergens such as pollen is self-evident, but less well-recognized factors such as air pollution and cold dry environments should also be considered. Similarly, repeated sprinting, such as occurs during many team games, could result in symptoms during activity (the EIA response normally manifests 5–15 minutes post-exercise), which could limit participation in these sports. In contrast, participation in, say, continuous running or cycling may be unaffected. However, if EIA is well controlled with medication, bronchoconstriction should not be triggered, and if it is, it should be readily reversible during the activity by administering a bronchodilator. Furthermore, patients will only adhere to activities that they find enjoyable, so it is far better to spend time identifying the optimal pharmacological management regimen than to encourage patients to undertake less 'asthmogenic' activities.

About half of people with asthma experience what is known as a 'refractory period' following a 10- to 15-minute bout of moderate-intensity exercise (50–60% maximum heart rate), or 'warm-up'. For up to 2 hours after the 'warm-up', this subgroup can exercise (even intensely) and not experience EIA (McKenzie et al 1994). The precise mechanisms for refractoriness remain unknown, but it can be used to manage EIA in those who show refractoriness.

SUMMARY

The functional ability of patients with COPD is the most important predictor of both morbidity and mortality, making it an extremely worthwhile therapeutic target. There is now ample evidence to support the promotion of exercise training in patients with COPD and asthma, especially in COPD. Indeed, Troosters and colleagues conclude that, 'The current programs improve health-related quality of life and exercise tolerance to a greater extent than any other intervention available for patients with COPD' (Troosters et al 2005). Similarly, the benefits of exercise for adults and children with asthma are well supported, and have wide-reaching implications for long-term health. The important issues that remain to be resolved over the coming years are how to:

1. optimize the modality, intensity and duration of exercise training programmes
2. identify the optimal combination of inpatient, outpatient and domiciliary settings for initial training and maintenance
3. optimize the use of resistance training both as a stand-alone intervention and in combination with endurance exercise
4. identify the optimal role for inspiratory muscle training.

KEY POINTS

1. Around 14% of the UK's population live with some form of respiratory illness, which is the most common reason for emergency admission to hospital.
2. Asthma and COPD are the two most common respiratory illnesses.
3. COPD is primarily a smoking-related illness of later life.
4. COPD is a systemic disease in which widespread muscle myopathy is a feature.
5. Exercise limitation in COPD is primarily linked to dyspnoea, but the underlying aetiology of dyspnoea is complex.
6. Patients with COPD have very low levels of aerobic fitness and muscle strength.
7. A major contributor to dyspnoea is the increased inspiratory muscle work that is a direct consequence of lung hyperinflation due to expiratory flow limitation.
8. Although the inspiratory muscles of patients with COPD exhibit functional adaptations in response to increased inspiratory muscle work, these are not sufficient to restore normal dyspnoeic sensation, or to protect the inspiratory muscles from fatigue.

9. The peripheral and respiratory muscles of patients with COPD adapt to appropriate training stimuli.
10. The functional ability of patients with COPD is the most important predictor of both morbidity and mortality.
11. Asthma is an inflammatory disease causing airway narrowing that can strike at any age.
12. In the presence of airway narrowing, exercise limitation in asthma is related to dyspnoea.
13. A major contributor to dyspnoea in asthma is the increased inspiratory muscle work that is a direct consequence of lung hyperinflation due to expiratory flow limitation (a consequence of airway narrowing).
14. Patients with asthma have low levels of aerobic fitness; this has worrying implications for the long-term health of young people with asthma.
15. Exercise is the most common trigger for bronchoconstriction, for which the major trigger is airway drying.
16. Exercise training in respiratory disease is normally part of a holistic programme of pulmonary rehabilitation.
17. Exercise training is more common in COPD than in asthma; furthermore, the evidence base is stronger and more extensive for COPD.
18. Patients with lung disease respond to exercise training with meaningful effect sizes for the most important outcome variables (exercise tolerance, dyspnoea and health-related quality of life).
19. There are special considerations for exercise training in asthma because of the influence of exercise and environmental factors upon airway function.
20. Specific inspiratory muscle training targets dyspnoea directly and can be used as both a stand-alone treatment, and as part of a rehabilitation programme; it has the advantage of very few contraindications.

Conflict of interest declaration

AKM acknowledges a beneficial interest in the POWERbreathe® inspiratory muscle trainer (www.powerbreathe.com) in the form of a royalty share on licence income to the University of Birmingham. She also acts as a consultant to Gaiam Ltd.

References

AACVPR 2004 Guidelines for pulmonary rehabilitation programmes. Human Kinetics, Champaign, IL

ACCP/AACVPR 1997 Pulmonary rehabilitation: joint ACCP/AACVPR evidence-based guidelines. ACCP/AACVPR Pulmonary Rehabilitation Guidelines Panel. American College of Chest Physicians. American Association of Cardiovascular and Pulmonary Rehabilitation. Chest 112:1363–1396

Ambrosino N, Strambi S 2004 New strategies to improve exercise tolerance in chronic obstructive pulmonary disease. European Respiratory Journal 24:313–322

ATS 1999 Pulmonary rehabilitation-1999. American Thoracic Society. American Journal of Respiratory and Critical Care Medicine 159:1666–1682

ATS/ERS 1999 Skeletal muscle dysfunction in chronic obstructive pulmonary disease. A statement of the American Thoracic Society and European Respiratory Society. American Journal of Respiratory and Critical Care Medicine 159:S1–S40

Beckerman M, Magadle R, Weiner M et al 2005 The effects of 1 year of specific inspiratory muscle training in patients with COPD. Chest 128:3177–3182

Bellofiore S, Ricciardolo F L, Ciancio N et al 1996 Changes in respiratory drive account for the magnitude of dyspnoea during bronchoconstriction in asthmatics. European Respiratory Journal 9:1155–1159

Belman M J, Kendregan B A 1981 Exercise training fails to increase skeletal muscle enzymes in patients with chronic obstructive pulmonary disease. American Review of Respiratory Disease 123:256–261

Bernard S, LeBlanc P, Whittom F et al 1998 Peripheral muscle weakness in patients with chronic obstructive pulmonary disease. American Journal of Respiratory and Critical Care Medicine 158:629–634

Britton M 2003 The burden of COPD in the UK: results from the Confronting COPD survey. Respiratory Medicine 97(Suppl C):S71–S79

BTS 2000 The burden of lung disease. Online. Available: http://www.brit-thoracic.org.uk/reports.html

BTS 2001 Pulmonary rehabilitation. Thorax 56:827–834

BTS/BLF 2003 Joint report on pulmonary rehabilitation in the UK. Online. Available: http://www.brit-thoracic.org.uk/reports.html

Casaburi R 1995 Mechanisms of the reduced ventilatory requirement as a result of exercise training. European Respiratory Journal 5:42–46

Casaburi R, Patessio A, Ioli F et al 1991 Reductions in exercise lactic acidosis and ventilation as a result of exercise training in patients with obstructive lung disease. American Review of Respiratory Disease 143:9–18

Celli B R 1995 Pathophysiology of chronic obstructive pulmonary disease. Chest Surgery Clinics of North America 5:623–634

Connors A F Jr, Dawson N V, Thomas C et al 1996 Outcomes following acute exacerbation of severe chronic obstructive lung disease. The SUPPORT investigators (Study to Understand Prognoses and Preferences for Outcomes and Risks of Treatments). American Journal of Respiratory and Critical Care Medicine 154:959–967

Decramer M, de Bock V, Dom R 1996 Functional and histologic picture of steroid-induced myopathy in chronic obstructive pulmonary disease. American Journal of Respiratory and Critical Care Medicine 153:1958–1961

Decramer M, Gosselink R, Troosters T et al 1997 Muscle weakness is related to utilization of health care resources in COPD patients. European Respiratory Journal 10:417–423

Decramer M, De Benedetto F, Del Ponte A et al 2005 Systemic effects of COPD. Respiratory Medicine 99(Suppl 2):S3–S10

Dickinson J W, Whyte G P, McConnell A K et al 2005 Impact of changes in the IOC-MC asthma criteria: a British perspective. Thorax 60:629–632

Emtner M, Hedin A, Stalenheim G 1998 Asthmatic patients' views of a comprehensive asthma rehabilitation programme: a three-year follow-up. Physiotherapy Research International 3:175–193

Franssen F M, Broekhuizen R, Janssen P P et al 2005 Limb muscle dysfunction in COPD: effects of muscle wasting and exercise training. Medicine and Science in Sports and Exercise 37:2–9

Gigliotti F, Coli C, Bianchi R et al 2003 Exercise training improves exertional dyspnea in patients with COPD: evidence of the role of mechanical factors. Chest 123:1794–1802

Gigliotti F, Coli C, Bianchi R et al 2005 Arm exercise and hyperinflation in patients with COPD: effect of arm training. Chest 128:1225–1232

Gosselink R A, Wagenaar R C, Rijswijk H et al 1995 Diaphragmatic breathing reduces efficiency of breathing in patients with chronic obstructive pulmonary disease. American Journal of Respiratory and Critical Care Medicine 151:1136–1142

Hajiro T, Nishimura K, Tsukino M et al 1999 A comparison of the level of dyspnea vs disease severity in indicating the health-related quality of life of patients with COPD. Chest 116:1632–1637

Helenius I, Haahtela T 2000 Allergy and asthma in elite summer sport athletes. Journal of Allergy and Clinical Immunology 106:444–452

Holguin F, Folch E, Redd S C et al 2005 Comorbidity and mortality in COPD-related hospitalizations in the United States, 1979 to 2001. Chest 128:2005–2011

Horowitz M B, Littenberg B, Mahler D A 1996 Dyspnea ratings for prescribing exercise intensity in patients with COPD. Chest 109:1169–1175

Huiart L, Ernst P, Suissa S 2005 Cardiovascular morbidity and mortality in COPD. Chest 128:2640–2646

Kyroussis D, Polkey M I, Keilty S E et al 1996 Exhaustive exercise slows inspiratory muscle relaxation rate in chronic obstructive pulmonary disease. American Journal of Respiratory and Critical Care Medicine 153:787–793

Lacasse Y, Brosseau L, Milne S et al 2002 Pulmonary rehabilitation for chronic obstructive pulmonary disease. Cochrane Database Systematic Review CD003793

Levine S, Kaiser L, Leferovich J et al 1997 Cellular adaptations in the diaphragm in chronic obstructive pulmonary disease. New England Journal of Medicine 337:1799–1806

Levine S, Nguyen T, Kaiser L R et al 2003 Human diaphragm remodeling associated with chronic obstructive pulmonary disease: clinical implications. American Journal of Respiratory and Critical Care Medicine 168:706–713

Lindberg A, Jonsson A C, Ronmark E et al 2005 Prevalence of chronic obstructive pulmonary disease according to BTS, ERS, GOLD and ATS criteria in relation to doctor's diagnosis, symptoms, age, gender, and smoking habits. Respiration 72:471–479

Lotters F, van Tol B, Kwakkel G et al 2002 Effects of controlled inspiratory muscle training in patients with COPD: a meta-analysis. European Respiratory Journal 20:570–577

Lougheed M D, Lam M, Forkert L et al 1993 Breathlessness during acute bronchoconstriction in asthma. Pathophysiologic mechanisms. American Review of Respiratory Disease 148:1452–1459

Lougheed D M, Webb K A, O'Donnell D E 1995 Breathlessness during induced lung hyperinflation in asthma: the role of the inspiratory threshold load. American Journal of Respiratory and Critical Care Medicine 152:911–920

McConnell A K, Romer L M 2004a Dyspnoea in health and obstructive pulmonary disease: the role of respiratory muscle function and training. Sports Medicine 34:117–132

McConnell A K, Romer L M 2004b Respiratory muscle training in healthy humans: resolving the controversy. International Journal of Sports Medicine 25:284–293

McConnell A K, Romer L M, Weiner P 2005 Inspiratory muscle training in obstructive lung disease; how to implement and what to expect. Breathe 2:38–49

McKenzie D C, McLuckie S L, Stirling D R 1994 The protective effects of continuous and interval exercise in athletes with exercise-induced asthma. Medicine and Science in Sports and Exercise 26:951–956

Magadle R, Berar-Yanay N, Weiner P 2002 The risk of hospitalization and near-fatal and fatal asthma in relation to the perception of dyspnea. Chest 121:329–333

Maltais F, LeBlanc P, Jobin J et al 2000 Peripheral muscle dysfunction in chronic obstructive pulmonary disease. Clinics in Chest Medicine 21:665–677

Martinez-Moragon E, Perpina M, Belloch A et al 2003 Determinants of dyspnea in patients with different grades of stable asthma. Journal of Asthma 40:375–382

Montes de Oca M, Torres S H, De Sanctis J et al 2005 Skeletal muscle inflammation and nitric oxide in patients with COPD. European Respiratory Journal 26:390–397

Moy M L, Woodrow Weiss J, Sparrow D et al 2000 Quality of dyspnea in bronchoconstriction differs from external resistive loads. American Journal of Respiratory and Critical Care Medicine 162:451–455

Mungall I P, Hainsworth R 1980 An objective assessment of the value of exercise training to patients with chronic obstructive airways disease. Quarterly Journal of Medicine 49:77–85

NHLBI/NIH 1992 International consensus report on diagnosis and treatment of asthma. National Heart, Lung, and Blood Institute, National Institutes of Health. Bethesda, MD 20892. Publication no. 92-3091, March 1992. European Respiratory Journal 5:601–641

NICE 2004 Chronic obstructive pulmonary disease. National clinical guideline on management of chronic obstructive pulmonary disease in adults in primary and secondary care. Thorax 59(Suppl 1):1–232

O'Donnell D E 2001 Ventilatory limitations in chronic obstructive pulmonary disease. Medicine and Science in Sports and Exercise 33:S647–655

O'Donnell D E, McGuire M, Samis L et al 1998 General exercise training improves ventilatory and peripheral muscle strength and endurance in chronic airflow limitation. American Journal of Respiratory and Critical Care Medicine 157:1489–1497

Oga T, Nishimura K, Tsukino M et al 2000 The effects of oxitropium bromide on exercise performance in patients with stable chronic obstructive pulmonary disease. A comparison of three different exercise tests. American Journal of Respiratory and Critical Care Medicine 161:1897–1901

Orozco-Levi M 2003 Structure and function of the respiratory muscles in patients with COPD: impairment or adaptation? European Respiratory Journal (Suppl 46):41s–51s

Pastva A, Estell K, Schoeb T R et al 2004 Aerobic exercise attenuates airway inflammatory responses in a mouse model of atopic asthma. Journal of Immunology 172:4520–4526

Porszasz J, Emtner M, Goto S et al 2005 Exercise training decreases ventilatory requirements and exercise-induced hyperinflation at submaximal intensities in patients with COPD. Chest 128:2025–2034

Pride N B, Macklem P T 1986 Lung mechanics in disease. In: Fishman A P (ed) Handbook of physiology, Section 3, Vol III, Part 2. American Physiological Society, Bethesda, MD, pp 659–692

Puhan M A, Schünemann H J, Frey M et al 2005 How should COPD patients exercise during respiratory rehabilitation? Comparison of exercise modalities and intensities to treat skeletal muscle dysfunction. Thorax 60:367–375

Ram F S, Wellington S R, Barnes N C 2003 Inspiratory muscle training for asthma. Cochrane Database Systematic Review CD003792

Ram F, Robinson S, Black P et al 2005 Physical training for asthma. Cochrane Database Systematic Review CD001116

Redelmeier D A, Bayoumi A M, Goldstein R S et al 1997 Interpreting small differences in functional status: the Six Minute Walk test in chronic lung disease patients. American Journal of Respiratory and Critical Care Medicine 155:1278–1282

Ries A L, Kaplan R M, Myers R et al 2003 Maintenance after pulmonary rehabilitation in chronic lung disease: a randomized trial. American Journal of Respiratory and Critical Care Medicine 167:880–888

Rosimini C 2003 Benefits of swim training for children and adolescents with asthma. Journal of the American Academy of Nurse Practitioners 15:247–252

Rundell K W, Jenkinson D M 2002 Exercise-induced bronchospasm in the elite athlete. Sports Medicine 32:583–600

Sandland C J, Singh S J, Curcio A et al 2005 A profile of daily activity in chronic obstructive pulmonary disease. Journal of Cardiopulmonary Rehabilitation 25:181–183

Satta A 2000 Exercise training in asthma. Journal of Sports Medicine and Physical Fitness 40:277–283

Satta A, Migliori G B, Spanevello A et al 1997 Fibre types in skeletal muscles of chronic obstructive pulmonary disease patients related to respiratory function and exercise tolerance. European Respiratory Journal 10:2853–2860

Schols A M 2003 Nutritional and metabolic modulation in chronic obstructive pulmonary disease management. European Respiratory Journal (Suppl 46):81s–86s

Schols A M, Buurman W A, Staal van den Brekel A J et al 1996 Evidence for a relation between metabolic derangements and increased levels of inflammatory mediators in a subgroup of patients with chronic obstructive pulmonary disease. Thorax 51:819–824

Troosters T, Gosselink R, Decramer M 2000 Short- and long-term effects of outpatient rehabilitation in patients with chronic obstructive pulmonary disease: a randomized trial. American Journal of Medicine 109:207–212

Troosters T, Casaburi R, Gosselink R et al 2005 Pulmonary rehabilitation in chronic obstructive pulmonary disease. American Journal of Respiratory and Critical Care Medicine 172:19–38

Vogiatzis I, Nanas S, Roussos C 2002 Interval training as an alternative modality to continuous exercise in patients with COPD. European Respiratory Journal 20:12–19

Vogiatzis I, Nanas S, Kastanakis E et al 2004 Dynamic hyperinflation and tolerance to interval exercise in patients with advanced COPD. European Respiratory Journal 24:385–390

Weiner P, Suo J, Fernandez E et al 1990 The effect of hyperinflation on respiratory muscle strength and efficiency in healthy subjects and patients with asthma. American Review of Respiratory Disease 141:1501–1505

Weiner P, Azgad Y, Ganam R et al 1992 Inspiratory muscle training in patients with bronchial asthma. Chest 102:1357–1361

Weiner P, Berar-Yanay N, Davidovich A et al 2000 Specific inspiratory muscle training in patients with mild asthma with high consumption of inhaled beta(2)-agonists. Chest 117:722–727

Weiner P, Magadle R, Beckerman M et al 2002a The relationship among inspiratory muscle strength, the perception of dyspnea and inhaled beta2-agonist use in patients with asthma. Canadian Respiratory Journal 9:307–312

Weiner P, Magadle R, Massarwa F et al 2002b Influence of gender and inspiratory muscle training on the perception of dyspnea in patients with asthma. Chest 122:197–201

Welsh L, Kemp J G, Roberts R G 2005 Effects of physical conditioning on children and adolescents with asthma. Sports Medicine 35:127–141

Further reading

AACVPR 2004 Guidelines for pulmonary rehabilitation programs. Human Kinetics, Champaign, IL

ACCP/AACVPR 1997 Pulmonary rehabilitation: joint ACCP/AACVPR evidence-based guidelines. ACCP/AACVPR Pulmonary Rehabilitation Guidelines Panel. American College of Chest Physicians. American Association of Cardiovascular and Pulmonary Rehabilitation. Chest 112:1363–1396

Chapter **5**

Arthritis and low back pain

Alan Leigh, Helen Mitchell and Paul Firth

CHAPTER CONTENTS

Learning objectives   119
Introduction   120
Osteoarthritis   121
   Epidemiology   121
   Pathophysiology   122
Rheumatoid arthritis   123
   Epidemiology   123
   Pathophysiology   124
Exercise for osteoarthritis and
   rheumatoid arthritis   124
   Primary prevention   124
   Secondary prevention   125
   Aerobic activity   125
   Flexibility exercise   127
   Proprioceptive exercise   130
   Strength training for osteoarthritis
      and rheumatoid arthritis   134
   Water-based resistance training   137
   Summary on exercise and
      arthritis   139
Low back pain   139
   Epidemiology   139
   Pathophysiology   140
Exercise for low back pain   141
   Exercise for acute low back pain   142

Case study: acute low back
   pain   142
Case study: exercise programme
   development   144
Case study: special considerations
   for exercise programme
   development   146
Chronic low back pain – aerobic
   exercise   148
Chronic low back pain – spinal
   stabilization exercise
   (core stability)   148
Chronic low back pain and the
   exercise dose response   149
Case study: resistance training for
   chronic low back pain   150
Psychological considerations when
   working with individuals with
   musculoskeletal injury and
   pain   151
Conclusion   152
Future research   152
Key points   153
References   154
Further reading   159

LEARNING OBJECTIVES

After studying this chapter, you should be able to:

- Understand the epidemiology and pathophysiology of osteoarthritis, rheumatoid arthritis and low back pain.

- Understand the features that identify the differences between acute symptoms and chronic symptoms in the above three musculoskeletal conditions.
- Identify the supporting evidence and the gaps in the evidence on the efficacy of exercise adapted for individuals with osteoarthritis, rheumatoid arthritis and low back pain.
- Understand how to apply issues of graded exposure and pacing to an exercise programme for osteoarthritis, rheumatoid arthritis and low back pain.

INTRODUCTION

Arthritis is an umbrella term that includes over 200 different conditions. These are divided into three categories: non-inflammatory arthritis (osteoarthritis), inflammatory arthritis (rheumatoid arthritis), and connective tissue disorders such as systemic lupus erythematosus (Arthritis Care 2006). Within this chapter, the two most common types of arthritis (osteoarthritis and rheumatoid arthritis) will be covered, as will low back pain. These three conditions are collectively amongst the most common musculoskeletal conditions that cause individuals to seek medical help (Chard et al 2005, Kaaria et al 2006). The benefits of exercise for such individuals have been shown to be both biophysical and psychosocial (Brosseau et al 2003, Minor & Kay 2003, Vuori 2001). The associated cost of healthcare treatment for people suffering from osteoarthritis, rheumatoid arthritis and low back pain runs into many billions of pounds (Maetzel et al 2004, Rat & Boissier 2004, Stone 1984). This economic burden has numerous facets including loss of work and productivity, physical and psychological therapy in addition to the more easily identifiable costs of pharmaceutical prescriptions which on their own account for £400 million per annum (Prescription Pricing Authority: www.ppa.org.uk). A good starting point to access general information on arthritis is the website www.arthritiscare.org.uk, which relates to data collected by the NHS Centre for Reviews and Dissemination, University of York, UK.

Reduced physical fitness is consistently identified as a key parameter associated with musculoskeletal disorders such as arthritis and back pain (Minor & Kay 2003). These findings identify the potential value in increasing physical activity in those with musculoskeletal disorders who are less active, sedentary or those who have traditionally been discouraged from engaging in many forms of physical activity and exercise. Questions are therefore raised regarding the most appropriate types of therapeutic exercise and physical activity and their role in reducing the impact on disease status and the course of these conditions (Hayden et al 2005a, 2005b). In the past, controversy has existed over the long- and short-term consequences of osteoarthritic, rheumatoid arthritic and low back pain patients participating in exercise (Minor & Hewett 1995). The controversy has related to the potential exacerbation of disability, pain and joint swelling and increases in joint damage which could occur from exercise (Minor 1996, Minor & Lane 1996). Partly in response to these issues, but also because of the multifaceted nature of the three conditions, the research has focused on measures of psychological, physical and subjective outcomes brought about through exercise (Ottawa Panel Members 2004, 2005, Van Baar et al 1999, Van den Ende et al 1998, Westby 2001). However, there is still a paucity of evidence on the type and role of therapeutic exercise in reducing the burden.

The effect of muscle and joint disorders leading to inactivity cascades into the development of numerous health conditions that have been discussed throughout this book. Crucially, there appears to be increasing evidence that symptom reduction and improved management may occur with participation in regular exercise (Ottawa Panel Members 2004, 2005, Richardson et al 1999).

The most direct advantage of exercise to individuals with osteoarthritis, rheumatoid arthritis and low back pain lies in reducing the negative effects on a whole host of physical and psychological health conditions (chronic and acute) related to inactivity (Minor & Kay 2003). Reduced fitness only serves to magnify symptoms and consequences of musculoskeletal disorders. Factors such as inflammation, swelling and pain decrease activity levels. Correspondingly, there is an increase in the biomechanical and metabolic cost of activities (Minor & Kay 2003), which only heightens the individual's perception that activity within daily life is an increasing challenge. To reverse such effects, appropriate physical fitness parameters (and psychological issues) need to be addressed by taking an approach of graded exposure to exercise to boost individual physical capacity and confidence, reduce fear of exacerbating the condition and aid independent living (Hayden et al 2005b, Lindstrom et al 1992, Vlaeyen et al 2001). The evidence to support such an approach is increasing and has shown that there are also further benefits of symptom reduction and improved management from participation in regular exercise (Griffin & Guilak 2005, Richardson et al 1999, Vuori 2001, Westby 2001). This evidence indicates varying degrees of efficacy of activities such as walking, aerobic aquatic exercise, dance, stationary cycling, tai chi, and exercises specifically focused on joint flexibility, muscular strengthening and trunk core stability.

In order to assess more closely the issues raised so far, it is first important to review the relevant epidemiology and pathophysiology of the musculoskeletal conditions in question. Following this, the recommendations found within the evidence and any related guidelines for developing exercise protocols for these populations will then be evaluated in order to best answer the question: does exercise truly help with the suffering caused by osteoarthritis, rheumatoid arthritis and low back pain? Finally, from the best available evidence and the authors' experience of applying such evidence, a framework and examples of exercise prescription will be given.

OSTEOARTHRITIS

Osteoarthritis presents either with observable physical changes but without symptoms or with physical changes that elicit signs and symptoms (pain, swelling, weakness). Because of the natural ageing process, most if not all individuals will have physical changes to the joint structure without any symptoms. The process of physical changes (whether signs and symptoms are present) is more properly known as osteoarthrosis.

Epidemiology

It is estimated that 8.5 million (~15%) people in the UK have osteoarthritis and it is the single most common form of musculoskeletal disease (Arthritis Care 2002). It can potentially affect any joint but most commonly it affects the knees, hips, hands and spinal zygapophyseal joints (Hall 1983). Changes in joint tissue, where osteoarthrosis is identified by radiological assessment, often begin to show from the second decade of life but only 20% of individuals will complain of any related symptoms. Once individuals are over the age of 55 years, up to 85–90% will present with changes identified by radiological assessment. Similar to younger individuals, however, only about 10–20% of those with radiological evidence of changes will present with actual symptoms (Chard et al 2005, D'Ambrose 2005). Pain and suffering can vary greatly, from those who suffer continually to those with brief episodes of pain followed by periods of little or no pain (Birrell 2004). Many benefits can be gained during the periods when there are fewer or no symptoms, such as improving flexibility or strength. Despite the progressive nature of osteoarthritis that can be identified by radiology, this progression is not necessarily evidenced by any corresponding increase in pain and symptoms (Birrell et al 2005). It is only when there are extensive tissue changes that symptoms of pain tend to correspond more closely with actual physical deterioration to the joint structures.

Pathophysiology

Whilst the majority of changes related to osteoarthritis are to the hard elements of the joint (cartilage and bone), all joint structures can be affected, including the capsule, extracapsular ligaments and the supporting musculature (Felson 2004, Kidd 2006). In addition to these elements, it is important to bear in mind two points previously noted:

1. that the correlation between structural changes and joint symptoms is poor (Felson 2004), and
2. pain correlates poorly with degenerative changes found on radiological assessments (Rosen 1994).

Darby (1998) has summarized the progression of tissue changes associated with osteoarthritis (Fig. 5.1). The first changes seen are fissuring or hairline splits of the hyaline cartilage with a progressive loss, at highly variable rates, of the cartilage. Such progressive loss eventually exposes the subchondral bone. The loss of cartilage affects various elements of joint function, including normal weight-bearing capabilities of the articular surface and movement capabilities of the joint. With the progressive loss of articular cartilage, the exposure of bone produces a disturbance in bone remodelling activity and results in joint crepitus, discomfort and possibly pain. Other changes to the articular surfaces include cystic development, sclerosis and osteophytes or bony hooks usually at the joint margins.

Felson (2004) has noted the related soft tissue changes, which include:

- synovial swelling (synovitis), with thickening and capsular adhesions
- loss of articular cartilage (loss of joint space as shown on X-ray), and
- ligament laxity through swelling or degenerative changes, which may produce progressive joint instability.

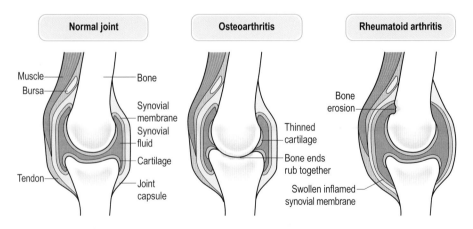

Figure 5.1   Changes in osteoarthritic and rheumatoid arthritic joints. With permission from www.medicinenet.com.

Other soft tissue changes can include progressive muscular wastage due to periods of pain-related enforced inactivity and/or inhibition of the motor units. Distinctive patterns of movement loss caused by tightening of tendons, connective tissue and capsular ligaments are also likely developments. Examples of typical movement impairment that correspond with signs of osteoarthritis include loss of extension in the knee and loss of internal and external rotation at the hip and shoulder (Felson 2004).

Osteoarthritis can be divided into three distinct types:

1. Primary generalized osteoarthritis that attacks apparently normal joints.
2. Secondary osteoarthritis where a number of factors actually cause the onset of joint tissue changes, including:
   - A history of trauma either related to sprained ligaments or a fracture adjacent to a joint; this leads to an alteration of bone angulation that disturbs the normal joint mechanics and produces muscular weakness.
   - Repeated excessive loads to the joint such as jumping, throwing or running, or a sudden impact that damages the joint surfaces. All of these may affect the ability of the joint to maintain normal lubrication and nutrition or prevent ideal distribution of pressure over the articular surface. Not included here is the consequence of altered articular nutrition.
   - Congenital deformity.
   - Infection or virus – within one or more joints
   - Autoimmune responses.
   - Genetic factors.
   - Ageing.
   - Obesity.
   - Postmenopausal decline particularly of the knee joint.
   For further reading on articular biomechanics, nutrition and adaptation see: Woo & Buckwalter (1987) and Martin et al (1998).
3. Osteoarthrosis – this third pattern relates to the asymptomatic state with changes seen frequently on X-ray. The person is functionally healthy and pain-free.

RHEUMATOID ARTHRITIS

Epidemiology

There is a generally consistent prevalence of rheumatoid arthritis of between 0.5 and 1% in Western populations. However, there do appear to be some populations that show raised occurrence such as American Indians (Eberhardt & Fex 1998, Silman & Pearson 2002). Conversely, there is low occurrence among Chinese and Japanese. In addition, in a study of rural South African and Nigerian populations there were no recorded cases at all (Brighton et al 1988, Silman et al 1993). There is some evidence of protection with populations migrating to other countries; MacGregor et al (1994) found that when Nigerians moved to the UK, their incidence of rheumatoid arthritis remained unchanged.

As with many chronic diseases there is good evidence to show that genetics also plays a role in the occurrence of rheumatoid arthritis (Silman & Pearson 2002). Pregnancy has also been shown to increase the risk of rheumatoid arthritis, particularly after the first birth, due to some hormonal influence (Nelson & Ostensen 1997). Autoimmune conditions including type 1 diabetes and possible infective agents such as the Epstein–Barr virus and the Parvovirus act as triggers of rheumatoid arthritis

(Silman & Hochberg 2001). Various bacteria have been reported as being implicated in rheumatoid arthritis, although some studies have shown that there is little direct evidence that this is the case (Silman & Hochberg 2001).

Pathophysiology

Rheumatoid arthritis is an autoimmune and systemic condition presenting as a symmetrical polyarthritis of particularly the hands, feet and knees (Hall 1983, Kasper et al 2004). Unlike osteoarthritis, the first changes in rheumatoid arthritis appear as an acute inflammation of the synovial membrane. In addition, unlike osteoarthritis the patient may initially present feeling unwell, tired, feverish or with weight loss. Interestingly the individual may present initially without any joint aches; this may be due to the autoimmune nature of rheumatoid arthritis and may be associated with a virus attack in the first place prior to any joint changes (Hall 1983, Kasper et al 2004). There is a progressive thickening of the synovium, fluid exudes into the joint space and there are also other inflammatory signs of heat and pain (Darby 1998). Proliferation of synoviocytes and macrophages causes thickening of the synovial lining and, together with lymphocytes, plasma cells and mast cells, this develops into pannus. A pannus is a sheet of invasive cellular tissue that is continuous with the synovial lining. Because of the higher proportion of synoviocytes and macrophages, pannus causes erosion of bone and cartilage at a joint's margins. Fibroblasts lay down collagen and fibrin, resulting in scarring with adhesions. Prostaglandins and leukotrienes further amplify the inflammatory and pain response (Hall 1983, Kasper et al 2004). Rupturing of ligaments and tendons is also possible with ongoing inflammation. Disuse-related atrophy of muscles also contributes to the typical deformities seen in rheumatoid arthritis (Fig. 5.1) (Hall 1983, Kasper et al 2004).

There are a number of other variants of rheumatoid arthritis that will not be discussed in this chapter:

1. juvenile rheumatoid arthritis (Still's disease)
2. Felty's syndrome
3. Sjögren's syndrome.

EXERCISE FOR OSTEOARTHRITIS AND RHEUMATOID ARTHRITIS

The range and severity of symptoms that an individual has will commonly fluctuate throughout a short time span and requires the exercise or therapy practitioner to be fully aware of each individual's specific requirements.

The recommendations made in this section assume that a thorough subjective and objective assessment of the client is made. This assessment should include the length of time the person has lived with osteoarthritis or rheumatoid arthritis, the range of symptoms suffered, activities that exacerbate or improve symptoms, the barriers to activities and the client's health behaviour towards the disease (assess psychosocial aspects). It is therefore particularly important to be able to assess the client's perception of how the disease has impacted on their life.

Primary prevention

Moderate, regular exercise can be beneficial, potentially bolstering joint integrity (Manninen et al 2001, Ottawa Panel Members 2005). Conversely, high volumes of exercise over numerous years have been shown to contribute to osteoarthritis and rheumatoid arthritis (Manninen et al 2001). Examples include the continuous and concentrated joint loading of competitive running and the torsional joint loading activities such as rugby, football (soccer), jumping, throwing and weightlifting (Manninen et al 2001). Occupational joint loading (e.g. farming, mining) also increases the probability of developing osteoarthritis (Vuori 2001). However, it is difficult to ascertain any dose–response relationships between physical activity and the development of osteoarthritis due to possible genetic factors, relevant injury history as well as personal and individual lifestyle factors (Vuori 2001).

Secondary prevention

The efficacy of exercise in the secondary management of osteoarthritis and rheumatoid arthritis is becoming clearer. Aerobic endurance activities, stretching, neuromuscular (coordination, proprioception) and functional strengthening exercises have consistently shown benefits in both groups (Ottawa Panel Members 2004, 2005, Van den Ende et al 1996, Vuori 2001). Many affected individuals are capable of exercising frequently and at intensities that stimulate beneficial effects (Brosseau et al 2003). Fundamentally, individuals may not experience further injury or exacerbate disease activity (Minor & Kay 2003), but as in the case of osteoarthritis, exercise could potentially reduce further joint damage (Ottawa Panel Members 2005).

Establishing the limitations of a specific type of aerobic or any other mode of exercise requires further clarity. Future research should strive to address the following shortcomings. Several types of exercise, sometimes in conjunction with other forms of treatment/manual therapy, are often included in the studies and it is difficult to determine the benefit directly related to the exercise type or exercise component of the treatment/therapy intervention. Specific details regarding the intensity, progression and types of exercises are often inconsistent, missing or poorly explained within guidelines and the scientific literature. The stage, grade or range of symptoms experienced by the participants in studies is often not stated.

Aerobic activity

Low/moderate-impact activities such as aquatic exercise, walking and stationary cycling have been examined and demonstrate modest, short-term improvements in the fitness of individuals with osteoarthritis and rheumatoid arthritis (Bilberg et al 2005, Ottawa Panel Members 2004, 2005). Furthermore, there is evidence of corresponding improvements in psychological and coping factors (Ottawa Panel Members 2004, 2005) and long-term benefits (Messier et al 1997) for both rheumatoid arthritis and osteoarthritis.

Minor et al (1989) assessed the efficacy of a 12-week programme that included low-impact aerobic walking, aerobic aquatics and non-aerobic range of movement (ROM) exercises. One hundred and twenty osteoarthritis (hip, knee and ankle) and rheumatoid arthritis patients were randomly assigned to one of the three groups. All groups performed co-interventions of stretching and strengthening. Those in the aerobic intervention groups performed the activity three times per week for 12 weeks at an intensity of 60–80% of heart rate maximum. Results for the osteoarthritis patients indicated that walking and aquatics elicited significant improvement in aerobic capacity, time to walk 50 feet and physical activity compared to the control group. Psychological/emotional benefits were also noted in reduced depression and anxiety. Benefits for rheumatoid arthritis individuals assigned to aerobic activities included reduced joint swelling, reduced pain and improved physical function (including increased aerobic capacity). These observations may indicate that the interventions prompted a beneficial localized biochemical and/or circulatory effect on joint inflammatory pathways (Minor & Lane 1996). The aquatic exercise group reported greater improvement in the number of clinically active joints, a decreased duration of morning stiffness and greater grip strength compared with the aerobic walking group. This indicates that aquatic based exercise may be a more appropriate therapy for some rheumatoid arthritis patients. Minor et al (1989) concluded that the low-impact activities of aerobic walking and aerobic aquatics were successful and potentially safe methods for increasing the fitness parameters for individuals with osteoarthritis and rheumatoid arthritis.

More recently, findings similar to those of Minor et al (1989) have emerged. Evcik & Sonel (2002) and Messier et al (1997) considered the effects of aerobic exercise in osteoarthritis patients and Noreau et al (1995) in rheumatoid arthritis patients. These trials examined aerobic activities undertaken for a frequency of two to three times per week and ranging between 12 weeks (Evcik & Sonel 2002, Noreau et al 1995) and 18 months (Messier et al 1997). Many interventions reported assessment periods of less than 6 months, which raises questions regarding long-term benefits, adverse reactions and patient adherence. The longer-term study by Messier et al (1997) illustrated that benefits continued as long as the exercise continued. The more recent evidence continues to support the above findings and there is a consistent pattern emerging that aerobic exercise demonstrates effects that go beyond just the physical benefits (Ottawa Panel Members 2004, 2005, Vuori 2001). These more holistic effects that arise are thought to help offset the extensive multidimensional consequences of both types of arthritis (Fifield et al 1996).

What is still missing, as noted earlier, is a consensus statement as to the most effective mode of aerobic activity for either osteoarthritis or rheumatoid arthritis patients. This probably reflects the wide diversity in symptoms, joint involvement and individual differences of the people affected. Minor & Kay (2003) suggest a combination of low/moderate-impact activities (cross-training) combining appropriate intervals of weight-bearing (e.g. walking), partial weight-bearing (semi-seated stepping machines) and non-weight-bearing activity (e.g. cycling, swimming). In the authors' experience, cross-training (using a variety of low-impact aerobic activities, flexibility and appropriate resistance exercise) and interval type activity facilitate active rest periods, which aid in reducing joint impact, strain and tissue overuse and decrease the potential for biomechanical dysfunction as a result of postural fatigue. This flexible approach to exercise planning and programming is felt to offer greater opportunities and variety (less boredom) for individualized prescription and progression with activities that can easily be reassessed and graded.

The aerobic exercise interventions reviewed by the Ottawa Panel Members (2004, 2005) were of durations of 5 or more minutes and a frequency from one to three times per week. The recommended frequency of exercise for arthritis groups is similar to that recommended for healthy individuals by the American College of Sports Medicine (ACSM 1998, Minor & Kay 2003). Indications are that individuals with inflammatory joint disease typically respond to a training stimulus in a similar manner to healthy non-affected populations. The difference may be that the expected physiological adaptations may occur at a slower rate due to a lower intensity at which the exercise can be performed. Joint movement limitations and older individuals are the main reasons for the need to work at a lower intensity. The exercise movements need to consider the disease-limiting factors of reduced joint mobility, reduced coordination and balance and the influence of any related neurological deficits. The main implications are that when planning each exercise phase, goals and strategies should reflect both the direct and indirect effects on the exercise dose to compensate for reduced mobility.

A variety of methods to set the intensity of aerobic exercise have been recommended. These include 40–70% of heart rate reserve (Mangion et al 1999), ratings of perceived exertion of 11 to 16 (light to hard on Borg's RPE scale, 1998) and 60–80% of age-predicted maximal heart rate (Minor & Kay 2003). In applying such intensities, no ill effects were reported. Mangion et al (1999), for example, examined the effects of low- and high-intensity stationary cycling on 39 patients with osteoarthritis of the knee. The study participants were divided into two groups and carried out 10 weeks of cycling, three times per week for 25 minutes. The high- and low-intensity groups exercised respectively at 70% and 40% of maximum heart rate reserve. Both groups improved aerobic capacity, function and gait and had reduced pain levels.

Low-impact, low-intensity exercise (such as static cycling) for rheumatoid arthritis patients is specifically advised by the Ottawa Panel Members (2004). Minor & Kay (2003) suggest that during an active inflammatory stage of rheumatoid arthritis, low-intensity aerobic activity combined with stretching is desirable. The underpinning belief is that exercise becomes part of the self-management strategy for affected individuals. Optimizing this, however, involves regular adherence to an exercise programme. Adherence to exercise has been established as closely related to reductions in pain, depression and awareness of arthritis (Perlman et al 1990). A key component to empowering the individual is to grade exposure to activity and ensure goals are attainable by establishing the correct type, duration and frequency of activities during periods of disease inactivity (Vlaeyen et al 2001). During periods of disease activity, the individual then becomes more physically, emotionally and psychologically capable of self-management (Minor & Brown 1993).

From the authors' experience, the use of RPE to monitor subjective exercise intensity is desirable. During the initial phases of the activity programme, the inexperienced participant may find it more in keeping with lowered states of self-efficacy to exercise to preferred levels of exertion, enabling them to work at their own pace (Parfitt et al 2006). Once exercise confidence has been gained, the use of target heart rates and RPE to set the appropriate physiological training thresholds can be employed to meet newly established goals.

The data available indicate that aerobic exercise has the capacity to favourably alter functional and fitness deficits. In turn, this can enhance several dimensions of health and promote self-management, particularly for individuals with rheumatoid arthritis and osteoarthritis of the knee. The effects of exercise on disease characteristics remain active areas of current research. Indications are that various forms of aerobic activity are safe and offer a number of benefits. Importantly they do not lead to increased disease activity for people with osteoarthritis and rheumatoid arthritis.

Box 5.1 summarizes recommended aerobic exercise in osteoarthritis and rheumatoid arthritis.

Flexibility exercise

Joint flexibility or range of movement exercise is often prescribed to reduce pain/discomfort and contractures in tissues surrounding joints and to improve soft tissue function, encouraging correct joint movement (Minor & Kay 2003). Reduced range of movement due to degenerative or inflammatory disease in any joint will affect

---

Box 5.1   Summary of recommended aerobic exercise in osteoarthritis and rheumatoid arthritis

- **Goals/Special considerations:** Initially allow the individual to have option to control own pace below typical physiological target thresholds. Duration rather than speed and distance goals may provide for more psychological achievement. Extremely deconditioned individuals may require a conditioning programme of flexibility, proprioception and strength prior to commencing aerobic activities.
- **Mode:** combinations of (low/moderate-impact) weight-bearing, non-weight-bearing and partial weight-bearing large muscle activities: walking, stationary cycling, aerobic aquatics.
- **Frequency:** Two to five times per week.
- **Duration:** Aim for 5 minutes per session initially progressing duration towards the recommended 20-minute goal, then frequency to three or more times per week and then consider achieving appropriate intensity targets.
- **Intensity:** Progress towards 40–70% $\dot{V}O_2$max (60–80% heart rate maximum, 40–70% heart rate reserve and/or RPE 11–14).

---

the biomechanical functioning of adjacent joints (Minor & Kay 2003). However, in the major weight-bearing joints gait abnormalities may occur, muscle strength can become compromised and impaired balance can result from related declines in neuromuscular competence (Minor & Kay 2003). This is likely to enhance pain and stiffness and promote disability whilst increasing the risk of falls, particularly in the older person (Lord et al 1991, Petrella et al 1997).

Several studies within the Ottawa Panel Members review (2004, 2005) included range of movement interventions. These were performed at a frequency of twice a day, one to five times per week for periods up to 12 weeks. Increases in joint range were at times apparent but it was not clear if these arose from the stretching exercises or other interventions in the trials. For example, Petrella (2000) assessed the benefits of a progressive dose of stretching and strengthening exercises compared with a non-progressive programming. The progression group consisted of 91 patients and the non-progression group 88 patients, both with osteoarthritis. Both groups started exercises that consisted of two repetitions per session for one to three exercise sessions per week. Over an 8-week period the progression group worked up to five repetitions performed over five sessions per week. The non-progression group maintained two repetitions of exercise per session for one to three sessions per week. The results indicated a significant clinical benefit in knee range of movement for the progression group in comparison to the non-progression group. Although this trial did not specifically establish that stretching alone could increase joint range, it did indicate that individuals with knee osteoarthritis tolerate progressive exercise. It has also provided some evidence for beneficial stretching and strengthening exercise doses that can be used.

It is not clear from the evidence available which exercise frequency is the most efficacious. Minor & Kay (2003), for instance, also recommend that flexibility exercises are performed one to two times per day, and particularly so during an inflammatory stage of rheumatoid arthritis. Personal experience of the authors has found that some patients benefit from two to three stretching sessions a week and others from daily sessions. In general, the aim is to gain relief (i.e. pain reduction) using a range of stretching exercises to improve perceived joint stiffness, soft tissue contractures or muscle tightness. Again, there is little consensus within the evidence to recommend the most beneficial frequency.

The variation in the prescription of stretching exercises may be based on the belief that stretching per se does or does not induce long-term (i.e. >24 hours) positive effects on joint range of movement. In addition, some reduction in the development of contractures may be gained from continuation of the activity during a rheumatoid arthritis 'flare-up'. There is some evidence that for older and non-affected populations there are some lasting effects from flexibility exercises (Feland et al 2001, Harvey et al 2002). It remains questionable that this assumption can be applied to patients with inflammatory joint disease.

There is still a lack of consensus on the length of time for which a stretch should be held in order to be beneficial. Feland et al (2001) evaluated the benefits of stretching for 15, 30 and 60 seconds in a group of non-affected older people and found the greatest benefit with the 60-second stretch. However, Petrella (2000) found that affected individuals with arthritis may experience discomfort in maintaining a static position for this timescale and advised two to three repetitions of a given stretch for 10 to 15 seconds. This may also reduce the probability of incorrect performance if the patient becomes weary from maintaining the same position over an extended period. The authors have also found the advice of Petrella (2000) to be more suitable and more achievable than that of Feland et al (2001).

Patients may find that stretches for the lower limb (e.g. the calf and hamstring muscle groups) are best performed in the seated position. Furthermore, active and not ballistic stretches are advised. Minor & Kay (2003) found that ballistic stretching increases the likelihood of exceeding the pain-free range of movement. This may provoke tissue damage or possibly spontaneous rupture, particularly in the rheumatoid arthritis patient who has had the disease for a long time and/or who has received steroid injections, both of which can alter bone and soft tissue integrity.

In addition to stretching exercises, other activities have been shown to equally augment joint range of movement for arthritis patients, including: walking, tai chi, yoga and strength training (Han et al 2004, Ottawa Panel Members 2004, 2005). Han et al (2004) reviewed four studies and concluded that tai chi did not exacerbate symptoms of rheumatoid arthritis but demonstrated benefits for ankle, knee and hip range of movement. It is therefore possible that for some patients who regularly participate in such activities, because they develop strength, mobility and balance, beneficial improvements can occur without the need for specific stretching exercises. Such thinking is based on the idea that in some patients the primary cause of reduced joint range of movement is bony changes (e.g. osteophyte development) and not soft tissues, which can literally be stretched. It is therefore necessary to establish during the assessment process which tissues are causing the reduced range of motion: hard bony end-points or potentially malleable soft tissues. Such an assessment may need to include both physiotherapeutic and radiological examinations. Where necessary, adaptations to prescribed range of movement exercises should be made in order to minimize risks associated with overstretching.

Similar to aerobic activity interventions, there is no established consensus statement on the evidence for prescribing stretching exercises. Flexibility exercise is seldom studied in isolation and greater information regarding number of repetitions, sets and exercise specifics is required. Given that general aerobic activities such as tai chi and yoga have improved joint range, and that the true value of stretching exercise remains somewhat unclear, the best evidence available is to prescribe the former. Furthermore, there are other health benefits (as noted in the other chapters of this book) to be gained from activities that are aimed at improving endurance, strength, balance and coordination.

Box 5.2   Summary of recommended range of movement exercise for osteoarthritis and rheumatoid arthritis

- **Goals/Special considerations:** Decrease pain and stiffness. Improve gait. Facilitate programme progression. Maintain or increase range of joint movement. Ensure correct skill acquisition.
- **Mode:** Active range of movement exercise and muscular stretches and/or specific activities including tai chi, yoga and regular walking.
- **Frequency:** For individual movements one to three repetitions; one to two times per day; three to five times per week.
- **Duration:** Individual movements 5-8 seconds.
- **Intensity:** Within pain-free range of movement progressing towards graded exposure to pain, stiffness and mobility limitations.

Box 5.2 summarizes recommended range of movement exercise for osteoarthritis and rheumatoid arthritis.

Proprioceptive exercise

Proprioceptive exercise is utilized to improve neuromuscular coordination, thus promoting functional stability and correct joint dynamics (Lephart et al 1997). Proprioception declines with advancing age but this decline can be accentuated by inactivity, joint disease and injury (Swanik et al 2000). The deterioration in the proprioceptive sensitivity and the fine motor control of muscle tissue are of importance as they compound muscle weakness. This is particularly apparent in the quadriceps muscle group for people with rheumatoid arthritis and osteoarthritis of the knee (Bearne et al 2002, Hortobágyi et al 2004). Neuromuscular limitations (or 'steadiness' of motor unit recruitment) during the eccentric phase of a quadriceps movement, for example, have particular relevance for joint stability, disease progression (due to mal-alignment) and ultimately for independent living (Bearne et al 2002, Hortobágyi et al 2004).

The inclusion of balance training for individuals with knee instability due to ligament damage appears to enhance the effectiveness of rehabilitation programmes (Fitzgerald et al 2000, Swanik et al 2000). Similar training techniques also have benefits for rheumatoid arthritis and knee osteoarthritis (Bearne et al 2002, Fitzgerald et al 2000). Bearne et al (2002) investigated the efficacy and safety of a 5-week rehabilitation regimen on patients with rheumatoid arthritis. The programme of simple dynamic exercises increased quadriceps sensorimotor function and decreased lower limb disability without exacerbating pain or disease activity.

The regimen implemented by Bearne et al (2002) consisted of individually prescribed functional, dynamic coordination (e.g. step-ups), balance (e.g. wobble-board) and isometric strength exercises each performed for 1–5 minutes. Exercise progressions included improving the quality of movement during the performance of a given activity. Correct motor skill acquisition optimizes joint balance and stability training and in combination with supervised practice in a controlled environment, further enhancement of patient confidence will occur (Fitzgerald et al 2002). It is suggested that proprioception exercises should commence early in an exercise regimen and also be complemented by a well-rounded exercise programme which focuses in the initial stages on building strength and flexibility (Table 5.1; Lephart et al 1997).

Table 5.1 Example of a gymnasium and equipment-based exercise programme undertaken by a patient with bilateral osteoarthritis of the knee (exercise progressions occurred throughout each 3- to 4-week stage)[a]

Weeks	Main strength and aerobic exercises	Balance and proprioceptive exercises (can be performed separately or used for active rest between main strength and aerobic exercises)
1	3 days per week Static cycle ergometer Limit range of movement on stepping machine Seated resistance exercises with resistance bands Seated stretch	6 × heel and toe raises 6 × heel to toe weight transfers with available hand support 6 × sit-to-stand 2 minutes of unidirectional balance board activity with available hand support
2 to 3	Repeat of week 1 activities but perform resistance and stretching exercises in standing Add home-based strength and aerobic exercises on non-gym days	10 × heel and toe raises – wide stance 10 × heel-toe weight transfers with less use of hand support 10 × sit-to-stand 3 to 4 minutes of unidirectional balance board activity with available hand support
4 to 7	Repeat previous week's activities but Increase duration of cycling Introduce further aerobic activities Either perform resistance exercise more slowly and/or increase amount of resistance Progress to using fixed-weight resistance machines	10 × heel-toe exercises, narrow stance with reduced use of hand supports Heel-toe exercise incorporated into a walk (6 to 10 strides of 2 to 3 sets) 8 to 12 sit-to-stand exercises but with a slow eccentric phase on alternate repetitions 3 to 4 minutes of unidirectional balance board activity with reduced use of hand support; progressing challenge by adding gentle head turns
8 to 11	Repeat previous week's activities but Progress unsupervised home exercise to include balance activities, including: the heel-toe exercise incorporated into a walk (6 to 10 strides of 2 to 3 sets – with support down hallway) Practising standing with one foot in front of the other (tandem) when performing basic domestic tasks such as peeling vegetables or brushing teeth	2 sets × 6 single side steps using a hand support 8 to 10 sit-to-stand exercises but with both a slow rise and brief stop halfway through the movement and the same on the downward eccentric phase 2 to 4 minutes of round multidirectional 'wobble-board' activity with available hand support
12 to 15	Continue with previous week's exercises both in the gym and at home	2 sets × 10 single side steps, incorporating a head turn progressing from open to closed eyes but with available hand support

(Continued)

Table 5.1 Example of a gymnasium and equipment-based exercise programme undertaken by a patient with bilateral osteoarthritis of the knee (exercise progressions occurred throughout each 3- to 4-week stage)[a]—Cont'd

Weeks	Main strength and aerobic exercises	Balance and proprioceptive exercises (can be performed separately or used for active rest between main strength and aerobic exercises)
		10 to 15 sit-to-stand exercises as above but with balance-challenge pad under one foot then repeat with the balance pad under the other foot
		4 minutes of round-multidirectional 'wobble-board' activity with reduced hand support and progressing towards the use of head turns with open then closed eyes

[a]These proprioceptive and balance activities are also used as part of a falls prevention programme. Instructors or therapists should refer to more detailed training and course material cited and recommended in Chapter 6.

Rationale of the practical aspects of an exercise programme

Many areas within the evidence base lack an agreed approach to the actual 'coaching' or instruction of a client within an exercise programme. This is certainly an area within clinical exercise therapy that needs further work; hence the approaches that therapists take often involve as much 'art' as they do 'science'. The recommendations to follow are therefore subject to the individual interpretation of the evidence by the authors. The programme outlined in Table 5.1 provides examples of activities prescribed to develop proprioception. The guidance and recommendations for practice in this section are based on the best available evidence (Bearne et al 2002, Fitzgerald et al 2000), which at present still requires much more research. The examples given also aim to illustrate supplementary exercises that may help to address coexisting fitness deficits typical of the deconditioned arthritis patient and some may be utilized to progress sensorimotor skills. Proprioception exercise can be planned with a specific focus on improving joint sensorimotor feedback; for example, 'wobble-board' performed with eyes open and then closed. It may also be addressed within functional exercises, for example repeated bouts of sit-to-stand activities. These type of exercises develop balance and coordination and when progressed may require the inclusion of a slow eccentric phase that is aimed to further enhance neuromuscular efficiency and strength (Bearne et al 2002).

The initial week (days 1 to 3) of a programme should focus on continual assessment, safety, the client learning about why they need to exercise, and the therapist gaining an appreciation of the client's behaviour or attitude towards exercise. This time period also aims to help the client achieve the appropriate skill acquisition and confidence for effectively performing the exercises. The client is exposed to basic proprioception or balance exercises that alternate between seated resistance and flexibility activities. At this point aerobic-type activities are minimized. With the exception of flexibility exercise, in order to minimize intra-articular pressure and soft tissue exertion, particular care should be taken to avoid use of the same muscle group in successive activities. This, however, can be a useful strategy for increasing exercise intensity in the later stages of a programme. Alternating the programme components in this way is aimed at improving the long-term carry-over of proprioception. Once an exercise 'dose' has been tried and its effects evaluated as safe and the proprioception activities have been mastered, other 'graded activities' may gradually be introduced.

Grading exercise progressions so that proprioception abilities can continue to be enhanced may take many forms. For example, performing resistance exercises in standing (more in-depth discussion and guidelines concerning resistance training follow) represents a practical method of increasing task difficulty which then facilitates the automatic activation of sensorimotor skills. Note that the option to include an activity while seated should always be considered at any stage in a session or exercise regimen depending on fluctuating disease status, changes in symptoms and confidence. Programme progression can also be achieved by: decreasing the speed with which an activity is performed, increasing repetitions and sets, altering the base of support, varying foot configuration, challenging/altering visual input and distracting the patient during the exercises. Perturbation training (Fitzgerald et al 2000, 2002), using 'wobble-boards', is specific and an easily graded technique for addressing joint proprioception deficits. Home-based exercises can be introduced once basic skills have been mastered and progressed within the safety of the clinical environment. Whether performed at home or in the clinic, exercise task complexity needs to be increased and integrating proprioceptive skills into activities of daily living needs to be encouraged.

To date there are no known research-based guidelines available regarding the most advantageous frequency, duration and intensity of proprioception exercise. It has been indicated that twice-weekly training for durations greater than 5 minutes can provide an adequate stimulus to improve proprioception (Bearne et al 2002, Fitzgerald et al 2002). More research is needed to identify whether increased frequency of daily practice can enhance acquisition of proprioception. Intensity of the activity has not been researched so the authors' current practice dictates that patients not exceed 12 to 13 on Borg's RPE scale to prevent fatigue, which can be detrimental to motor skill acquisition. Assessing intensity in terms of task difficulty remains an ongoing challenge. Verbal feedback, visual analogue scales for pain and objective visual assessment may all prove helpful.

Box 5.3 provides a summary of proprioception exercise for osteoarthritis and rheumatoid arthritis.

Box 5.3   Summary of proprioception exercise for osteoarthritis and rheumatoid arthritis

- **Goals/Specific considerations:** Increase joint proprioception. Improve joint stability and gait. Facilitate programme progression. Increase patient confidence.
- **Mode:** Dynamic coordination and balance activities. Perturbation training.
- **Frequency:** 1–2 times per day to 3–5 times per week.
- **Duration:** 5 minutes +
- **Intensity:** Patient feedback. Rating activity difficulty using visual analogue scale. Observation.

Strength training for osteoarthritis and rheumatoid arthritis

When considering resistance training for the management of osteoarthritis and rheumatoid arthritis, the present evidence does not seem to highlight any disease-specific differences in terms of recommendations for exercise prescription guidance. Therefore, the following discussion will consider the evidence and practice for pre-scribing resistance exercise for osteoarthritis and rheumatoid arthritis concurrently.

As with the other components of fitness previously discussed, Fransen et al (2001) concluded that:

> *There were insufficient data to provide useful guidelines on optimal exercise type or dosage. Supervised exercise classes appeared to be as beneficial as treatments provided on a one-to-one basis.*

One of the problems associated with establishing optimal exercise type and dosage is the multifaceted nature of arthritis (e.g. severity of symptoms, type of disease, age, perceptions of condition and quality of life). However, strength training has been shown to be beneficial for individuals with and without arthritis as a means of main-taining functionality in daily life. The authors have therefore chosen to reflect on the best available evidence in light of their own experiences from which the reader may be able to corroborate exercise prescriptions specific to the patients with whom they work.

Modes of resistance training

The mode of resistance training can include using one's own body mass (e.g. a wall press) or equipment such as elasticated bands, fixed weight machines, free hand weights, dumbbells and barbells. It is prudent to move through these common exercise tools in the order in which they have been listed. The reasons behind this are as follows:

- Exercises performed using the *client's own bodyweight* (either with individual limbs or in non-, partial- or full-weight-bearing situations) allow for movements that reflect activities in daily life and are also a useful means of coaching the correct exercise techniques required when using the subsequent resistive exercise equipment.
- *Resistance bands* are helpful as they move with the individual and can be secured to wrists if the hands are affected. They are also somewhat less intimidating.
- *Fixed weight machines* typically are fully adjustable with regard to the seat and movement arm, which can be extremely helpful when determining a pain-free range of motion and then adjusting the machine to fit this.
- The exercise movements utilized in *free weights* training most resemble functional movements. The risk of injury, however, is also greater and fully supervised ses-sions to maintain technique are highly recommended.

Table 5.2 shows a selection of available exercises in these three categories – resis-tance bands, fixed weight machines and bodyweight/free weight; in all of these the movements can initially be performed without the resistive equipment.

There are many more exercises than those listed in Table 5.2, as the choice of avail-able equipment will vary between exercise facilities or clinical settings. These are purely as a guide and tool to stimulate thought. Consequently, a certain amount of

Table 5.2   An example of typically used land-based strength exercises

Resistance bands	Fixed weight machines	Free weights or use of bodyweight
Punching (seated or standing)	Incline bench press	Wall press
Seated leg push	Leg press	Squat (using stability ball placed between the back and a wall)
Row (seated or standing)	Seat row using a low pulley	Upright row
Lateral or front deltoid raise	Shoulder press machine	Dumbbell lateral or front deltoid raise
Biceps curl	Seated pulley arm curl	Alternate dumbbell biceps curl
Seat overhead elbow extension	Triceps pushdown	Modified bench triceps dips

original and innovative thinking is required to devise a programme for this client group. Along with the type of equipment to be used, the actual form (e.g. isometric, isotonic) of the resistance training needs to be considered.

Isometric training

Isometric resistance training has proved a popular and successful mode with researchers, particularly for those clients with osteoarthritis and rheumatoid arthritis who are most affected (Hurley & Scott 1998, Van den Ende et al 2000). Factors to consider when applying this type of training are that gains will occur at the specific joint angle exercised and 20° on either side of this angle (Wathen & Roll 1994). Therefore, different starting angles need to be employed to develop muscular strength and endurance in a joint's full range of movement. An important objective in exercise training for arthritis is to increase functional movement. Isometric exercises tend to be lacking in this area and consequently isotonic movements may supersede this technique as progress is achieved.

Isotonic training

If isotonic movements become the mainstay of the exercise programme, the range of movement that causes no pain or minimal pain should be ascertained. Movement should be restricted to this pain-free range, slowly increasing further as pain or discomfort diminishes.

As noted previously, no differences have been found between the different forms of resistance training (Bennell & Hinman 2005). What seems most important is that the exercise prescription is specific to the individual.

Frequency

Frequency of exercise sessions is a critical factor from the perspective of pain management. It is advisable that the arthritic sufferer should not exercise if pain from the previous exercise session is still being experienced in a joint (Bearne et al 2002). This approach can be problematic as it is to be expected that a certain amount of pain, joint or muscle stiffness may well be experienced, especially in the initial stages of the exercise programme. Post-exercise discomfort should be similar to that experienced by other novice exercisers and should follow the same pattern. Individuals who endure pain on a regular basis are generally well aware of their pain and its particular characteristics. Consequently, it is vital to have knowledge of this to effectively distinguish between their 'normal' pains and new but unacceptable exercise-induced pain.

As discussed, osteoarthritis may only be present in specific joints while other joints are free of the disease. This means that exercise can and should continue to be performed using the non-affected joints. As rheumatoid arthritis typically affects all joints during an exacerbation, the frequency of physical activity may need to be reduced; in many cases, complete rest is advised during this period. Hakkinen et al (2001) found that it was practicable to get clients to perform resistance training exercise 1 to 2 times per week, as it needed to be incorporated into a programme with the other components of fitness (e.g. aerobic and flexibility work).

Intensity

Intensity most commonly relates to the load lifted and typically is determined by using a percentage of a maximum effort lift, typically the one repetition maximum (1-RM). From experience, this way of establishing a resistance training intensity for arthritic clients is likely to be inappropriate. When establishing the exercise intensity, attempting to attain a 1-RM may be inadvisable due to variability of symptoms, pain experienced and an individual's preconception of the potential drawbacks or benefits of exercise. The aims for a client are likely to include either improving functional movements to enhance their quality of life with a reduction in the pain experienced or no increase in their 'usual' pain. An initial starting load just below the level at which joint pain occurs is a potential way of establishing a safe intensity. The Borg CR-10 scale is particularly helpful in this regard, as it was designed to assess sensations specific to an area of the body. However, graded exposure needs to occur over time in order to create useful hard and soft tissue adaptations and improved functionality even if there is no improvement in pain experience. This trial and error approach may seem unscientific and possibly even simplistic. However, such a method adheres to processes applied within the evidence base; such as specificity (a pain free movement around a specific joint), progression (an increase in load maybe from no load to a load) and goal-setting (a decrease in pain or increased functional movement).

Repetitions

Many studies fail to publish the exact training programmes used. The American College of Sports Medicine (1998) presently recommends performing one set of 12–15 repetitions for healthy individuals. Thomas et al (2002) utilized 20 repetitions in arthritic individuals. These differences illustrate that more than one approach can be effective. It is felt that having a flexible approach to exercise prescription is essential in this population, particularly for long-term adherence (Fransen et al 2001). This means that initially concepts of instruction, good technique and getting used to the feel of resistance training are just as important as attempting to achieve a target

---

Box 5.4   Key points for resistance training

- Use a mixture of the options available to suit the client's particular stage of disease.
- Be aware of the particular risks of each equipment mode.
- Be imaginative in exercise prescription while still keeping the goals of the exercise programme in mind.
- Schedule frequency of training sessions to coincide with an absence of joint pain. This will vary between individuals; although twice weekly should be a goal.
- Determine training load by aiming for pain-free movement.
- Repetition ranges of between 5 and 15 have proven to be effective.
- A variety of exercises, preferably multi-joint, should be utilized.

---

prescription (e.g. one set of 12–20 repetitions). For example, it may be advisable to start the client with one set of five repetitions, as it seems to be an achievable and non-threatening goal. From experience, it has been observed that increasing repetitions (up to 12 to 15) rather than the load is more acceptable to clients, allowing them to feel a sense of achievement/mastery and confidence in the early stages of rehabilitation. Interestingly, these numbers of repetitions correspond to everyday tasks such as climbing stairs (12 to 15 steps) and using a tin opener (12 to 15 turns). It is felt that if clients can see the relationship of the exercise to actual activities in daily life, they may be more compliant in performing the exercise programme. Wherever possible, joint overuse and strain needs to be avoided; exercises that use multiple joints (e.g. 'lat' pull, leg press, shoulder press actions), as opposed to those which use single joint actions (e.g. simple knee extension/flexion, elbow extension/flexion), should be prescribed first.

Feigenbaum & Pollock (1999) concluded that, for populations with chronic disease, one set of an exercise is just as effective as multiple sets. In any therapeutic exercise programme it is important to consider increasing fitness in the non-affected parts of the body, as these may have to take up the strain of the affected parts. For those non-affected areas, the strength training can be performed using guidelines for healthy individuals (ACSM 1998).

Box 5.4 summarizes the key points for resistance training.

Water–based resistance training

Water-based exercise has been shown to be a workable alternative for this population (Wyatt et al 2001). Firstly, the aspect of buoyancy reduces joint loading and the warm water provides a soothing sensation to the joints and muscles. Such features may be very attractive for those severely affected and in the initial stages of rehabilitation exercise. The resistance created by the water behaves in a pseudo isokinetic manner. Moving a limb slowly through water provides a low resistive stimulus but by increasing speed, there is a curvilinear increase in resistance. Within such a resistance gradient, a sufficient and controllable stimulus can be found for individuals who are weak or with muscle or joint pain. Wyatt et al (2001) found that although the physiological benefits were similar when comparing water to land-based exercise, lower subjective pain ratings were reported when exercising in water, therefore removing one of the barriers to exercise. Table 5.3 gives suggestions for various water-based exercises.

Table 5.3 An example of water-based mobility and strength exercises

	Muscle group	Brief description
Lower body: lying		
Prone leg kicks	Hip extensors/flexors, quadriceps, hamstrings, gluteal, trunk	Float on front, holding poolside, leg kick for front crawl, progress to using kick-board
Supine leg kicks	Hip extensors/flexors, trunk, quadriceps, hamstrings, gluteal	Floating on back, holding on poolside kicking for back-stroke, progress to using kick-board
Lower body: standing		
Squats	Quadriceps, hamstrings, gluteal, trunk	Feet hip width apart, bend legs as though sitting, return to start
Lunges	Quadriceps, hamstrings, gluteal, trunk	Step forward bending front leg, forcibly return to start
Hip extensions	Hip extensors, gluteal	Keeping leg straight, move leg backwards from hip
Hips	Adductor/abductor	Keeping leg straight, move leg out to side and back past midline
High knee lifts	Hip flexors	Bend legs, bringing knees up in front as high as possible
Walking		In contact with floor of shallow end or in deep water with buoyancy jacket
Jogging		In contact with floor in shallow end or in deep water with buoyancy jacket
Upper body		
Shoulder raises	Shoulders	Lift arms above head either in front or to side
Rows (+ with ball)	Back, forearm flexors	With arms out in front pull hands forcibly back to waist
Punching	Chest, triceps, elbow extensors	Alternate hands, varying direction of punches
Arm stroke actions	All upper body muscles	Simulate swimming strokes
Ball dunk	Back, chest, elbow extensors	Using medium size rubber ball push down into water with arms straight or bent
Shoulder push	Shoulders, triceps, elbow extensors	Push hands directly upwards, straightening arms
Biceps curl	Forearm flexors	Bend and straighten arms with elbows tucked into the sides
Ball pushes	Chest, forearm extensors	With ball at chest push arms forcibly forwards
Trunk rotations	Trunk	Rotate at waist keeping feet flat, extend arms for more resistance

Box 5.5   **Key points for water-based resistance exercise**

- Resistance exercise in a swimming pool is useful for those most affected.
- Pain may be decreased and therefore motivation increased.
- Balls and other equipment can be introduced to aid in progression.
- General principles previously described are suitable.

Box 5.5 summarizes the key points for water-based resistance exercise.

Summary on exercise and arthritis

Aerobic, strength training, flexibility and proprioceptive exercise have been shown to be safe for patients with osteoarthritis and rheumatoid arthritis. The chosen activities do require tailoring to the individual client's needs in light of symptoms and functional capacity. Ultimately, regular participation in exercise has therapeutic benefits, such as improved functional ability, reduced pain and improved coping strategies. It has not yet been demonstrated which mode of exercise (aerobic, strength, flexibility, proprioceptive) is the most beneficial. However, it is felt that, as in any other health-based activity, arthritis exercise prescription should contain elements of all these different modes in order to reflect the demands of daily life and the ageing process. The extreme range of symptoms and multifaceted nature of osteoarthritis and rheumatoid arthritis demand a flexible approach to prescription. The role of exercise in preventing or reducing the chronicity of episodes is yet to be proven. However, it should not be forgotten that in engaging such clients in physical activity the aim is more than just trying to rectify the specific musculoskeletal condition. It is about increasing physical activity that can counter many other health conditions brought on by enforced inactivity resulting from arthritis.

Providing the exercise intensity is sufficient, the physiological training benefits for those with arthritis mirror those for healthy individuals and this can often be achieved without detrimental effects (Minor & Kay 2003). It has been established thus far that aerobic endurance, flexibility, neuromuscular (proprioception) and strengthening exercise may benefit both clinical groups (Fisher 2002, Van Baar et al 1999, Van den Ende et al 1998, Vuori 2001). The challenge to setting an individualized exercise programme is establishing the limitations of specific forms of aerobic or any other mode of activity. The main gap in the evidence is what individual type (aerobic, strength, flexibility, proprioceptive) or mixture of exercises brings about an optimal benefit.

LOW BACK PAIN

Epidemiology

There is no evidence of any change in low back pathology or prevalence of low back pain related to modern sedentary lifestyle; however, there is an exponential increase in disability associated with low back pain (Waddell 1998). Papageorgiou et al (1995) of the epidemiology research unit at the University of Manchester concluded that the prevalence of low back pain in the UK population was 35–37%. The prevalence does not appear to have altered in recent decades. For the USA, Deyo et al (2006) and

Manchikanti (2000) have reported a prevalence of about 25%. The Bandolier review group cited the Clinical Standards Advisory Group (CSAG; Rosen 1994) that in Britain back pain is a growing problem. The prevalence includes 16 million sufferers, resulting in three to seven million GP (family doctor) consultations each year.

It needs to be appreciated that acute low back pain and chronic low back pain are quite different and the approaches to therapy in each condition need to be addressed separately (Waddell 1998). The University of York NHS Centre for Reviews (2000) estimated the annual cost of acute and chronic low back pain as between £265 million and £383 million. Parroy (2005) stated that in the UK, 500 million working days are lost each year, with healthcare costs amounting to £653 million. More recent data from Sleed et al (2005) quote costs of £3.84 billion for adolescent populations with chronic pain including low back pain.

Pathophysiology

Low back pain is characterized by a range of symptoms such as stiffness, pain, muscle tension or muscle spasms that may appear in the low back area or be referred to the lower limbs (University of York NHS Centre for Reviews 2000). Referred pain in the leg does not automatically imply impingement of or damage to a nerve (e.g. sciatica). All tissues in the human body are capable of referring pain some distance away from the actual location of the problem, which is ultimately registered as an unpleasant sensation within the brain referred to as pain (Gifford 1997, Gifford & Butler 1997, Main & Spanswick 2000). In a Finnish study the conclusion was that low back pain had a recurrence rate of 65–88% (Kaaria et al 2006).

Various tissues are thought to be possible sources of low back pain, including:

- muscle fibre – strains, tears, instability (hyperflexibility) and dysfunction or imbalance of muscle groups
- ligaments – strains and tears
- discs – strains, bulges, protrusions or ruptures
- facet joint strains – inflammation and stiffness
- nerves – inflammation, entrapment and encroachment
- injuries to the vertebral column – including fractures and subluxations.

Injuries, stresses and strains to one or any combination of the above structures may give rise to the diagnosis of spinal pain of unknown or uncertain origin (Merskey & Bogduk 1994) often referred to as mechanical low back pain, simple back pain or non-specific back pain (Waddell 1998). It should be remembered that there are more sinister causes of low back pain such as infections, tumours, aortic aneurysms and abdominal organ pathologies that are capable of presenting themselves in the form of back pain as the sole symptom (Waddell 1998). Suffice to say, a completely satisfactory term to accurately describe low back pain is not available. There is often a lack of pathophysiological evidence of tissue changes that underpin the causation of low back pain.

Acute low back pain is defined as a period of complaint of up to 6 weeks (University of York NHS Centre for Reviews 2000). There may or may not be a causal link to an event or incident of trauma, with many people describing their back problem as occurring for no apparent reason. Classic examples of patients reporting the onset of back pain might include descriptions such as 'I only bent down to get a pencil' or 'I turned to wave to a friend and suddenly I was in terrible pain'.

Box 5.6   **Differences between acute and chronic pain**

- Acute and chronic pains are different.
- Low back pain, osteoarthritis and rheumatoid arthritis may well have periods of acute pain but are either chronically constant or chronically recurring.
- Pain has several facets: sensory, cognitive, emotional and affective. The proportions of each vary from person to person and from one episode to another.
- Low back pain, osteoarthritis and rheumatoid arthritis are episodic in nature.

Sources: Main & Spanswick (2000), Eberhardt & Fex (1998).

The clinical definition of *chronic low back pain* is largely agreed to be where symptoms are present for longer than 3 months. The term chronic low back pain may also be applied in those individuals who have short-lived recurrent attacks that appear as acute (new) episodes several times in a year and often for many years.

In our experience, patients often use the terms acute and chronic with a different meaning to the medical definition. Medically, 'acute' means a new and recent onset of symptoms. It is important to qualify whether the sufferer is using the word acute to imply the severity or the impact of the pain and not necessarily the recent onset of symptoms. Therefore, it is important to clarify such terminology with the patient before embarking on an assessment and a treatment plan that includes exercise. Acute pain often has a simple relationship with tissue damage and pain intensity and has a natural tendency to recover and respond to physical treatments. Whereas with chronic (long-standing) pain there may be little evidence of any remaining or related tissue damage. Pain appears to be self-sustaining and cannot be treated with a purely biomechanical, biomedical or tissue-orientated approach; the pain may indeed have little biological meaning or purpose (Sternback 1974, Waddell 1998). However, there are some low back pain conditions that may exist for far longer than 3 months, which then resolve spontaneously irrespective of any therapeutic intervention. Spinal disc problems can resolve with time and the associated pathology is well described in other texts (Adams & Hutton 1983, 1985, Masui et al 2005).

It does appear that most problems start with some physical cause that is often relatively trivial or occurs during commonplace movements (Waddell 1998). In the chronic pain sufferer there appears to be a strong relationship with psychosocial issues including fear of re-injury, lack of a diagnosis, or conflicting diagnoses and psychological aspects related to work (Vlaeyen & Linton 2000). Pain is a personal experience and is often unrelated to the disease state that has been evaluated by radiological assessment (Bogduk 2004, Rosen 1994). The pain can be created by such issues as fear of movement, further injury or outstanding concern in the mind of the patient (e.g. 'what the future may hold') (Vlaeyen & Linton 2000).

Box 5.6 summarizes the differences between acute and chronic pain.

EXERCISE FOR LOW BACK PAIN

The symptoms and causes of low back pain are so widely varied, often with little or no relationship between 'cause and effect', that developing a useful physical activity programme can be a challenge (Simmonds & Dreisinger 2003, Vuori 2001). The next sections will look at exercise for both acute and chronic low back pain.

Exercise for acute low back pain

Research into acute episodes of back pain demonstrate no sound evidence that commonly prescribed flexibility and strengthening exercises are any more useful than an individual continuing with simple activities like a daily walk (Smidt et al 2005, Vuori 2001). Cholewicki et al (1997) argue that spinal flexion or extension exercises may exacerbate the problem, promoting further trunk muscle co-activation where excessive contraction or muscle spasm already exists. Hagen et al (2004) concluded that the latent risks associated with bed rest alone justified a prescription for remaining physically active. In support of this, Vuori (2001) contends that continuing with low-stress (low-impact) aerobic activities (walking, cycling, swimming) during the first 2 weeks of an episode of acute back pain appeared to facilitate recovery and reduce the likelihood of disability.

Case study: acute low back pain

There is a mixture of opinion concerning the evidence that specific strengthening exercises provide a significant benefit over general graded exercise programmes for either acute or chronic low back pain. The case study in Box 5.7 provides an illustration of the individualized nature of recommending exercise for back pain. Table 5.4 shows the timeline of rehabilitation, highlighting significant points and exercise programme progressions for the case study outlined in Box 5.7.

In the early stages of the case study's rehabilitation programme (Box 5.8), advice on how to progress was taken from a variety of sources. This leads to an extremely important point, that rehabilitation is typically a multidisciplinary endeavour requiring input from a variety of health professionals, e.g. therapists, exercise specialists and medical practitioners.

Prior to the case client (Box 5.7) performing a desired gym-based portion of his rehabilitation, an exercise test was performed using the Åstrand–Rhyming cycle ergometer protocol (ACSM 2000). The results of this are displayed in Table 5.5. The main reason for this test was not so much to estimate aerobic capacity but more importantly to remove the guesswork in setting an appropriate intensity for the subsequent gymnasium exercise sessions. It is clear from the table that the majority of heart rate reserve (HRR) percentages are below 40%, the threshold recommended by the ACSM for improvements in cardiorespiratory fitness. During the initial stages of rehabilitation, the client was not psychologically ready to work at the required target physiological training thresholds recommended by the ACSM. Consequently, intensity levels were set at the heart rate, RPE and metabolic equivalents (METs) that related to the highest level at which the client was confident to work. It is important that exercise physiologists consider the person and their psychological status before focusing on the simpler goals of increasing fitness. For many patients, simply focusing on simple goals (e.g. walking further without pain and having the strength and skill to get out of the bath) will be far more rewarding than attaining any specific physiological target (Biddle & Mutrie 2001).

Box 5.7   Case study (acute back pain)

- 35-year-old man, no previously reported incidences of low back pain and no other relevant medical history.
- Exercise history predominantly strength training and power-lifting, supplemented by aerobic conditioning, 6 days per week.
- First back pain experienced a day after a strength training session. Advice sought from physiotherapist who identified a prolapsed disc at L4/L5.
- All exercise, except for walking, ceased. Regular walking for 2 weeks after the initial pain.
- Two weeks after the initial onset of symptoms, a dramatic increase in pain and abnormal neurological symptoms (pins and needles, numbness and loss of tendon reflex) occurred. It is important to note that this was not related to the modified exercise programme but rather a progression of the original injury (nucleus pulposus protrusion).
- Emergency operation to remove an intervertebral disc was performed; hospitalized for 8 days.
- Post-surgery advice from orthopaedic surgeon was to curtail all activity for 6 weeks except for basic activities of daily living and physiotherapy to aid recovery, particularly for the persistent neurological symptoms (numbness in lower limbs, abnormal muscle recruitment patterns).

Table 5.4   The timeline of rehabilitation for 35-year-old man (Box 5.7) with acute back trauma and surgery, highlighting main exercise progression targets[a]

Week	Event
0 to 2	Day 0: Onset of injury
	Day 1: Onset of pain (receipt of advice)
	Days 2 to 14: Exercise training ceased except for daily walking
2 to 3	Progression of injury and admission to hospital for emergency surgery
4	Hospital discharge
5 to 11	Physiotherapy treatment to manage mobility, pain, numbness and abnormal leg muscle recruitment
12 and 13	Daily walking
14 and 15	Daily walking plus use of static cycle ergometer
16 to 19	Daily walking plus addition of modified use of stepping and rowing machines
20 to 23	Increased total cardiovascular exercise duration up to 20+ minutes and introduced fixed resistance machines (upper body)
24 to 27	Cardiovascular exercise intensity increased to recommended physiological thresholds and lower body fixed resistance exercise machines added
28 to 31	Maintained intensity and duration of cardiovascular exercise, increased resistance training intensity towards recommended thresholds
32 weeks onwards	Exercise programme considered that of a healthy individual without back problems

[a]Throughout this programme the average time for each main progression of either intensity or duration or both was about 4 weeks. Physiotherapy treatment, including ball stability exercises, was integral within the timeline of activities either to progress mobility and/or to manage any arising symptoms.

Table 5.5   Early rehabilitation submaximal cycle ergometer test results for case study example (see Box 5.8 and Table 5.4); resting heart rate 75 beats/min; body mass 85 kg; age 35 years

Work rate (watts)	Estimated METs	Heart rate (beats/min)	% Maximal heart rate reserve	Perceived exertion (Borg 6–20)
60	3.5	94	18	9
60	3.5	95	18	9
90	5.2	108	30	12
90	5.2	112	34	12
120	6.9	118	39	14
120	6.9	129	50	15

Case study: exercise programme development

The rehabilitation timeline (Table 5.4) shows that once the initial 6-week stage of rehabilitation had taken place, walking was reintroduced as the main form of exercise both in and out of the gym. This applies the recommendations of Vuori (2001). Exercise bouts were limited to a maximum of 5 minutes, and speeds that elicited perceived exertion ratings of 11–13 on the Borg scale were advised. At the end of 2 weeks into the rehabilitation programme, the client was achieving 30 minutes of walking two to three times per week (10 minutes around home and 20 minutes on the treadmill). This type of programming is helpful as it gives both the therapist and the client a measure of ability in daily life and in the rehabilitation setting. From a general health perspective, the aim of achieving a total of 30 minutes of physical activity per day meets the recommendations of the Chief Medical Officer for England and the US Surgeon General (Department of Health 2004, Centers for Disease Control and Prevention 1996).

In weeks 14–15, a second mode of cardiovascular equipment, the upright exercise cycle ergometer, was introduced as a programme progression. In addition to walking, 10 minutes of cycle ergometry was the initial goal, divided into two bouts of 5 minutes. The treadmill and cycle were alternated with rest periods determined by the time it took for pain and stiffness to be relieved. Intensity remained at 11–13 (Light to Somewhat Hard) on Borg's RPE scale. This is prudent as it not only makes a limited programme more interesting but moving from weight-bearing to non-weight-bearing activities also gives the lower back musculature an interval of rest. The upright cycle was chosen to focus on posture. However, it is just as acceptable in the initial stages to use a recumbent cycle (seat and backrest) to support the torso if required, especially if it is found to be more comfortable.

The client grew in confidence as his fear of re-injury decreased. After negotiation, other gym activities such as the cross-trainer, stepping machine and the rowing ergometer were added to the programme. Progressions were attempted as all three factors of physical function, confidence and symptoms permitted. As more pieces of equipment were added, the duration on each was manipulated to attain at least 20 minutes of aerobic exercise (ACSM 1998), with the total session time being 45 minutes. Eventually, once such an achievement was obvious, the client was happy to exercise at the recommended physiological intensities (>50% $\dot{V}O_2$max; 65% HRmax and RPE 13–14; McArdle et al 2006) Attendance at the gym decreased in frequency from 5 days to 3 days and structured home-based walking was increased to 2 days per week. This

Case study: exercise programme development—Cont'd

reflected a more realistic exercise plan that aimed to fit into the individual's daily pattern of living.

As mentioned in Box 5.8, this individual's previous history exercise was dominated by strength training. As this was an activity that the patient enjoyed, from a psychological perspective it was important to reintroduce it. In this case it occurred once aerobic fitness had improved and good functional and stable mobility had been achieved (20 weeks post injury). A variety of exercise modes were employed using fixed resistance weights machines. Table 5.6 highlights the stages of the gym exercise programme for the case client (Box 5.8).

Table 5.6 Exercise programme and progressions for case study in Box 5.8

	Exercise	Number of bouts[a]	Time per bout (min)[a]	Total time (min)	Machine setting	METs
Progression 1	Treadmill	2–4	5	10–20	4 kph	3.6
Progression 2	Treadmill	4	5	20	4 kph	3.6
	Upright cycle	2	5	10	80 watts	4.6
Progression 3	Treadmill	4	5	20	4–4.5 kph	3.6–3.8
	Upright cycle	2	5	10	80–90 watts	4.6–5.2
	Rowing ergometer	1	3	3	3:00 min/ 500 m	4.3
	Cross-trainer	1	3	3	4–4.5 METs	4–4.5
	Stepping machine	1	3	3	4 METs	4
Progression 4	Treadmill	4	5	20	4.5–5 kph	3.8–4.3
	Upright cycle	2	5	10	90–100 watts	5.2–5.7
	Rowing ergometer	2	3	6	3:00 min/ 500 m	4.3
	Cross-trainer	1	3	3	4–4.5 METs	4–4.5
	Stepping machine	1	3	3	4 METs	4
Progression 5	Treadmill	3	5	15	5 kph	4.3
	Upright cycle	2	5	10	100 watts	5.7
	Rowing ergometer	3	3	9	3:00 min/ 500 m	4.3
	Cross-trainer	1	4	4	4–4.5 METs	4–4.5
	Stepping machine	1	4	4	4 METs	4
Progression 6	Treadmill	3	5	15	5–5.5 kph	4.3–4.6
	Upright cycle	2	5	10	100 watts	5.7
	Rower ergometer	3	3	9	2:55 min/ 500 m	5
	Cross-trainer	1	5	5	4–4.5 METs	4–4.5
	Stepping machine	1	5	5	4 METs	4
Progression 7	Treadmill	3	5	15	5.5 kph	4.6
	Upright cycle	2	5	10	100–110 watts	5.7–6.3

(Continued)

Table 5.6 Exercise programme and progressions for case study in Box 5.8—Cont'd

	Exercise	Number of bouts[a]	Time per bout (min)[a]	Total time (min)	Machine setting	METs
	Rowing ergometer	3	3	9	2:55 min/ 500 m	5
	Cross-trainer	1	5	5	4–4.5 METs	4.5–5
	Stepping machine	1	5	5	4–5 METs	4–5
	Fixed resistance	4	1.5 (15 reps)	6	–	–
Progression 8	Treadmill	3	5	15	5.5–6 kph	4.6–5.1
	Upright cycle	2	5	10	100–110 watts	5.7–6.3
	Rowing ergometer	3	3	9	2:55–2:50 min/ 500 m	5.3
	Cross-trainer	1	5	5	4.5–5.0 METs	4.5–5
	Stepping machine	1	5	5	4–5 METs	4–5
	Fixed machine; strength training	8	(15 reps)	12	–	–
Progression 9	Progress towards settings which elicit 70% max heart rate reserve and/or RPE 13 to 14. Introduce free weights exercises as confidence increased					

[a]Each bout of exercise is interspersed with lower-intensity, smaller muscle group muscular endurance or mobility exercises.

Case study: special considerations for exercise programme development

1. Treadmill   Walking on the treadmill was conducted without an incline as it was felt that this might increase trunk flexion and related tension/compression on the spinal area that was traumatized. This is most likely due to a change in the centre of gravity experienced when walking uphill that effectively throws the bodyweight forwards. This puts extra stress on the stabilizing muscles of the lower back as well as increasing the pressure between the intervertebral discs (Rao et al 2002). Exercise duration was progressed up to 20 minutes before an increase in walking speed (exercise intensity) with the aim of ensuring a stable gait and correct neuromuscular coordination. This individual exhibited signs of neurological dysfunction in the lower limbs (foot drop, loss of control of foot inversion/eversion) due to the prolapse having pressed on the L4/5 nerve roots of the lumbar spine. An increase in speed might have placed stress on a bodily system ill equipped to cope at this time.

Case study: special considerations for exercise programme development— Cont'd

2. Rowing ergometer   With reference to the rowing ergometer, this needs to be approached with caution when a lower back pathology is concerned. Not only is the lower back required in the maintenance of lumbar posture, but the muscles also have to stabilize the thoracic spine from which the shoulder and arm muscle gain their foundation for movement (Secher 1993). With an increase in arm work, there will be a proportional increase in work of the back; typically much more than in aerobic exercise involving only the legs. Therefore, the machine resistance should be minimal and a slow controlled speed advised to begin with, ensuring correct technique. Symptoms and quality of movement should be continually assessed both during and days after the introduction of this mode of activity. Prior to injury, this individual performed 2000 m in 8 minutes (an average 500 m split time of 2 minutes). An initial exercise duration for the rehabilitation programme was set at 3 minutes, where the patient achieved 500 m. This time point was the longest period sustainable before an unacceptable level of back fatigue set in as subjectively evaluated by the patient. Borg's CR-10 scale was used as a means of specifically assessing the degree of low back fatigue with a rating of 5 (strong or heavy levels of fatigue) used as the threshold for termination. Following this exercise session and 2 days later, the physiotherapist assessed back mobility, strength and function to see if this exercise brought on any noticeable negative changes.

As shown in Table 5.6, one 3-minute bout of rowing ergometry per session was originally advised during each of the three weekly exercise visits. The duration and intensity of rowing was increased over the next 12-week period as the client's physical function, confidence and symptoms permitted.

3. Fixed resistance machines   The aim of these machines is to remove much of the balance aspect of free-weight training, allowing the user to concentrate more on technique. The client was required to implement the core stability processes during resistance training as recommended in previous sections of this chapter (Kasai 2006, Richardson et al 1999). At this early stage and once appropriate core stability skills were achieved, the client proceeded to perform one set of 15 repetitions. This number of repetitions is the upper limit for loads to elicit a strength benefit (ACSM 1998). Any greater number of repetitions will require a lowered level of resistance, which is more related to developing muscular endurance. Some examples of how the exercises were adapted include:

- Leg press (recumbent 'squat') being performed unilaterally, as compared to normal bilateral leg usage. This was used to both challenge the client using lower loads and to introduce proximal trunk stabilizing to the routine.
- Bench press was performed in a semi-recumbent position and with the feet placed on a small box at a height of 25 cm in order to limit hyperextension of the back and allow for better posture control.
- Exercises that required the biomechanical moment arm to move substantially from the centre of gravity were avoided, i.e. leg extension, leg curl and biceps curl.

As previously recommended, localized muscular fatigue was monitored using Borg's CR-10 scale with the muscular exercise being limited to a rating of 5.

Chronic low back pain – aerobic exercise

Therapeutic exercise is as effective as standard physiotherapy techniques such as manipulation and electrotherapy in the management of chronic low back pain (Goldby et al 2006, Hayden et al 2005b, Smidt et al 2005). However, there is little evidence to support aerobic exercise as a 'stand-alone' therapy for chronic low back pain (Hayden et al 2005a). Simmonds & Dreisinger (2003) have demonstrated, and we have found in our own clinical experience, that the inclusion of aerobic exercise in a patient's programme not only maintains but can eventually enhance the ability to perform activities in daily life.

Example of applied clinical practice

Aerobic exercise can also be included as part of the 'active rest periods' during an exercise session that involves strength and spinal stabilization exercises. This may be very useful during more intense exercise sessions. Aerobic exercise helps to vary the movement patterns during a given exercise session, which may prevent or at least delay the onset of postural and/or spinal muscle fatigue. The theory of using active rest periods in an interval style approach is aimed at enabling the patient to exercise for longer in total as compared to continuous exercise. The drawback of this approach is that the total exercise session has to be longer compared to a continuous session. These active rest periods may well include periods of gentle seated activity of the non-affected limbs, while such therapies as heat or ice are used to soothe painful areas. The exercise session may be carried out at home or within a location that provides supervised structured exercise. The lighter aerobic exercise employed as a means of active rest can also be used on its own as part of more gentle exercise sessions during periods of heightened pain or disease progression.

A moderate to more vigorous aerobic exercise programme may well need to involve a combination of weight-bearing, partial weight-bearing and non-weight-bearing activities to enable the patient to achieve appropriate physiological thresholds (e.g. $>50\%$ $\dot{V}O_2max$ or $>65\%$ HRmax) so as to avoid pain being the limiting factor to exercise intensity. Specific attention needs to be paid to factors such as static positions or movement patterns that exacerbate back pain, or activities that are perceived as potential barriers to commencing and maintaining the exercise programme. Movements and activities will need introducing in a graded fashion in order to improve both working within the physical limitations of the spinal structures while correspondingly at levels where the patient feels confident.

In chronic conditions, as discussed earlier, pain frequently does not relate to further damage or progression of a disorder (Felson 2004). Similar to rheumatoid arthritis, low back pain can have periods of peaks and troughs in symptoms that make performing exercise a challenge. The patient may have to commence an exercise programme with as little as 2 to 4 minutes of ergometer cycling from which graded progressions can be planned. It may be that such short-term aerobic exercises simply provide a means for important psychosocial processes that are necessary in the management of back pain. Once physical function and confidence have improved, a secondary goal focusing on improving cardiovascular fitness, using standard guidelines for developing cardiorespiratory fitness (as noted in the section below on dose response), allows aerobic exercise to be increased and new health and fitness goals set.

Chronic low back pain – spinal stabilization exercise (core stability)

Hayden et al (2005a, 2005b) have shown that individually designed strengthening and spine-stabilizing routines were effective in reducing pain and improving function. There is a growing body of research that supports the concept of spinal stabilization or 'motor control retraining' for the back pain population (Goldby et al 2006, Panjabi 1992, Richardson et al 1999). Dysfunctional neuromuscular control of the deep local muscles of the spine, for example the lumbar multifidus and transversus abdominis, have been consistently identified in low back pain patients (Richardson et al 1999). These findings have resulted in the development of core stability training or 'spinal segmental stabilization exercises'. The aim is to rehabilitate patients using a motor control re-education strategy that will reactivate the muscles by enhancing or recovering motor control and proprioception. The theory is that these muscles can then operate adequately in their role of supporting the spine. The assumption is that a strong, stable spinal core is required for healthy and effective movement of the peripheral joint segments. By implementing these muscle re-education exercises early in the treatment plan, muscle control can be a part of the goal to control pain (Hides et al 1996). The process for attaining such a goal is that the patient first acquires the skill associated with isolating and contracting the deep muscles (gently drawing the lower abdomen inward and away from the waist band); practising the skill; and then integrating the skill into low-level functional activities (e.g. walking, moving from sitting to standing). Such skill can then be gradually progressed to higher-level activities (e.g. jogging, stair climbing, resistance training, and other more vigorous daily activities such as lifting and gardening). Richardson et al (1999) provide a fuller set of guidelines on the above recommendations.

Core stability exercises often employ activities that challenge stability (e.g. use of stability balls). These exercises aim to enhance spinal stability, because they are more likely to enhance correct neural activation following periods of dysfunctional muscular activation (Lehman et al 2005). However, the use of stability balls may not be justified, as trunk muscle rehabilitation research has shown mixed results (Lehman et al 2005). As much if not more evidence supports the use of ground-based exercise (e.g. mat work or a stable exercise bench).

Chronic low back pain and the exercise dose response

It is difficult to standardize dose response and exercise guidelines for individuals with low back pain. The condition itself warrants a truly individualized approach to prescription (Hayden et al 2005b). Each patient needs to be exposed to graded activities from which the responses of pain and symptoms are monitored and intensity and range of movement is graduated. It may be advisable with aerobic exercise that intensity in the range of 40–50% $\dot{V}O_2$max (RPE 11–13 or heart rate of 50–65% maximum) and progressing over time to 50–70% $\dot{V}O_2$max (RPE 14–15 or heart rate 65–80% maximum) is practicable. Barker and colleagues (2003) used RPE to assess the physiological benefits to a chronic low back pain population and found that it was possible to achieve aerobic benefits although for some individuals their pain was a limiting factor. Simmonds & Dreisinger (2003) and Vuori (2001) recommend that exercise programming should aim to attain guidelines for the general healthy and older population (ACSM 1998, 2000) whilst allowing for appropriate condition-related adjustments (e.g. pain and symptoms).

Box 5.8 summarizes aerobic and spinal stabilization exercise for chronic low back pain.

Box 5.8 Summary of aerobic and spinal stabilization exercise for chronic low back pain

- **Goals and specific considerations:** Enhance motor control and muscle strength and endurance. Improve spinal stability and gait. Increase patient confidence and facilitate positive coping strategies. Programme progression. Facilitate return to work and improve functional capacity. Ensure correct posture throughout.
- **Modes:** A combination of weight-, partial- and non-weight-bearing aerobic large muscle group activities implemented as intervals with focused abdominal muscle strength/endurance and postural coordination exercise.
- **Frequency:** Three to five times per week.
- **Duration:** Aerobic activity progressing from as little as 2-minute bouts with seated or active rest up to the required 20 minutes. The aim, however, is to have the patient consider postural control at all times.
- **Intensity:** 40–70% $\dot{V}O_2$max RPE 11–14; 40–70% maximum heart rate reserve.

Box 5.9 Case study (chronic back pain)

- Client was a 74-year-old man, with previously reported incidences of low back pain over a 40-year period.
- Self-reported problems during military career and since retirement. Client accredits damage to army lifestyle.
- Advice sought from physiotherapist, who identified general wear and tear of spinal structure, otherwise non-specific.
- Pain cyclic in nature ranging from no pain to severely limiting activities of everyday life.
- Recent exercise history of regular walking and activities of daily living (e.g. gardening).
- Client's primary goal is to decrease frequency and severity of pain.

Case study: resistance training for chronic low back pain

The initial resistance programme for the case described in Box 5.9 was based on ACSM (1998) recommendations for older people with adaptations to accommodate the chronic low back problem. These recommendations include: one set of 12–15 repetitions performed on 8–12 different muscle groups, two or more times per week. This client did not have any specific limitations (functional and range of movement), although caution was taken similar to that with the acute case study regarding exercise selection and execution. Table 5.7 displays the initial programme, as well as the specific equipment used. This also highlights the need for a range of equipment to bring variety to the programme.

The exercises and progressions outlined in Table 5.7 were chosen not just for their suitability for chronic lower back pain, but also to address issues common in this age group (e.g. protracted physiological adaptation and the likely existence of co-pathologies).

Table 5.7 Chronic back pain resistance programme (for case in Box 5.9) with progressions

Exercise	Equipment	Progression 1	Progression 2
'Lat' pull down	Fixed machine	Increase repetitions to 20	Increase load and decrease repetitions
Ball squat[a]	Bodyweight	Hold a dumbbell in each hand	Move to one-legged squats without dumbbells
Seated alternate punches	Resistance band	Switch to performing with both arms simultaneously	Perform alternate punching in standing
Rear deltoid	Fixed machine	Pause briefly in contracted position	Increase repetitions to 20
Unilateral leg press	Fixed machine	Slow movement to emphasize control	Switch to standard two-legged version
Wall press	Bodyweight	Lean on stability ball instead of wall	Stand on one leg while doing exercise
Seated row	Resistance band	Move to front of seat so torso semi-supported	Perform in standing with one foot in front of the other
Seated unilateral arm raises	Resistance band	Perform with both arms simultaneously	Perform in standing
Partial chair dips	Bodyweight	Increase range of motion	Take one foot off the ground
Seated biceps curls	Resistance band	Perform in standing	Move to next level of resistance band

[a]Ball squat requires placing a large Swedish exercise ball between the client's back and a wall.

PSYCHOLOGICAL CONSIDERATIONS WHEN WORKING WITH INDIVIDUALS WITH MUSCULOSKELETAL INJURY AND PAIN

Although this text focuses on the physiology of exercise, it is paramount to include a small section on the psychology related to muscle and joint problems that involve stiffness, pain and discomfort. Exercise progression needs to be a balance between biophysical function and psychological readiness. If an individual is in pain and has a fear that movement will increase this pain, avoidance of leisure activities including exercise is likely (Picavet et al 2002).

In the acute case study presented (Box 5.8), the client faced a dilemma in that a speedy return to strength training using free weights was a prominent goal and yet fear of re-injury was constantly present. A graded exposure approach was used where the client was gradually put in situations that challenged the perception of re-injury. Using this technique the client rated movements based on expected levels of pain/re-injury. Together with the practitioner, small goals are agreed, tackling lower rated items first. Vlaeyen et al (2001) found this technique to be even more helpful than graded physical activity in those with chronic back pain. Figure 5.2 shows the generic concept.

In the first case study (acute back pain), fear originated from a lack of confidence in the ability of the lower back to cope with loads placed upon it, which previously had been taken for granted. This individual did not perceive cardiovascular exercises or core stability work to be threatening so these were implemented first. The

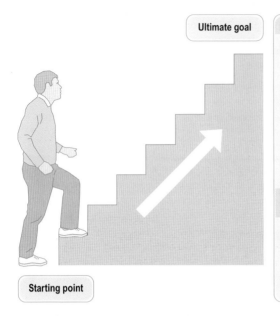

Ultimate goal	Every step is planned by considering:
	• Which activities are chosen
	• The intensity of the activity
	• The duration of each session
	• Rest intervals within each session
	• The frequency of the sessions
	• The expected after-effects (pain, stiffness etc.) of the session in order to provide the patient with advance notice
	• The expected time (days, weeks) at which all the above will be progressed, so as to plan the next step

Each step should graduate the patient towards

a. Initially achieving the exercise recommendations for the individuals with musculoskeletal disorders (Vuori 2001), then towards

b. The exercise recommendations for healthy adults (ACSM 1998)

Starting point

Figure 5.2 The graded exposure staircase.

introduction of fixed weight machines, using higher repetitions, lower loads and adapted technique instigated a return to strength training without the individual having to perform this activity outside his psychological comfort zone. Crombez et al (2002) found that the positive effects of exposure to one movement may not have a carry-over effect to others, indicating that a variety of exercises should be included. This generic template summarized in Figure 5.2 can also be applied to the client with chronic lower back pain or arthritis if the steps are made specific.

CONCLUSION

A well-controlled, specifically tailored exercise programme should aim to provide functional improvement and symptomatic relief as well as an improved sense of well-being. Ultimately, improvement in one's quality of life, through increased physical activity, may be achieved despite little or no alteration in pain: this is a more honest likelihood in the case of osteoarthritis, rheumatoid arthritis and chronic low back pain (Klaber-Moffett et al 1999). It is essential to the prescribing of exercise to acknowledge the suffering and anguish associated with these three conditions as essential ingredients of *being* in pain as well as the sensory experience of pain but also the associated stiffness, weakness and impact on overall functionality (Box 5.10).

FUTURE RESEARCH

Future research is required in assessing the longer-term effects of regular aerobic exercise versus proprioception and range of movement activities. With regard to the modes of exercise, studies showing the integration of various modes (aerobic, strength, flexibility and proprioception) versus the use of any of these modes

> **Box 5.10   Summary of points for the management of multifactorial conditions that involve osteoarthritis, rheumatoid arthritis and low back pain**
>
> - Pain (acute or chronic) is a personal experience that can be influenced by coinciding (acute) physical events or continuing (chronic) perceived significant social and psychological events in one's life. Pain, especially chronic pain, is not necessarily well correlated with the amount of tissue damage present or pathophysiology.
> - An exercise programme should be graded and flexible so that it can be adapted to deal with recurring peaks and troughs in function, pain, stiffness, inflammation and any other related symptoms. Patient progress should be evaluated on a 'stock market analysis style approach' by attempting to determine the general benefit (setback) trend in and amongst various peaks and troughs.

singularly are required. There is still much study required to establish more specific guidelines on the dose (frequency, intensity, duration and mode) of exercise required to achieve the best outcomes for reducing disease progression and the frequency of clinical signs and/or symptoms associated with arthritis and back pain.

KEY POINTS

- Each client will have specific and individualized needs and preferences, which will affect potential adherence to an exercise plan.
- Close attention has to be paid to monitoring exercise intensity and its relation to pain/discomfort levels, particularly in the early stages of rehabilitation/exercise. This promotes confidence on a number of levels.
- Implement the use of RPE and pain scales; typically Borg's 6–20 scale for aerobic exercise and Borg's CR-10 scale for resistance/strength training and pain, in order to differentiate between aspects of exertion (muscle fatigue and breathlessness) and muscle/joint pain that limit exercise ability.
- Very-low-impact, low-intensity, shorter duration activities should be used during the initial stages of a programme. For example, one may need to start with just 2–5 minutes of aerobic exercise and alternate between full-weight-, partial- and non-weight-bearing activities (e.g. treadmill walking, seat-supported stepping and stationary cycling)
- Assess the client's fitness and symptoms regularly, and progress with caution every 2 to 6 weeks. Extend the exercise duration, then frequency and finally intensity with aerobic endurance activities.
- Unless advised otherwise by a registered physiotherapist, have the client work within pain-free ranges of movement.
- In any given session, paying attention to the balance between rest and activity is key. If possible, use low-intensity active-rest periods between more vigorous therapy activities and ensure rest days are taken between exercise therapy days.
- Performing exercises with correct skill acquisition and posture is essential to reduce negative biomechanical, intra-articular and musculoskeletal stresses.
- Aerobic activities, upper and lower body resistance training, proprioception and flexibility exercise can be utilized in an interval and active-rest training format.
- Clients should be advised that they may have post-exercise muscle and joint stiffness, particularly during the early stages of a conditioning programme. Confirm that this would be normal in any individual who has had a sustained period of

inactivity, whether injured or not. However, specific consideration should be given to any changes in medication usage and perceptions of pain. Most clients will learn to know 'usual' pain from 'bad' pain, where alterations in exercise intensity and/or exercise mode are needed to accommodate the latter.

- Caution is advised during an inflammatory stage of rheumatoid arthritis. Any increases in swelling, pain and disability will occur with associated psychological and emotional consequences. Increases in rheumatoid arthritis symptoms and joint disease should merit making alterations in the prescription of exercise. Additional advice and support during a 'flare-up' of rheumatoid arthritis is vital to promote the development of positive management strategies.

References

Adams M A, Hutton W C 1983 The effects of fatigue on the lumbar intervertebral disc. Journal of Bone and Joint Surgery 65-B(2):199–203

Adams M A, Hutton W C 1985 Gradual disc prolapse. Spine 10(6):524–531

American College of Sports Medicine 1998 Position stand on exercise and physical activity for older adults. Medicine and Science in Sports and Exercise 30(6):992–1008

American College of Sports Medicine 2000 ACSM's guidelines for exercise testing and prescription (Franklin B A, Whaley M H, Howley E T, eds) 6th edn. Lippincott Williams & Wilkins, Philadelphia

Arthritis Care 2002 1 in 5: The prevalence and impact of arthritis in the UK. Online. Available: www.arthritiscare.org.uk

Arthritis Care 2006 Fact Sheet: The impact of arthritis (statistics). Revised. Online. Available: www.arthritiscare.org.uk

Barker K L, Dawes H, Hansford P et al 2003 Perceived and measured levels of exertion of patients with chronic low back pain in a hydrotherapy pool. Archives of Physical Medicine and Rehabilitation 84:1319–1323

Bearne L M, Scott D L, Hurly M V 2002 Exercise can reverse quadriceps sensorimotor dysfunction that is associated with rheumatoid arthritis without exacerbating disease activity. Rheumatology 41(2):157–166

Bennell K, Hinman R 2005 Exercise as a treatment for osteoarthritis. Current Opinion in Rheumatology 17(5):634–640

Biddle S J H, Mutrie N 2001 Psychology of physical activity: determinants, well-being and interventions. Routledge, London

Bilberg A, Ahlmen M, Mannerkorpi K 2005 Moderate intensity exercise in a temperate pool for patients with rheumatoid arthritis: a randomised controlled study. Cochrane Central Register of Controlled Trials. Issue 3

Birrell F N 2004 Patterns of joint pain: lessons from epidemiology. Rheumatology 43:408–409

Birrell F N, Lunt M, Macfarlane G et al 2005 Association between pain in the hip region and radiographic changes of osteoarthritis; results from a population-based study. Rheumatology 44(3):337–341

Bogduk N 2004 Clinical update: management of chronic low back pain. Medical Journal of Australia 180(2):79–83

Borg G 1998 Borg's perceived exertion and pain scales. Human Kinetics, Champaign, IL

Brighton S W, de la Harpe A L, van Staden D J et al 1988 The prevalence of rheumatoid arthritis in a rural African population. Journal of Rheumatology 15:405–408

Brosseau L, Macleay L, Robinson V A et al 2003 Intensity of exercise for the treatment of osteoarthritis. Cochrane Database of Systematic Reviews

Centers for Disease Control and Prevention (CDC) 1996 Physical activity and health. A report of the Surgeon General. Atlanta, GA

Chard J, Lohmander S, Smith C 2005 Osteoarthritis of the knee. Clinical Evidence 14:1–16

Cholewicki J, Panjabi M M, Khachatryan A 1997 Stabilizing function of trunk flexor-extensor muscles around a neutral spine posture. Spine 22:2207–2212

Crombez G, Eccleston C, Vlaeyen J W et al 2002 Exposure to physical movements in low back pain patients: restricted effects of generalization. Health Psychology 21(6):573–578

D'Ambrose R D 2005 Epidemiology of osteoarthritis. Orthopaedics 28(2 Suppl):s201–s205

Darby A J 1998 Bone and joint pathology In: Tidswell M (ed) Orthopaedic physiotherapy. Mosby, London, pp 3–14

Department of Health 2004 At least five a week: Evidence on the impact of physical activity and its relationship to health. A report from the Chief Medical Officer. Department of Health, London

Deyo R A, Mirza S K, Martin B I 2006 Back pain prevalence and visit rates: estimates from US national surveys. Spine 31(23):2724–2727

Eberhardt K, Fex E 1998 Clinical course and remission rate in patients with early rheumatoid arthritis: relationship to outcome after 5 yrs. British Journal of Rheumatology 37:1324–1329

Evcik D, Sonel B 2002 Effectiveness of a home-based exercise therapy and walking programme on osteoarthritis of the knee. In: Ottawa Panel Members et al 2005 Ottawa panel evidence-based clinical practice guidelines for therapeutic exercises and manual therapy in the management of osteoarthritis. Physical Therapy 85(9):907–971

Feigenbaum M S, Pollock M L 1999 Prescription of resistance training for health and disease. Medicine and Science in Sports and Exercise 31(1):38–45

Feland J B, Myrer J W, Scuthies S S et al 2001 The effect of duration of stretching of the hamstring muscle group for increasing range of motion in people aged 65 years or older. Physical Therapy 81(5):1110–1117

Felson D T 2004 An update on the pathogenesis and epidemiology of osteoarthritis. Radiology Clinics of North America 42(1):1–9

Fifield J, Reisine S, Sheehan T et al 1996 Gender, paid work, and symptoms of emotional distress in rheumatoid arthritis patients. Arthritis and Rheumatism 39(3):427–435

Fisher N M 2002 Osteoarthritis, rheumatoid arthritis and fibromyalgia. In: Myers J N, Herbert W G, Humphrey R (eds) ACSM's resources for clinical exercise physiology: Musculoskeletal, neuromuscular, neoplastic, immunologic and haematologic conditions. Lippincott Williams & Wilkins, Philadelphia

Fitzgerald G K, Axe M J, Snyder-Mackler L 2000 The efficacy of perturbation training in non-operative anterior cruciate ligament rehabilitation programs for physically active individuals. Physical Therapy 80:128–140

Fitzgerald G K, Childs J D, Ridge T M et al 2002 Agility and perturbation training for a physically active individual with knee osteoarthritis. Physical Therapy 82(4):372–382

Fransen M, McConnell S, Bell M 2001 Exercise for arthritis of the hip or knee. The Cochrane Database of Systematic Reviews: Issue 2

Gifford L S 1997 Pain. In: Pitt-Brooke J, Reid H, Lockwood J, Kerr K (eds) Rehabilitation of movement: theoretical bases of clinical practice. Saunders, London, pp 196–232

Gifford L S, Butler D S 1997 The integration of pain sciences into clinical practice. Hand Therapy 10(2):86–95

Goldby L J, Moore A P, Doust J et al 2006 A randomised controlled trial investigating the efficiency of musculoskeletal physiotherapy on chronic low back pain. Spine 31 (10):1083–1093

Griffin T M, Guilak F 2005 The role of mechanical loading in the onset and progression of osteoarthritis. Exercise and Sports Science Reviews 33(4):195–200

Hagen K B, Hilde G, Jamtvedt G et al 2004 Bed rest for acute low-back pain and sciatica. The Cochrane Database of Systematic Reviews

Hakkinen A, Tuulikki S, Kontaniemi A, Hannonen P 2001 A randomised two year study of the effects of dynamic strength training on muscle strength, disease activity, functional capacity, and bone mineral density in early rheumatoid arthritis. Arthritis and Rheumatism 44(3):515–522

Hall H (ed) 1983 Rheumatology, Volume 1. The new medicine: an integrated system of study. MTP Press

Han A, Judd M G, Robinson V A et al 2004 Tai chi for treating rheumatoid arthritis. Cochrane Database of Systematic Reviews. Online. Available: http//www.pubmed. gov 25 Sept 2006

Harvey L, Herbert R, Crosbie J et al 2002 Does stretching induce lasting increases in joint ROM? A systematic review. Physiotherapy Research International 7(1):1–13

Hayden J A, van Tulder M W, Malmivaara A V, Koes B W 2005a Meta-analysis; exercise therapy for non-specific low back pain. Annals of Internal Medicine 142(9):765–775

Hayden J A, van Tulder M W, Malmivaara A, Koes B W 2005b Exercise therapy for treatment of non-specific low back pain. Cochrane Database of Systematic Reviews 2005, Issue 3

Hides J A, Richardson C, Jull G A 1996 Multifidus muscle recovery is not automatic following resolution of acute episode low back pain. In: Richardson C, Jull G, Hodges P et al 1999 Therapeutic exercise for spinal segmental stabilization in low back pain. Churchill Livingstone, Edinburgh

Hortobágyi T, Garry J, Holbert D, Devita P 2004 Aberrations in the control of quadriceps muscle force in patients with knee osteoarthritis. Arthritis and Rheumatism (Arthritis Care and Research) 51(4):562–569

Hurley M V, Scott D L 1998 Improvements in quadriceps sensorimotor function and disability of patients with knee osteoarthritis following a clinically practicable exercise regime. British Journal of Rheumatology 37:1181–1187

Kaaria S, Luukkonen R, Riihimaki H, Kirjonen J, Leino-Arjas P 2006 Persistence of low back pain reporting among a cohort of employees in a metal corporation: A study with 5-, 10-, and 28-year follow-ups. Pain 120(1–2):131–137

Kaplan F S, Nixon J E, Reitz M et al 1985 Age related changes in joint proprioception and sensation of joint position. Acta Orthopaedica Scandinavica 56:72–74

Kasai R 2006 Current trends in exercise management for chronic low back pain: comparison between strengthening exercise and spinal segmental stabilization exercise. Journal of Physical Therapy Science 18:97–105

Kasper D, Branwald E, Fauci A et al (eds) 2004 Harrison's principles of internal medicine, 16th edn. McGraw Hill, Maidenhead

Kidd B 2006 Osteoarthritis and pain. Pain 123(1–2):6–9

Klaber-Moffett J, Torgerson D, Bell-Seyer S et al 1999 Exercise for low back pain: clinical outcomes, costs and preferences. British Medical Journal 319:279–283

Lehman G J, Gordon T, Langley J 2005 Replacing a Swiss ball for an exercise bench causes variable changes in trunk muscle activity during upper limb strength exercises. Dynamic Medicine 3;4:6. Online. Available: http//www.pubmed.gov 25 Sept 2006

Lephart S M, Pincivero D M, Giraldo J L et al 1997 The role of proprioception in the management and rehabilitation of athletic injuries. American Journal of Sports Medicine 25(1):130–137

Lindstrom I, Ohlund C, Eek C et al 1992 The effect of graded activity on patients with subacute low back pain; a randomised prospective clinical study with an operant conditioning behavioural approach. Physical Therapy 72:279–291

Lord S R, Clark R D, Webster I W 1991 Physiological factors associated with falls in an elderly population. Journal of the American Geriatrics Society 39:1194–1200

McArdle W D, Katch F I, Katch V L 2006 Exercise physiology. Lippincott Williams & Wilkins, Philadelphia

MacGregor A J, Riste L K, Hazes J M W, Silman A J 1994 Low prevalence of rheumatoid arthritis in black-Caribbeans compared with whites in inner city Manchester. Annals of the Rheumatic Diseases 53:293–297

Main C J, Spanswick C C 2000 Models of pain. In: Pain management. An interdisciplinary approach. Churchill Livingstone, Edinburgh, pp 3–18

Manchikanti L 2000 Epidemiology of low back pain. Pain Physician 3(2):167–192

Mangion K K, Gloviak A, McCully K et al 1999 The effects of high-intensity and low-intensity cycle ergometry in older adults with knee osteoarthritis. In: Vuori I M 2001 Dose–response of physical activity and low back pain, osteoarthritis, and osteoporosis. Medicine and Science in Sports and Exercise 33(6):s551–s586

Manninen P, Riihimaki H, Heliovaara M et al 2001 Physical exercise and risk of severe knee osteoarthritis requiring arthroplasty. Rheumatology 40:432–437

Masui T, Yukawa Y, Nakamura S et al 2005 Natural history of patients with lumbar disc herniation observed by magnetic imaging for a minimum of 7 years. Journal of Spinal Disorders and Techniques 18(2):121–126

Maetzel A, Li L, Pencharz J et al 2004.The economic burden associated with osteoarthritis, rheumatoid arthritis and hypertension: a comparative study. Annals of the Rheumatic Diseases 63:395–401

Martin R B, Burr D B, Sharkey N A 1998 Skeletal tissue mechanics. Springer, New York

Merskey H, Bogduk N (eds) 1994 Classification of chronic pain. Descriptions of chronic pain syndromes and definitions of pain terms, 2nd edn. IASP Press, Seattle

Messier S P, Ettinger M H, Thompson C D 1997 Effects of long-term aerobic or weight training regimens on gait in an older, osteoarthritic population. In: Ottawa Panel Members et al 2005 Ottawa panel evidence-based clinical practice guidelines for therapeutic exercises and manual therapy in the management of osteoarthritis. Physical Therapy 85(9):907–971

Minor M A 1996 Arthritis and exercise: the times they are a-changin. Arthritis Care and Research 9(2):79 81

Minor M A, Brown J D 1993 Exercise maintenance of persons with arthritis after participation in an exercise experience. Health Education Quarterly 20(1):83–95

Minor M A, Hewett J E 1995 Physical fitness and work capacity in women with rheumatoid arthritis. Arthritis Care and Research 8(3):146–153

Minor M A, Kay D R 2003 Arthritis. In: Durstine J, Moore G (eds) American College of Sports Medicine's exercise management for persons with chronic diseases and disabilities, 2nd edn. Human Kinetics, Champaign, IL, pp 210–216

Minor M A, Lane N E 1996 Recreational exercise in arthritis. Rheumatic Disease Clinics of North America 22(3):563–577

Minor M A, Hewett J E, Webel R R et al 1989 Efficacy of physical conditioning exercise in patients with rheumatoid arthritis and osteoarthritis. Arthritis and Rheumatism 32:1396–1405

Nelson J L, Ostensen M 1997 Pregnancy and rheumatoid arthritis. Rheumatic Disease Clinics of North America 23:195–212

Noreau L, Martineau H, Roy L et al 1995 Effects of a modified dance-based exercise on cardiorespiratory fitness, psychological state and health status of persons with rheumatoid arthritis. In: Ottawa Panel Members et al 2004 Ottawa panel evidence-based clinical practice guidelines for therapeutic exercises in the management of rheumatoid arthritis. Physical Therapy 84(10):934–937

Ottawa Panel Members et al 2004 Ottawa Panel evidence-based clinical practice guidelines for therapeutic exercises in the management of rheumatoid arthritis. Physical Therapy 84(10):934–972

Ottawa Panel Members et al 2005 Ottawa Panel evidence-based clinical practice guidelines for therapeutic exercises and manual therapy in the management of osteoarthritis. Physical Therapy 85(9):907–971

Panjabi M M 1992 The stabilizing system of the spine. Part 1. Function, dysfunction, adaptation, and enhancement. Journal of Spinal Disorders 5:383–389

Papageorgiou A C, Croft P R, Ferry S et al 1995 Estimating the prevalence of low back pain in the general population. Evidence from the South Manchester Back Pain Survey. Spine 20(17):1889–1894

Parfitt G, Rose E A, Burgess W M 2006 The psychological and physiological responses of sedentary individuals to prescribed and preferred intensity exercise. British Journal of Health Psychology 11(Pt 1):39–53

Parroy S 2005 Joint effects. The impact of allied health professionals on orthopaedic and musculoskeletal service change in Scotland. Rheumatology 43:408–409

Perlman S G, Clark A, Connell K J et al 1990 Dance-based aerobic exercise for rheumatoid arthritis. Arthritis Care and Research 3(1):29–35

Petrella R J 2000 Is exercise effective treatment for osteoarthritis of the knee. British Journal of Sports Medicine 34:326–331

Petrella R J, Lattanzio P J, Nelson M G 1997 Effect of age and inactivity on knee joint proprioception. American Journal of Physical Medicine and Rehabilitation 76(3): 235–241

Picavet H S J, Vlaeyen J W S, Schouten J S 2002 Pain catastrophizing and kinesiophobia: predictors of chronic low back pain. American Journal of Epidemiology 156(11):1028–1034

Rao R D, Wang M, Singhal P et al 2002 Intradiscal pressure and kinematic behavior of lumbar spine after bilateral laminotomy and laminectomy. Spine Journal. 2(5):320–326

Rat A C, Boissier M C 2004 Rheumatoid arthritis: direct and indirect costs. Joint Bone Spine 71(6):518–524

Richardson C, Jull G, Hodges P et al 1999 Therapeutic exercise for spinal segmental stabilization in low back pain. Churchill Livingstone, Edinburgh

Rosen M 1994 Back pain. Clinical Standards Advisory Group. Chaired by Professor Michael Rosen. 57. HMSO, London

Royal College of Radiologists 1998 Making the best use of a department of radiology: guidelines for doctors, 4th edn. RCR, London

Secher N H 1993 Physiological and biomechanical aspects of rowing; implications for training. Sports Medicine 15(1):24–42

Silman A J, Hochberg M C 2001 Rheumatoid arthritis. In: Silman A J, Hochberg M C (eds) Epidemiology of the rheumatic diseases. Oxford University Press, Oxford, pp 31–71

Silman A J, Pearson J E 2002 Epidemiology and genetics of rheumatoid arthritis. Arthritis Research 4(Suppl 3):S265–S272

Silman A J, Ollier W, Holligan S et al 1993 Absence of rheumatoid arthritis in a rural Nigerian population. Journal of Rheumatology 20(4):618–622

Simmonds M J, Dreisinger T E 2003 Lower back pain syndrome. In: Durstine J, Moore G (eds) American College of Sports Medicine's exercise management for persons with chronic diseases and disabilities, 2nd edn. Human Kinetics, Champaign, IL, pp 217–221

Sleed M, Eccleston C, Beecham J, Knapp M, Jordan A 2005 The economic impact of chronic pain in adolescence: methological considerations and a preliminary cost-of-illness study. Pain 119:183–190

Smidt N, Henrica C W, Bouter L M et al 2005 For the Exercise Therapy Group. Effectiveness of exercise therapy; a best-evidence summary of systematic reviews. Australian Journal of Physiotherapy 51:71–85

Sternback R A 1974 Pain patients: traits and treatment. Academic Press, New York

Stone C E 1984 The lifetime economic costs of rheumatoid arthritis. Journal of Rheumatology 11:819–827

Swanik C B, Rubash H E, Barrack R L et al 2000 The role of proprioception in patients with DJD and following total knee arthroplasty. In: Lephart S M, Fu F H (eds) Proprioception and neuromuscular control in joint stability. Human Kinetics, Champaign, IL, pp 323–338

Thomas K S, Muir K R, Doherty M et al 2002 Home based exercise programme for knee pain and knee osteoarthritis: randomised controlled trial. British Medical Journal 325:752–756

University of York NHS Centre for Reviews and Dissemination 2000 Effective health care: Acute and chronic low back pain. November, Vol 6, number 5

Van Baar M E, Assendelft W J, Dekker J et al 1999 Effectiveness of exercise therapy in patients with osteoarthritis of the hip or knee. A systematic review of randomised clinical trials. Arthritis and Rheumatism 42:1361–1369

Van den Ende C H M, Hazes J M W, le Cessie S et al 1996 Comparison of high and low intensity training in well controlled rheumatoid arthritis: results of a randomised clinical trial. Annals of Rheumatology and Disability 55:798–805

Van den Ende C H M, Vliet Vlieland T P M, Munneke M et al 1998 Dynamic exercise therapy for treating rheumatoid arthritis. The Cochrane Database of Systematic Reviews 1998, Issue 4

Van den Ende C H M, Breedveld F C, le Cessie S et al 2000 Effect of intensive exercise on patients with active rheumatoid arthritis: a randomised controlled trial. Annals of the Rheumatic Diseases 59:615–621

Vlaeyen J W, Linton S J 2000 Fear-avoidance and its consequences in chronic musculoskeletal pain: a state of the art. Pain 85:317–332

Vlaeyen J W, de Jong J, Geilen M et al 2001 Graded exposure in vivo in the treatment of pain related fear: a replicated single case experimental design in four patients with chronic low back pain. Behaviour Research and Therapy 39(2):151–166

Vuori I M 2001 Dose response of physical activity and low back pain, osteoarthritis, and osteoporosis. Medicine and Science in Sports and Exercise 33(6):s551–s586

Waddell G 1998 Pain and disability. In: The back pain revolution. Churchill Livingstone, London, pp 27–44

Wathen D, Roll F 1994 Training modes and methods. In: Baechle T R (eds) Essentials of strength training and conditioning. Human Kinetics, Champaign, IL, pp 403–415

Westby M D 2001 A health professional's guide to exercise prescription for people with arthritis: a review of aerobic fitness activities. Arthritis Care and Research 45(6):501–511

Woo S L-Y, Buckwalter J (eds) 1987 Injury and repair of the musculoskeletal soft tissue. American Academy of Orthopaedic Surgeons Symposium

Wyatt F B, Milam S, Manske R C et al 2001 The effects of aquatic and traditional exercise programs on persons with knee osteoarthritis. Journal of Strength and Conditioning Research 15(3): 337–340

Further reading

Buckley J P, Eston R 2005 Perceived exertion. In: Winter E M, Mercer T, Bromley P D, Davison R C (eds) Sport and exercise physiology testing guidelines: exercise and clinical testing, Vol 2. BASES Sport and Exercise Science. Routledge, London

Hall H (ed) 1983 Rheumatology, Volume 1. The new medicine: an integrated system of study. MTP Press

Kasper D, Branwald E, Fauci A et al (eds) 2004 Harrison's principles of internal medicine, 16th edn. McGraw Hill, Maidenhead

Martin R B, Burr D B, Sharkey N A 1998 Skeletal tissue mechanics. Springer, New York

Refshauge K, Gass E Musculoskeletal physiotherapy. Clinical science and evidence-based practice. Butterworth-Heinemann, Oxford

Waddell G 1998 The back pain revolution. Churchill Livingstone, London

Woo S L-Y, Buckwalter J (eds) 1987 Injury and repair of the musculoskeletal soft tissue. American Academy of Orthopaedic Surgeons Symposium

Chapter 6

Ageing and older people

Dawn A Skelton and Susann M Dinan-Young

CHAPTER CONTENTS

Learning objectives 162
Introduction 162
Ageing is not a disease 163
Definitions of ageing – when is 'old'? 163
The ageing process 164
Quantitative aspects of ageing 166
The 'greying' of the population 167
Theories of ageing 167
Quality of life 169
Successful ageing 169
Can the ageing process be slowed? 169
Impact of ageing on major physiological systems and performance 170
Cardiovascular and respiratory systems 170
Musculoskeletal system 171
Endocrine system 176
Falls and fall-related injuries 177
Psychological function 178
Impact of chronic disease and sedentary lifestyle on progressive age-related decline 178
The evidence for effects of exercise training and physical activity in older people 180
Effects on the cardiovascular and respiratory systems 180

Effects on the musculoskeletal system 181
Effects on the nervous system 184
Effects on the endocrine system 185
Effects on falls and fall-related injuries 185
Effects on psychological function 186
Evidence-based guidance on the role and types of assessment 188
Screening and assessment principles 189
Assessment of ability to exercise 191
Assessment of physical activity 192
Assessment of functional ability 192
Evidence-based guidance on exercise training for older people 193
Exercise guidelines for older people 193
Adaptations to session structure 202
Motivation and adherence to exercise 204
Key points 207
References 210
Further reading 223

LEARNING OBJECTIVES

After studying this chapter, you should be able to:

1. Gain insight into the demographics of ageing.
2. Understand and distinguish between the current theories of ageing and the predictors of successful ageing.
3. Understand the impact of ageing on the major physiological systems.
4. Gain an insight into the impact of chronic disease and sedentary lifestyle on the progressive age-related physiological decline.
5. Understand the benefits of regular physical activity on age-related physiological changes, on disease, on function and on independence and quality of life in older people.
6. Gain an insight into the relationship between physical activity and cognition.
7. Gain an insight into the psychological and sociocultural aspects of physical activity in later life including the myths, stereotypes and the barriers to participation.
8. Understand the benefits of physical activity on self-efficacy, psychological well-being and quality of life.
9. Gain an insight into the appropriate adaptations when conducting pre-exercise and health screening and physiological, functional and psychological assessments for older people.
10. Gain an insight into the appropriate programming adaptations when prescribing exercise for older people, including goal setting, motivation and communication.
11. Gain an insight into the adaptations that need to be made in teaching, instructing, coaching and leadership skills when delivering physical activity and exercise to older participants.

INTRODUCTION

> *That which is used develops and that which is not used wastes away.*
> Hippocrates (Source of quote, Raric 1973)

With an ever-increasing older population, health and leisure professionals are now commonly dealing with patients who have poor functional mobility and co-morbidities commonly associated with an inactive lifestyle (Dinan 2001). A healthier old age requires less risk of disease, better physical and mental function, richer opportunities for social interaction and a greater sense of control over, and responsibility for, one's own health and well-being. Participation in regular physical activity or exercise contributes to all five of these interrelated determinants of health (WHO 1958). Regular physical activity that includes specific balance, aerobic and strength exercises has been shown to play an important part in enabling older people to remain above critical thresholds by preventing and managing disease, preserving and restoring function, reducing factors conducive to falling (falls risk factors) and maintaining an active, independent and functional later life (Skelton 2001, Taylor et al 2004, WHO 1997, Young 1997, 2001). The recent *National Service Framework for Older People* discusses the use of physical activity in the prevention and management of disease in five of its eight standards of care (Department of Health 2001).

AGEING IS NOT A DISEASE

Ageing is a natural, universal, complex and highly individual process, characterized by progressive declines in the function of most physiological and psychological systems, that leads to increasing frailty, a declining capacity to respond to stress, increasing incidence of disease and eventually death. Within a single individual, each biological organ and system ages at different rates and individual functional status depends not only on age and rates of ageing, but on gender, genetics, lifestyle, health behaviours and socioeconomic influences (Shephard 1997). Some people live longer and have a higher quality of life; they are more successful at ageing than others (Katz et al 1983, Spirduso et al 2005). Understanding something of the demographic trends and the processes and causes of ageing is fundamental to appreciating these differences and to recognizing that older people, far from being a homogeneous group, become increasingly diverse in their medical, psychological and physical status; physiological or 'body age' is as dubious a concept as chronological age (Young 1997). This understanding is also crucial in determining which interventions can delay or slow the ageing process, compress morbidity (physical dependence and poor health) and ensure enhanced quality as well as quantity of life.

Definitions of ageing – when is 'old'?

A consensus definition of ageing is 'a process or group of processes occurring in living organisms that begins with birth and, with the passage of time, leads to a loss of adaptability, functional impairment and eventually death' (Spirduso et al 2005). Definitions of 'ageing', 'old' and 'the older person' differ among nations and socioeconomic classes (Spirduso et al 2005). In many countries, demographers, insurers and employers have set the threshold of old age at 65 years, in others 55 years, yet, in contrast, geriatricians see their specialty as commencing at 75 years (Gill 2002). An increasingly popular way to describe older adults is as sexagenarians (60–69), septuagenarians (70–79), octogenarians (80–89), nonagenarians (90–99) and centenarians (100 and older) (Spirduso et al 1996). The term 'the elderly' is not helpful as it implies a uniformity that belies the considerable differences that result from a broad age range, inter-individual differences in the rate of ageing and a rising prevalence of chronic disease (Kirkwood & Young 2001). Spirduso's Age Categories descriptors are regarded as sufficiently generalizable and give an indication of the role of physical activity at different ages (Spirduso et al 1996; Table 6.1).

The term 'older' has changed its designation remarkably over the last 100 years; far from being in nursing care, many people over the age of 70 years are still in the

Table 6.1   Age categories and role of physical activity

Description	Age	Decade	Role of physical activity
Middle-aged	45–64	5th–7th	Self-esteem, maintenance (function, job)
Young old	65–74	7th–8th	Maintenance (mobility, job) recreation, social interaction
Old	75–84	8th–9th	Mobility, ADL, eating, bathing, dressing, walking, social interaction, IADL, cooking, washing clothes, gardening, shopping
Old old	85–99	9th–10th	Mobility, ADL, independent living
Oldest old	100+	11th	Mobility, ADL, independent living

Adapted from Spirduso et al (1996).

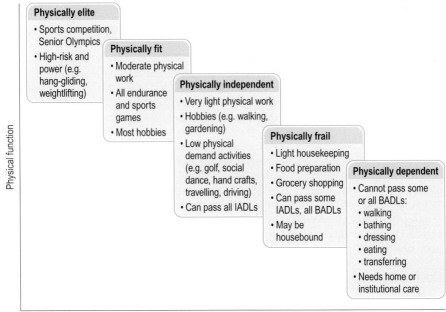

Figure 6.1   Functional ability in older people, as a function of physical activity. IADLs, instrumental activities of daily living; BADLs, basic activities of daily living. Adapted from Spirduso et al (1996) by kind permission of Human Kinetics.

workforce and some 85-year-old women have an aerobic endurance capacity appropriate to the 60–64 age category (Jones & Rose 2005, Malbut et al 2002, Puggaard et al 2000). Spirduso's hierarchy of physical function is highly regarded and effectively describes the diverse range of physical activity in older people, but it must be remembered that some older people defy categorization (Spirduso et al 1996; Fig. 6.1).

The ageing process

Ageing processes (primary ageing) differ from the process or syndrome of ageing (secondary ageing), but the interaction is strong (Kennie et al 2003). Primary ageing represents universal changes that occur with age within a population (e.g. puberty, menopause) and are independent of disease and environmental influence. Secondary ageing refers to clinical symptoms related to deterioration and includes the effects of environment and disease, which can accelerate the process and inherently increase vulnerability to further disease and environmental stress (Kennie et al 2003). Even in healthy individuals, the resulting progressive decline in the function of most physiological systems lowers the threshold of an individual's ability to respond effectively to any challenge and gradually narrows the safety margins between maximal function and critical threshold levels of function that were so generous in youth (Kirkwood & Young 2001, Young 1997). Examples include the decline of bone mineral content (towards a threshold for likelihood of fracture), of glomerular filtration rate (towards a threshold for susceptibility to clinical renal failure), or of physical capacity (e.g. maximal oxygen uptake towards a threshold necessary for everyday mobility; see Figs. 6.2A and 6.2B; Table 6.2) (Kirkwood & Young 2001, Skelton et al 1999).

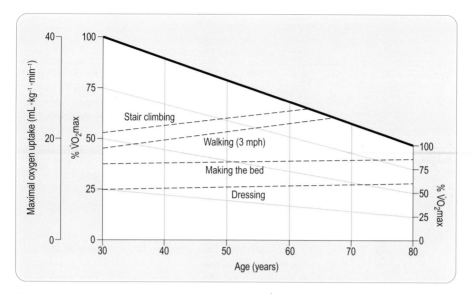

Figure 6.2A   Schematic representation of the loss of $\dot{V}O_2$max with age (between the ages of 30 and 80 years) and the relative percentage of $\dot{V}O_2$max used by an individual to perform everyday tasks. Translated and adapted from Saltin (1980).

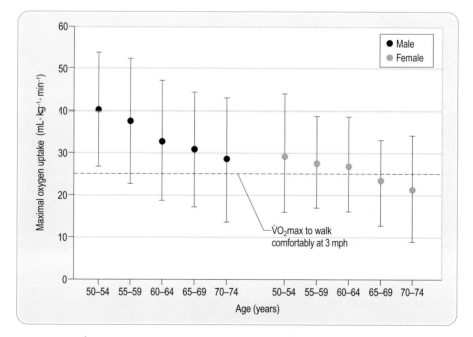

Figure 6.2B $\dot{V}O_2$max in a representative sample of older adults in the UK. The threshold of $\dot{V}O_2$max necessary for comfortable walking at 3 mph is illustrated by the dotted line. Many women over the age of 65 will get breathless walking at slow walking speeds purely because of unfitness. Adapted from Skelton et al (1999).

Table 6.2   Functional abilities of older people in the UK

Functional task	Ability within over 50-year-olds in the UK
Walking	• 9% of men and 38% of women could not be confident of walking comfortably at a 20 minute a mile pace (3 mph) • To illustrate the marked age effect, 35% of men and 80% of women aged over 70 would not be confident of walking comfortably at this pace with their current aerobic capacity
Step climbing or use of public transport	• 7% of men and 28% of women aged over 50 lacked the leg power to be confident to step 30 cm (some bus and train step heights) without having to use their arms • Age-related decline was evident in women, with 47% aged 70–74 having muscle power below the assumed threshold for climbing stairs without using their arms
Washing hair	• 14% of men and 20% of women aged over 50 do not have the flexibility in their shoulders to comfortably be able to wash their own hair
Getting out of a low chair or off the toilet	• 8% of men and 19% of women aged 70–74 were unable to get out of a low chair without using their arms

Adapted from Skelton et al (1999).

The result is that the older person becomes increasingly vulnerable to environmental threats such as extremes of heat and cold, fluctuations of blood sugar and circulatory disturbances associated with physical effort (Morgenthal & Shephard 2005, Skelton et al 1999). These will, inevitably, affect an older person's response to exercise.

Quantitative aspects of ageing

The *rate* of ageing is the change in the function of organs and systems over a unit of time. In normal ageing, these changes follow a linear sequence over the lifespan; however, males age steadily whereas females have periods of accelerated and slowed ageing rates (Ekonomov et al 1989). Disease and sedentary behaviour accelerate the rate of ageing. Restriction of calorie intake (Kinsella 1992, Walford & Crew 1989, Weindruch 1995), genetic manipulation (Shephard 1997) and regular general physical activity and moderate amounts of physical exercise (Taylor et al 2004, Young 2001) are the only three interventions that have been effective in changing the rate of ageing.

The maximum human lifespan potential is 115–120 years, based on Jeanne Calment who died aged 122 in 2000 (Spirduso et al 2005). The average biological human lifespan is limited to about 85 years with only 12% of the population exceeding that age and, unlike life expectancy (the average lifespan from birth), it has remained relatively stable (Fries 1980, Grundy 2003). Life expectancy, for both sexes and for most countries, has almost doubled since the beginning of the 20th century from 40 to approximately 80 years of age (Kinsella 1992, WHO 2002). The low, middle and high projections for life expectancy in 2050 are 74.8, 82.0 and 89.4 years, respectively (US Census Bureau 2001). It is different for different ages, cohorts (eg. 1946–1960 post World War II 'baby boomers'), genders and economic and geographical backgrounds, gender being the most significant. Worldwide, life expectancy for those born from 1946 is 73 for males and 79 for females (WHO 2002). Worldwide, women outlive men by 4–10 years; this gender gap is attributed to genetic, hormonal and social behavioural factors (Grundy 2003).

The 'greying' of the population

The demographic transition and permanent shift to an older age structure ('primary population ageing') is a consequence of long-term downward trends in fertility (Grundy 2003), alongside 25–30-year gains in average life expectancy, due to the reduction in infant and maternal mortality in the first half of the 20th century; advances in medicine, surgery and sanitation; improved availability of comprehensive healthcare and public health programmes; improved working conditions, nutrition and general hygiene; and a higher standard of living (Kinsella 1992, Shephard 1997). The resulting rapid growth in the ageing population is a global phenomenon (Grundy 2003). By 2050, in most European countries, the 85+ group will be 10% of the population, a projected increase of almost 70%, with the 60+ group constituting one in three of the population and outnumbering children under 15 by a ratio of 2.6 to 1 (Grundy 2003, ONS 2000, United Nations 2001). In poorer countries and continents the proportion of people aged 65 and over is small but increasing slowly and is resulting in unprecedented and significant growth in the absolute number of elderly people (Grundy 2003, United Nations 2001).

However, this increased quantity of years has not been accompanied by increased quality of life. The simultaneous deterioration in activity levels and increase in unhealthy lifestyles has resulted in increasing chronic disease, disability and morbidity (Close et al 2005, Kinsella 1992, Taylor et al 2004). This brings a number of major health, social and economic challenges for individuals, families and governments worldwide. In 1998–1999 the UK National Health Service spent approximately 40% and Social Services almost 50% of their budgets on older people (Kennie 2003, Taylor et al 2004). This is set only to increase.

Theories of ageing

There are three main theories of ageing: biological, psychological and sociological (Spirduso et al 2005). An understanding of them enables us to be more accurate in communication about how much of the process of ageing is within our control.

Biological theories

There are three main biological theories of ageing (Spirduso et al 2005):

- *Genetic theories* propose that cell death is in part a genetically controlled, programmed event designed to prevent over-population. They include: the extreme proposal of a 'death gene'; gene dictation of cellular ageing within the cell nucleus; the gradual breakdown of DNA (deoxyribonucleic acid) sequences causing incomplete cell reproduction and leading to chromosomal pathologies (Kirkwood & Young 2001); the accumulative influence of numerous genes on the development of diseases; the biological 'cell clock' or 'computer' theory where 'wear and tear' is programmed into each body cell and is turned on in middle age as in 'puberty' in youth (Hayflick 1997).

- *Damage theories* propose that irreversible, accumulative molecular defects are caused by internally produced reactive chemicals in response to both normal intrinsic body functions and extrinsic invading chemical pollutants (e.g. ultraviolet radiation (Shephard 1997), free radical, viral and traumatic damage, and tobacco smoking) (Spirduso et al 1995). Another proposal is the cross-linkage of proteins, where circulating glucose molecules are thought to randomly attach themselves to proteins in connective tissue, interfere with transport of nutrients and chemical messages and decrease the elasticity of muscles, ligaments and tendons, lung, kidney, vascular and gastrointestinal systems (Morgenthal & Shephard 2005).
- *Gradual imbalance theories* propose that the highly integrated central nervous, endocrine and immune systems begin to age at different rates and cause imbalances and failures in the regulation and integration of cellular and organ function in all biological systems (Finch 1976).

Genetic effects are believed to account for between 30–40% of 'ageing'. Epidemiological studies have shown that poor early growth in utero is associated with poor muscular strength and frailty (Sayer et al 1998), cardiovascular, immune and mental health diseases and poor cognitive function (Shenkin et al 2004, Taylor et al 2004), therefore suggesting that premature ageing is pre-programmed (Rowe & Kahn 1998).

Psychological theories

The psychological theories of ageing explore the psychological development of individuals, the degree of control and the psychological trials associated with successful ageing. There are three prominent psychosocial theories (Spirduso et al 2005):

- *Maslow's 'hierarchy of needs' theory* – the attainment of wisdom through a sense of completeness, realizing one's potential, together with assisting others (e.g. volunteering), is widely believed to be a predictor of successful ageing (Rowe & Kahn 1998).
- *Erickson's eight stages of psychosocial development of personality* are believed to enable the forging of close relationships and a productive family and/or work life and the ability to look back with pride and satisfaction on one's life.
- *Baltes and Baltes' 'optimization selective compensation' theory* promotes training in specific behavioural strategies to improve functional competence such as the ability of older adults to adapt to physical, mental and social losses in later life.

The psychological factors identified as determinants of how successfully we age include intelligence, cognitive capacity, self-efficacy, self-esteem, personal control, coping style and resilience (Spirduso et al 2005). Bandura positions self-efficacy as crucial for successful ageing as it impacts on thought patterns, emotional reactions, lifestyle choices and behaviours (Bandura 1997). Improving functional competence by developing and agreeing personally tailored, realistic, attainable goals, communicating respect and supporting new skills are regarded as crucial competencies when aiming to build self-esteem and self-efficacy in older adults (Jones & Rose 2005).

Sociological theories

There are two main sociological theories of ageing (Spirduso et al 2005):

- *The activity theory* promotes staying engaged in mental and physical activities of daily living throughout the lifespan (Atchley 1972, Fisher 1995).

- *The continuity theory* – people who carry positive health habits, preferences, lifestyles and relationships from mid to later life age most successfully (WHO 1997) and, conversely, inadequate environments are associated with an increase in mortality and morbidity and a decrease in overall health and well-being (Seeman et al 2002). In addition, positive cumulative social experiences and emotional supports are also associated with lower biological risk for morbidity and mortality (Seeman et al 2002).

Quality of life

Quality of life is a psychological construct that is most commonly defined as an individual's conscious judgement of satisfaction with his or her life and is the term used to describe a constellation of characteristics related to physical and psychological health (Spirduso et al 2005, Yardley et al 2003).

Extending years is only of value if quality of life can be maintained. Without improvement in health and health behaviours, we are increasing the potential for suffering one or more of the major chronic diseases that eventually lead to a morbid condition in which the individual is so physically and mentally disabled that he or she becomes immobile and dependent on the care of others. The challenge must be not just to delay mortality but to compress morbidity at the end of the lifespan (Spirduso et al 2005).

Many older individuals have multiple chronic pathologies and polypharmacy regimens. More than 75% of men and women over the age of 70 have one or more chronic medical conditions but chronic disease is predicted to rise by 50% by 2040 in the 65+ age group (Gill 2002). Only 16% have no chronic conditions (Gill 2002). This predisposes older individuals to very poor quality of life and may contribute to the significantly higher rate of suicide amongst these cohorts (65+ age group = 13% of population but 20% of all suicide deaths) (Spirduso et al 2005). The period of time in which individuals live in a state of morbidity can be compressed by adopting a healthy lifestyle earlier in the lifespan to maintain health and function and delay the onset of debilitating disease for as long as possible (Grundy 2003, Katz et al 1983).

Successful ageing

Active life expectancy, or the number of years an individual may expect to maintain the ability to perform the basic activities of daily living (ADLs) without significant disease or disability (Fries & Crapo 1981), is accepted as a key marker of physical, emotional and functional well-being and, therefore, of quality of life as we age (Katz et al 1983). The predictors of successful ageing include physical and mental health, functional and social competence, productivity, personal control and life satisfaction, and depend on the interplay of genetics, personal and social environment, lifestyle behaviours, attitudes, adaptability, social supports and certain personality characteristics (Rowe & Kahn 1998). Interestingly, there is a correlation between sleep quality, survival and successful ageing (Tafaro et al 2007). It is well known that older people who exercise regularly have better sleep patterns (Spirduso et al 2005). Successful ageing is in effect the difference between active living and just being alive (Spirduso et al 1996).

Can the ageing process be slowed?

Factors that influence the human survival curve are medical progress, reductions in levels of environmental pollutants, rates of smoking, drinking, drug abuse, rate of violent crime and increases in the number of people willing to make positive lifestyle changes (Grundy 2003). Increased longevity is associated with regular physical activity, good quality of life, independence, cognitive function and happiness (Spirduso et al 2005). Improving nutrition, decreasing total amount of food consumed and maintaining adequate general activity and moderate amounts of physical exercise have been identified as key to decreasing secondary ageing and increasing life expectancy (Spirduso et al 2005, Young 2001).

IMPACT OF AGEING ON MAJOR PHYSIOLOGICAL SYSTEMS AND PERFORMANCE

Most people, even without the effects of disease or sedentary behaviour, will live long enough to cross a functionally important threshold of fitness that will make an everyday task difficult (Saltin 1980, Young 1986). The effects of sedentary behaviour and disease will accelerate when they cross this functional threshold. Cardiorespiratory, musculoskeletal, endocrine and nervous systems play an important role in the maintenance of functional activities. Bodyweight will also impact on the crossing of such a threshold. Ageing is associated with an increase in percentage of body fat (Jackson et al 1995). In the absence of other changes, the accumulation of 15 kg of body fat in a man with an initial body mass of 70 kg reduces oxygen transport by some 18%, close to a half of the observed age-related loss (Shephard 1994).

For most body systems, the impact of ageing on everyday functional activities becomes noticeable from about the age of 30–40 years (Spirduso et al 2005).

Cardiovascular and respiratory systems

The practical consequences of ageing on the cardiovascular system are a progressive change in the *morphology* and *function* of the cardiovascular system and an increase in the number of age-related cardiovascular disorders (ACSM 1998, Shephard 1994).

The main *morphological* cardiovascular changes with ageing happen in the structure of cardiac tissue and chambers, in the conduction system, and in the coronary and elastic arteries (Shephard 1994). There is a reduction in mitochondrial volume and oxidative enzyme activity of cardiac muscle cells (Lakatta 1993). The reduced ability of the heart to supply the working muscles with sufficient oxygen (because of reduced maximal cardiac output and maximal stroke volume, a decrease in sympathetic sensitivity or outflow and some loss of intrinsic contractility) is a normal feature of ageing (ACSM 1998, Lakatta 1993). The heart becomes slightly hypertrophic and hyporesponsive to sympathetic (but not parasympathetic) stimuli, so that the exercise-induced increases in heart rate and myocardial contractility are blunted in older hearts (ACSM 2000, Hollenberg et al 2006). The aorta and major elastic arteries become elongated and stiffer, with increased pulse wave velocity, evidence of endothelial dysfunction, and biochemical patterns resembling early atherosclerosis (Ferrari et al 2003). Reflexes arising from cardiopulmonary vagal afferents are also blunted in aged individuals (Ferrari et al 2003). Blood pressures are generally higher in older individuals, especially during exercise (Stratton et al 1994).

But cardiac *function*, in healthy older people, is generally adequate to meet the body's needs, at least for submaximal activities (Shephard 1994). However, at the same relative work intensity, heart rate and, to a lesser extent, stroke volume is reduced, effectively producing a decreased cardiac output (Fleg et al 1995). Cardiac output is the product of heart rate and stroke volume. All three are reduced in older people, although it is difficult to isolate whether this is due to inherent processes of ageing, a decrease in habitual physical activity or cumulative pathological change (Brach et al 2004, Jackson et al 1995, Sesso et al 2000).

In terms of lung function, the maximum size of the lungs (total lung capacity) does not change with age, but functional residual capacity and residual volume both increase so that inspiratory capacity and vital capacity both decline with increasing age (Pride 2005). There is also a loss of elasticity of the tissues from greater cross-linkage between collagen molecules, giving rise to stiffness in the joints and changes in elasticity of lung alveoli (e.g. reduced vital capacity). There is a decline in static recoil pressure and also a tendency for the airways to close at small lung volumes (Chaunchaiyakul et al 2004, Pride 2005). The decline with increasing age in forced expiratory volume in one second (FEV_1), FEV_1/VC and in maximum flows at different lung volumes is of wider practical importance (Hollenberg et al 2006, Pride 2005). These changes are, in part, simply due to the smaller vital capacity, but this is not the whole explanation because FEV_1/VC also declines with age. Although this change is often attributed to 'occult' disease of the small airways, (undetected by resistance measurements) all the changes in maximum expiratory flow with increasing age in healthy subjects can be explained by a direct effect of the loss of static recoil pressure of the lungs due to decreased connective tissue elasticity within the lungs. This is without any effects of intrinsic narrowing of airways (Chaunchaiyakul et al 2004, Pride 2005). Recently, it has been found that expiratory flow limitation during resting tidal breathing is common in old age and this may further reduce the available ventilatory reserve during exercise (Pride 2005).

Taking the most readily accessible index of overall cardiorespiratory function (the maximal oxygen intake), values decline from young adult values of 42–50 mL · kg^{-1} · min^{-1} in males and 35–40 mL · kg^{-1} · min^{-1} in women to 25–30 mL · kg^{-1}· min^{-1} in both sexes at the age of 65 years (Shephard 1994). Additional losses are incurred during the 65 years, resulting in tasks that were previously untaxing taking a greater percentage of maximum reserve (Fig. 6.2A) (Paterson et al 1999, Saltin 1980, Young 1986). An elderly man would require greater physical effort than a younger woman to carry out an identical exercise using an absolute scale (Bell et al 1995, Fleg et al 1995, Paterson et al 1999, Stratton et al 1994) (Fig. 6.2A). This narrowing of safety margins, between normal function and the threshold values for functionally important activities, means that even a minor illness could render an elderly person unable to perform such tasks without assistance (Fig. 6.2A). The Allied Dunbar National Fitness Survey (ADNFS) suggested a threshold level of aerobic capacity to walk comfortably at a slow walking speed (3 mph = 4.8 km · h^{-1} = 1.3 m · s^{-1}) (Skelton et al 1999). The report suggested that 'comfortable' walking requires that the oxygen cost is less than 50% of maximal oxygen consumption. Nearly half of women and a significant proportion of men aged over 55 years do not have the aerobic capacity to walk comfortably at 3 mph (Fig. 6.2B). As people with overt disease were not included in the physical fitness tests, it paints a bleak picture of the nation's fitness (Skelton et al 1999). Indeed, much of the breathlessness associated with ill health in old age may well be due to lack of fitness.

Musculoskeletal system

Muscle

Sarcopenia, the loss of muscle mass associated with ageing, is one of the main causes of muscle weakness and reduced locomotor ability in old age (Bosco & Komi 1980, Young 1997). Although sarcopenia is mainly driven by neuropathic processes, other factors contribute to the decline, including nutritional, hormonal and immunological factors, as well as a reduction in physical activity (Young 1997, 2001). Apart from muscle loss, there is also specific weakness of the remaining muscle of around 20%, shown in comparisons of maximum force with muscle cross-sectional area in the adductor pollicis, particularly around the time of menopause (Phillips et al 1992). Much of the age-associated muscle atrophy and declining strength may be explained by motor unit remodelling, which appears to occur by selective denervation of muscle fibres with reinnervation by axonal sprouting from an adjacent innervated unit (Brooks & Faulkner 1994). Indirect estimates indicate a decrease in the total number of motor units and an increase in the size of the remaining motor units in elderly human muscles (Campbell et al 1973). The process of age-related denervation atrophy in old animals may be aggravated by an increased susceptibility of muscles to contraction-induced injury and by the impaired capacity for regeneration (Brooks & Faulkner 1994).

Sarcopenia alone, however, does not fully account for the observed muscle weakness, as the loss of force is greater than that accounted for by the decrease in muscle size. In addition, a reduction in the force per unit area, both at single fibre and at whole muscle level, is observed. Narici recently suggested that, at whole muscle level, this reduction in intrinsic force is the result of the combined effect of changes in (1) muscle architecture, (2) tendon mechanical properties, (3) neural drive (reduced agonist and increased antagonist muscle activity) and (4) single fibre-specific tension (Narici & Maganaris 2006). Whereas several studies support the role of the last two factors in the loss of intrinsic muscle force with ageing, alterations in muscle architecture and in tendon mechanical properties have also been shown to contribute to the above phenomenon. Indeed, sarcopenia of the human plantarflexors, represented by a 25% reduction in muscle volume, was found to be associated with a 10% reduction in fibre fascicle length and 13% reduction in pennation angle. These architectural alterations were accompanied by a 10% decrease in tendon stiffness, attributable to alterations in tendon material properties (Narici & Maganaris 2006). Most of these changes may be reversed by 14 weeks of resistive training but training has no effect on the estimated relative length–tension properties of the muscle, indicating that the effects of greater tendon stiffness and increased fascicle length cancel each other out. It seems that natural strategies may be in place to ensure that in old age the relative operating range of muscle remains unaltered by changes in physical activity (Narici & Maganaris 2006).

Muscle weakness (loss of strength and power) is one of the underlying mechanisms of poor function and correlates with several measures of functional status (Skelton et al 1994, Skelton 2001, Young 1997, 2001). The loss of quadriceps strength with age means that many older adults have strength close to the threshold level necessary to raise themselves out of a low chair without having to use their arms for help (Skelton et al 1994, 1999) (Table 6.2). Young, taking data from various sources and assuming a chair rise of less than 3 seconds, suggested that the healthy 80-year-old woman is at, or near to, the threshold value of quadriceps strength for rising from a low, armless chair (or lavatory) without having to use her arms (Young 1986) (Table 6.2). The ability to ascend and descend stairs, stand up from a chair, use a bath instead of a shower or use public transport can be significantly compromised (Brill et al 2000, Hyatt et al 1990, Skelton et al 1994). Low muscle mass is also associated with poor immune function and impaired temperature control (ACSM 1998).

After age 30 there is a progressive decline in the strength and power of skeletal muscle, which accelerates after the fifth decade and declines by 10–15% per decade after that (Skelton et al 1994). Critically, the reduction in strength with age is most notable in the weight-bearing lower limb muscles, and muscle power output (the ability to produce force quickly) declines more rapidly than strength (Skelton et al 1994). While cross-sectional data suggest that healthy women in their 70s retain

40–50% of the handgrip strength found in young adults (MacLennan et al 1980). They may retain as little as 26% of power, assessed by squat jumps (Bosco & Komi 1980). The decline in power is steeper than force because it is magnified by the loss of velocity due to the selective loss of both size and number of type II fibres with ageing (Bosco & Komi 1980, Lexell 1995). Especially vulnerable to immobilization and inactivity are the anti-gravity muscles of the lower extremities and the faster type II muscle fibres, especially in older people (Lemmer et al 2000).

Greater mitochondrial dysfunction is evident in muscles with higher type II muscle fibre content, which may be at the root of the preferential loss of type II fibres found in elderly people (Conley et al 2006).

Bone

At any one time approximately 10% of bone surface in the adult skeleton is undergoing active remodelling whereas the remaining 90% is quiescent. Bone mineral density (BMD) peaks at around the age of 25 years, at around the age of 30 the balance between bone formation and bone resorption is altered so that resorption begins to exceed deposition, and by the age of 50 progressive losses of calcium and deterioration in the organic matrix of bone occur (Morgenthal & Shephard 2005). Bone mass peaks between the ages of 20 and 40 years, with men achieving a greater peak bone mass (Rutherford 1999). After the age of 40, bone mass declines at a rate of 0.5–1% per year with an accelerated period of loss in women for 5–10 years after the menopause (Morgenthal & Shephard 2005). This accelerated bone loss occurs because of the decrease in the levels of the sex hormone oestrogen, which protects the female skeleton from excessive bone resorption (Eastell & Riggs 1988). In total, women lose about 25–30% of the cortical bone and 35–50% of the trabecular bone over a lifetime; men lose at about two-thirds this rate (Riggs et al 1981). This leaves thin cortical bone and thin or interrupted trabecular plates.

Bone density losses mirror losses in muscle strength, although strength declines well before bone density (Rutherford 1999). The muscular forces exerted on bone are probably one of the key factors in maintaining bone health (Rutherford 1999).

Changes in bone strength are both quantitative and qualitative in nature, and include (Kiebzak 1991, Spirduso et al 2005):

- alterations in the dynamics of bone cells, resulting in a change in the normal process of bone resorption and formation
- changes in bone architecture (e.g. rearrangement of trabecular struts) and cross-sectional geometry
- accumulation of microfractures
- localized disparity in the concentration of deposited minerals, with hypomineralization in some areas and hypermineralization in others
- changes in the crystalline properties of mineral deposits
- changes in the protein content of matrix material.

Fragility fractures, particularly those of the hip, vertebrae and distal forearm, constitute a major public health problem. The two ultimate determinants of fracture are bone strength and propensity to trauma. Bone strength depends not only upon bone mass but also upon a variety of qualitative aspects of bone structure (Cooper 1993). These include its architecture, the amount of fatigue damage it has sustained, and changes in its bulk material properties; indices that are collectively subsumed into the term 'bone quality' (Cooper 1993). Fragility fractures show differences in their patterns of incidence by age, sex, ethnic group, geographic area, and season. Many of these differences are currently unexplained and disorders of bone quality might contribute to them. There are two fracture sites at which evidence implicates bone quality more directly – the spine and proximal femur (Cooper 1993). Many vertebral compression fractures follow minimal trauma, and controlled studies suggest that vertebral microarchitecture contributes to fracture risk independently of vertebral bone mass. At the hip, observational studies have pointed to a role for disordered trabecular architecture, accumulation of microfractures (fatigue damage), and the accumulation of osteoids. The extent to which these phenomena act independently of bone mass, however, remains uncertain (Cooper 1993).

Serum parathyroid hormone (PTH) rises with age and production of the most active metabolites of vitamin D3 decreases (Visser et al 2003). It has been suggested that this rise may contribute to bone loss in postmenopausal women (Need et al 2004). This rise in PTH has been attributed to declining renal function, declining calcium absorption efficiency, and declining serum 25-hydroxyvitamin D levels (Need et al 2004). These hormonal changes undoubtedly affect the maintenance of normal bone homeostasis. Other important factors which can profoundly influence bone status in elderly are decreased physical activity and dietary inadequacies (particularly in calcium). Losses in bone density do not usually have a substantial effect until about the age of 70; however, when a person's BMD measurement is 2.5 standard deviations below that of a normal young adult, they will be diagnosed with osteoporosis (Rutherford 1999).

Flexibility

Loss of range of motion (ROM) or flexibility is inevitable as a result of ageing but the rate of decline appears to be joint specific (Bell & Hoshizaki 1981). Spinal extension declines on average by approximately 50% and hip extension and knee flexion range of movement (ROM) decline on average by 20% and 2%, respectively, between the second and seventh decades (Bell & Hoshizaki 1981, Einkauf et al 1987). Lower body ROM declines are more evident than upper body and this is consistent with declines in strength. Hamstring flexibility declines in both genders by approximately 14.5% (or one inch) per decade (Golding & Lindsay 1989) while losses of 15% (external rotation) and 11% (abduction) have been reported for the hip joints. Small but significant age-related changes have been reported in ankle dorsiflexion ROM. But ankle dorsiflexion strength has been shown to decrease by approximately 30% between middle age and 70 (Vandervoort et al 1992). Any reduction in ankle ROM and strength increases the likelihood of trips and falls during the swing phase of the gait.

Stiffness (the force required to move a joint through a specified ROM) increases with age in all joints and all muscle tissues and is probably the major cause of loss of ROM and the most common complaint of older adults. Even routinely used muscles (e.g. calf) show an increase in stiffness (McHugh et al 1999). A number of biological factors contribute to increased stiffness. These include an increase in the amount of inter- and intramuscular connective tissue, a change in chemical composition so that connective tissue is less extensible and more resistant to being reformed, a breakdown of articular cartilage that increases arthritis in major joint complexes, and a loss of muscle mass (Golding & Lindsay 1989). These changes make it more difficult to move freely with age.

Nervous system

Age is associated with a loss of neural function, slower complex reaction times and slower central processing (Schmidt & Lee 1999). In people without neurological disease, intellectual performance tends to be maintained until at least age 80. However, tasks may take longer to perform because of some slowing in central processing. Verbal skills are well maintained until age 70, after which some healthy elderly persons gradually develop a reduction in vocabulary and a tendency to make semantic errors (Schmidt & Lee 1999). These changes happen mostly because of a loss of neurons, which cannot be replaced, and also a loss of connective networks in the brain (Lexell 1997). There is preferential loss of distal large myelinated sensory fibres and receptors (Shaffer & Harrison 2007).

With normal ageing, the number of nerve cells in the brain decreases. Cell loss is minimal in some areas (e.g. brainstem nuclei) but is as great as 10–60% in others (e.g. hippocampus). Loss also varies within the cortex (e.g. loss is 55% in the superior temporal gyrus but 10–35% in the tip of the temporal lobe). From age 20 or 30 to age 90, brain weight declines about 10% (Schmidt & Lee 1999).

Problems can arise in the central processing of information despite normal sensory input and normal effector neuromuscular function (Spirduso et al 2005). With normal ageing, changes in neurotransmitter systems (enzymes, receptors and neurotransmitters) occur and cerebral blood flow decreases by about 20% on average, slowing processing times (Schmidt & Lee 1999). Free radicals may have a toxic effect on certain nerve cells (Schmidt & Lee 1999), affecting their function.

Evidence strongly suggests that after the age of 60, muscle undergoes continuous denervation and reinnervation, due to an accelerating reduction of functioning motor units (Lexell 1997), mediated through a loss of motor neurons in the spinal cord and hence of myelinated ventral root fibres. Initially, reinnervation can compensate for this denervation. However, as this process progresses, more and more muscle fibres will become permanently denervated and subsequently replaced by fat and fibrous tissue (Lexell 1997). Thus, an age-related degeneration of the nervous system is one of the main contributors to the gradual reduction in muscle volume and muscle strength that accompanies ageing (Lexell 1997).

There are also ageing changes to the sensory inputs into the nervous system. In a well-lit environment and with a firm base of support, healthy persons rely on somatosensory (70%), vestibular (20%) and visual (10%) information (Horak 2006).

Somatic sensation consists of the various sensory receptors that trigger touch or pressure, temperature (warm or cold), pain and the sensations of muscle movement and joint position including posture, movement and facial expression (collectively called proprioception). *Proprioceptive sensitivity* is reduced by age-related poor ankle flexibility and exacerbated by swelling in the feet or ankles due to disease or injury (Shaffer & Harrison 2007). Particularly common with increased age is impaired distal lower-extremity proprioception, vibration and discriminative touch (Shaffer & Harrison 2007). Diseases, such as arthritis, in weight-bearing joints may contribute to errors in foot placement, whilst distorted or painful feet and poorly fitting shoes may give misleading information on the nature of ground contact during walking. Cervical spine mechanoreceptors contribute to static postural sensation and to awareness of head and neck movements so degeneration of the cervical spine from ageing, disease or injury can disturb postural control (Sinaki 1982).

Vestibular abnormalities are an important cause of dizziness and postural instability in older people. An age-related decline in balance may also occur as a result of the accumulation of minute calciferous particles within the semicircular canals in the inner ear (Horak 2006). There appears to be an age-related loss of ciliated sensory cells and a thickening of the fluid in the semicircular canal of the inner ear and this will adversely affect vestibular sensitivity (Wright 1983). More than half of older people have deficits in their vestibulo-ocular reflex, causing potential dizziness when performing fast, voluntary head movements (Hirvonen et al 1997). Certain medications, prescribed commonly in the older population, may lead to vestibular dysfunction; these include aminoglycosides, aspirin, furosemide and quinine (Lysack et al 1998, Rybak 1985). Finally, major disturbances of the vestibular system are more common in older age (tinnitus, labyrinthitis, Ménière's disease) (Horak 2006).

Visual impairment with increasing age is associated with loss of strength in the eye muscles, a decreased elasticity in the lens, poor hydration of the eye and an observed increase in eye infections (Chaput & Proteau 1996). This can lead to an increased susceptibility to glare, and poor depth perception can lead to misinterpretation of the nature of ground surfaces or misjudgement of distance (Lord et al 2001, Schmidt & Lee 1999). During stair descent, poor eyesight is associated with increased foot clearance, allowing more space for perceptual error in the location of the edge of each step (Chaput & Proteau 1996, Lord et al 2001). There is also an increase in the incidence of structural eye disease in later life and many of the problems above are age related. Poor eyesight rates only a little lower than arthritis and heart disease as a cause of impaired physical function in those aged 70 years and above (Chaput & Proteau 1996).

Endocrine system

Decreasing levels of anabolic hormones and disruptions in hormone metabolism and control may be associated with musculoskeletal atrophy and decrease in function with ageing (Copeland et al 2004, Roubenoff & Hughes 2000, Visser et al 2003). In old age, the endocrine control systems work less efficiently and the output of many of the hormones is less well regulated. In addition some glands produce less of their hormone and sometimes the target tissues become less responsive. Overall, the endocrine system becomes more catabolic (Copeland et al 2004). Also, with increasing age, endocrine and metabolic diseases are more common and there is poorer local circulation. These changes will contribute to the muscle and bone loss and increasing frailty of the older person (Lamberts et al 1997).

The ageing process affects nearly every gland (Copeland et al 2004). The first to consider is the hypothalamus, which is responsible for releasing hormones that stimulate the pituitary gland. During ageing, there is either impaired secretion of some hypothalamic hormones or impaired pituitary response. These changes appear to influence the endocrine system's ability to respond to the body's internal environment. As a result, the body cannot respond as well to either internal or external stresses. Cortisol, produced in response to stress and inflammation, is produced more readily with increasing age and this has detrimental effects on muscle and bone and can also lead to depression (Copeland et al 2004). Increased secretion of cortisol is also significantly associated with impairment of cognitive function during ageing (Lupien et al 2005).

There is a progressive decline of growth hormone (GH) secretion with age, such that by the age of 60 most adults have total 24-hour secretion rates indistinguishable from those of hypopituitary patients (Savine & Sönksen 2000). Patterns of GH secretion in older people are similar to those in younger people but the pulses of GH are markedly reduced in amplitude. Sleep and exercise remain the major stimuli for GH secretion. Daytime sleepiness in older adults is associated with physical functional impairments and decreased exercise frequency (Chasens et al 2007). A short nap (30 minutes between 1300 and 1500 hours) and moderate exercise such as walking in the evening have been shown to increase sleep length and improve sleep quality (Tanaka & Shirakawa 2004). The fall in GH secretion seen with ageing coincides with changes in body composition and lipid metabolism that are similar to those seen in younger adults with clinical GH deficiency (Savine & Sönksen 2000). Physical activity might have an effect on hormone action as a result of changes in protein carriers and receptors (Copeland et al 2004). The effects of activity on the endocrine system are seen in ageing men, where regular moderate physical activity is associated with higher levels of insulin-like growth factor (IGF-1) and improved thyroid function (Ravaglia et al 2001).

Vitamin D deficiency is common both in geriatric patients (30–90%, depending on the deficiency definition) and in independent, community-dwelling older persons (2–60%) (Lips 2001). This is partly due to a lower sunshine exposure and a reduced capacity of the older skin to synthesize vitamin D3 under the influence of ultraviolet light (Lips 2001). Several cross-sectional studies have shown that low 1,25-hydroxyvitamin D (active form of vitamin D3) and low 25-hydroxyvitamin D (25-OHD) (blood calcium form of vitamin D3) are related to lower muscle strength, increased body sway, falls, and disability in older men and women (Lips 2001, Visser et al 2003). This is supported by vitamin D supplementation studies which have shown improvements in physical function and isometric knee extensor strength (Verhaar et al 2000).

Falls and fall-related injuries

Most cross-sectional studies show that with ageing gait patterns have a wider base, there is a slowing in sway, an increased time in double leg support phase of walking as well as a decrease in stride length, a decrease in trunk rotation and an increase in pain and discomfort that limits movement (Lord et al 2001, Skelton 2001). Sedentary older adults are also known to adopt a more cautious walking style with shorter step lengths and slower step velocities than active older adults. When required to increase walking speed, older people tend to increase their cadence rather than their stride length, whereas younger people do the reverse (Lord et al 2001, Rose 2003, Skelton 2001). Diseases such as peripheral neuropathy, arthritis and osteoporosis cause further gait adaptation. Other age-related effects also affect balance: the sensitivity of skin receptors is reduced (oedema, arthritis and medications), reflex speeds and reaction times slow, coordination gets worse (particularly hand/eye), and eyesight and vestibular function decline (often medication related) (Lord et al 2001, Skelton 2001).

Muscle weakness is associated with fall risk (Gillespie et al 2005). A recent meta-analysis observed a tripling of risk of recurrent falls in those with lower extremity weakness (Gillespie et al 2005). Slow reaction time and decreased functional ability owing to lack of practice and/or physical pain, inadequate strength of the muscle-tendon complex, decreased joint flexibility, and lower limb asymmetry in strength and power are considered the main muscle factors involved in postural instability, falls and fractures (Lord et al 1992, 1994, 2001, Skelton 2001, Skelton et al 2002).

Frequent fallers have a very poor prognosis, especially if they live alone and are likely to be waiting hours before they are found or can get attention (Tinetti et al 2003). One problem is often that people fall and, despite there being only a minor injury, they are not able to get up off the floor without help. If they cannot get up without help (long-lie), then they are more likely, on 21-month follow-up, either to have died, or at least to be hospitalized and to have suffered functional decline (Tinetti et al 1993). The role of exercise to maintain core body temperature whilst on the floor, to prevent hypothermia and other complications of a long-lie, should not be forgotten (Dinan & Skelton 2007, Skelton & Dinan 1999). Some of the difficulty of rising from the floor may be shock or injury but for many it is simply lack of familiarity, functional fitness and neuromuscular control and in these instances it can be retrained (Dinan & Skelton 2007, Skelton & Dinan 1999). People aged over 65 who have fallen account for the largest call-out for the London Ambulance, yet 40% of these people are not conveyed to hospital, merely picked up and made comfortable

(Close et al 2005, Skelton 2001). Fear of falling can also lead to avoidance of activities and further detraining and a spiral of inactivity that can lead to further falls and isolation (Yardley & Smith 2003).

Psychological function

The brain remains malleable throughout life and at any age can adapt in response to stimuli and activities. Grey matter can thicken, neural trunks can remyelinate, neural connections can be forged and refined and all these mechanisms can reinvigorate cognitive abilities (Mattson et al 2001, Verghese et al 2003). Cognitive function involves a combination of skills, including memory, attention, learning, goal setting, decision making and problem solving. In old age, poor health and disease impair cognitive performance (Chodzko-Zajko & Moore 1994). Impaired endocrine function, such as an increased production of cortisol, is associated with declining cognitive function, thereby illustrating the strong association between the nervous and endocrine systems (Lupien et al 2005). Natural age-related decline begins in the 30s and accelerates after 50. It is often characterized by memory lapses, slower thinking and growing difficulties in communicating with others (e.g. words sticking on the tip of the tongue, inability to recall telephone numbers). This functional decline is caused by negative brain plasticity (i.e. changes that slow or impede cognitive performance). Keeping the brain active has been shown to maintain cognitive fitness (Verghese et al 2003).

There are four components to the effects of ageing on cognitive functioning (Bao et al 2003):

- *Disuse* (lack of practice).
- *Noisy processing* where the older brain becomes 'noisier' (in the information theorists' sense that more meaningless pseudo-information is signalled) due to the deterioration of sensory inputs. The term has no specific connection with hearing. Nevertheless a specific example, which does concern hearing, is that as the inner ear deteriorates it sends the brain increasingly unclear signals about outside sounds. The brain adjusts its sampling rates and time constants and slows down to decipher these unclear signals. The result is poorer memory and less agile thinking.
- *Weakened neuromodulatory function* (reduced production of the brain chemicals that play vital roles in learning and memory).
- *Negative learning* (feeling less mentally sharp often leads to compensatory strategies that accelerate functional decline, e.g. paying less rather than closer attention).

Quality of life decreases with increasing age (Spirduso et al 2005), depression and anxieties increase (Chodzko-Zajko & Moore 1994) and social isolation occurs more frequently, due to death of spouse and friends and reduced physical activity (Spirduso et al 2005).

IMPACT OF CHRONIC DISEASE AND SEDENTARY LIFESTYLE ON PROGRESSIVE AGE-RELATED DECLINE

50% of the decline frequently attributed to physiologic aging is, in reality, disuse atrophy resulting from inactivity.
(Jette et al 1999)

Physical inactivity is a major under-recognized risk factor for chronic health problems, loss of functional reserve, and disability. It remains difficult to distinguish unavoidable effects of ageing from the consequences of chronic disease or sedentary behaviour (Shephard 1997). However, the impact of sedentary behaviour on an ever-broadening variety of health problems is clear, particularly in old age (ACSM 1998, CDC 1996, 2002, Department of Health 2001, NIA 1998, Nicholl et al 1994, WHO 1997).

The contribution of sedentary behaviour to prevalence and cost of chronic illnesses exacts a significant burden in terms of morbidity and mortality and is a contributing factor for extended hospital stay and/or need for subsequent post-hospital care in skilled nursing facilities (Department of Health 2001, Hoenig et al 1997, Inouye et al 1993, Kane et al 1996, Sager et al 1996).

If the predicted morbidity statistics prevail, there will be a 600% increase in health-care costs by 2040 (Guralnik et al 1993). One-third of the total healthcare expenditure is for older (65+) adults but the annual direct medical costs of physically inactive older adults (with no physical limitations) are significantly higher than those of their physically active peers (CDC 2002).

Conversely, regular physical activity is associated with significant reductions in average monthly Medicare expenditures ($196 over a 12-month period for walking or swimming; $241 for participating in active sports; and $162 for regular gardening over a 4-month period) (Stearns et al 2001). It has been estimated that if the whole population adopted the national guidelines for physical activity, healthcare costs for hip fractures alone could be reduced by about 50% (Nicholl et al 1994).

The effects of age vary from one individual to another and can be exacerbated by inactivity or ameliorated by regular physical activity. Unfortunately inactivity after middle age is prevalent. Forty per cent of people aged 50 or over in the UK perform less than half an hour of moderate activity in one session in a week (Skelton et al 1999). Over half of those people who are sedentary believe they are doing enough exercise to maintain adequate function. These people are likely to have 'inactivity determined' disability.

It is known that a few weeks of immobilization or disuse has a detrimental effect on muscle mass, muscle strength and power (Bloomfield 1997). The decrease in muscle strength is greatest, 3–4% per day, during the first week of immobilization and up to a 40% decrease in isokinetic muscle strength has been seen after 3 weeks of immobilization (Bloomfield 1997). Bed rest causes an increase in calcium excretion and bone mineral loss in the weight-bearing bones such as the calcaneus, iliac crest and lumbar spine (Whedon 1984). Prolonged periods of bed rest lead to the loss of 0.9% of bone mineral per week (Frost 1990, Krolner & Toft 1983). High rates of inactivity in older people, especially those in residential or nursing accommodation, will lead to an increased loss of bone with increasing age. Nursing home residents spend up to 90% of their time either sitting or lying down (Tinetti 1994). This will mean that extremely sedentary people will see an 'active' loss of bone and muscle over and above the 'ageing' loss.

The good news is that regular, appropriate exercise training has been shown to improve the functional abilities and psychological well-being of both healthy older people and patients with disabling symptoms common in old age. In older athletes, rate of decrease in maximal oxygen intake appears to be some 80% of that seen in sedentary individuals, peak heart rate 10 beats/min slower than in sedentary individuals, and muscle strength is similar to sedentary young adults (Pearson et al 2002, Shephard et al 1995). Therefore, it has been suggested that with a higher level of physical activity the rate of decline of $\dot{V}O_2$max could be reduced by half (Hagberg et al 1989).

THE EVIDENCE FOR EFFECTS OF EXERCISE TRAINING AND PHYSICAL ACTIVITY IN OLDER PEOPLE

Exercise of some kind or other is almost essential to the preservation of health in persons of all ages – but in none more so than in the old.
(MacLachlan 1863)

Physical health includes three components: *physical condition* (objective diagnosed health problems), *perceived physical condition* (subjective health status) and *physical function* (limitations in the ability to carry out basic activities of daily living (ADLs) such as self-care, dressing, washing, and instrumental activities of daily living (IADLs) such as shopping, gardening, cooking, going outside and taking part in hobbies, recreation, social activities) (Spirduso et al 2005). Even in frailer, older participants there is evidence that habitual physical activity can preserve *functional independence* by counteracting some of the age-related decline in performance, counteracting the effects of disease and increasing the sense of control over personal health and well-being (Spirduso et al 2005, WHO 1997, Young 1986, 2001).

Regular physical activity, more than any other intervention, has been shown to extend life, reduce disability, and improve quality of life in older adults (ACSM 1998, Buchner 1997, CDC 1996, Guralnik et al 1993, LaCroix et al 1993, Wagner 1997). Not only does it reduce risk for cardiovascular disease, osteoarthritis, osteoporosis, obesity, diabetes and insomnia but regular physical activity also significantly reduces risk for falls, depression and incontinence (ACSM 1998, CDC 1996, Coleman et al 1996, Gardner et al 2000, Nicholl et al 1994, Singh et al 1997). Because of the high prevalence of chronic conditions, frailer older people have the potential to gain most from regular physical activity (ACSM 1998, Buchner 1997, Buchner et al 1997, CDC 1996, Fiatarone et al 1990). Older adults with chronic illness can potentially reverse loss of mobility (ACSM 1998, CDC 1996, Young & Dinan 2005). Here exercise training takes on less of a disease prevention and more of a symptom alleviation role (Table 6.1) (Spirduso et al 1996, 2005).

Effects on the cardiovascular and respiratory systems

It is clear that the capacity of the cardiovascular and respiratory system to adapt to an endurance training load is not affected by age. Even women in their 80s and 90s can improve their $\dot{V}O_2$max as much as 17% after 24–32 weeks of aerobic training (Malbut et al 2002, Puggaard et al 2000). Aerobic endurance training also improves older adults' ability to sustain exercise at a fixed, submaximal level of energy expenditure. Similar increases in $\dot{V}O_2$max have been reported for young and old adults, with the magnitude of improvement (20–30%) being based on the intensity of the training stimulus and previous exercise history (Cress et al 1991, Malbut et al 2002). Interval endurance training has been suggested as more effective than continuous endurance training in older adults and in other special populations (Ahmaidi et al 1998, Bell 2001, Brooks 1997, Dinan 2001, Dinan et al 2004, Vogiatzis et al 2002). Interestingly, in older people, 12 weeks of strength training or combined strength and aerobic training are as effective as 12 weeks of aerobic training alone to improve relative $\dot{V}O_2$max (Aniansson & Gustafsson 1981) and 24 weeks of low- or high-intensity resistance training lead to similar improvements in aerobic capacity (DeVito et al 1997, Vincent et al 2002). Comparing modalities, walking is more effective than calisthenics at improving $\dot{V}O_2$max in women over the age of 70 years (Warren et al 1993).

Both resting heart rate and heart rate during submaximal activities can be reduced with aerobic training (DeVito et al 1997, Morey et al 1989, Spina 1999). Maximal voluntary ventilation and submaximal exercise ventilatory response are also improved with a low- and moderate-intensity aerobic programme (50–75% of heart rate reserve) after 12 weeks (DeVito et al 1997, Yerg et al 1985) in older men and women. In strength training, eccentric resistance exercises place less cardiopulmonary demands, and may be more suited for older people with low exercise tolerance, than concentric exercises (Vallejo et al 2006). A comparison between qigong and Tai Chi Chuan (TCC) practitioners in cardiorespiratory responses showed tai chi chuan, with its higher exercise intensity, to be more effective in terms of $\dot{V}O_2$max, but that qigong enhanced breathing efficiency due to the training effect on diaphragmatic breathing (Lan et al 2004).

The age-related decrease in cardiac mass and changes in composition of the myocardium are slowed but, probably, not abolished by regular physical activity (Saltin 1986). Regular physical activity can lead to an appreciable decrease in systemic blood pressure, particularly in individuals with hypertension, thus decreasing afterloading of the left ventricle (Shephard 1994). The degree of trainability appears to be unrelated to gender, although the mechanisms by which the change is produced are somewhat different. In older males any improvement in $\dot{V}O_2$max is a function of both central (enhanced β-adrenergic stimulation, enlarged ventricular chamber size) and peripheral changes (Ehsani et al 1991, Levy et al 1993, Ogawa et al 1992, Spina et al 1998), whereas in women improvements in $\dot{V}O_2$max occur exclusively due to changes in oxygen extraction at the tissue without any changes in cardiac function (Spina et al 1993). Exercise has been shown to improve endothelial-dependent relaxation of vascular smooth muscle in older people (Haykowsky 2005). This important exercise-induced effect on the endothelium has many potential clinical implications for older populations. Improved endothelial function can protect the blood vessel wall from the development of atherosclerosis and thrombosis, whereas dysfunctional endothelium can actively promote vascular damage and consequent plaque formation (Ross 1993, Taddei et al 1996). Therefore, by protecting the endothelium, physical activity may be responsible for the beneficial effect of exercise and the decreased risk of cardiovascular disease demonstrated in older people who walk further than 1.5 miles (2.4 km) per day and at a brisk pace (Manson et al 2002).

In general, the majority of studies suggest that following endurance training, there is a reduction in the concentration of total cholesterol, an increase in the concentration of high-density lipoprotein (HDL) cholesterol and a favourable modification of the total cholesterol:HDL ratio. However, there is greater ambiguity concerning the influence of training on the concentration of low-density lipoprotein (LDL) cholesterol (Hagberg et al 1989, Hurley 1989).

Effects on the musculoskeletal system

Muscle

An octogenarian's remaining muscle still shows a normal response to physical training. The improvements are equivalent to 10–20 years' 'rejuvenation' (Skelton et al 1995). Strength training has also provoked valuable enlargement of muscle fibres even though the age-related reduction in number of muscle fibres appears to continue (Aniansson & Gustafsson 1981). Skeletal muscle hypertrophy, or reversal of sarcopenia, requires at least 8–12 weeks of training in older adults (Aniansson & Gustafsson 1981, Brill et al 2000, Fiatarone et al 1990). For older individuals, the absolute resistance required to overload the musculoskeletal system is typically surprisingly low. So although strength training is traditionally performed in a gym environment with resistance exercise machines or free weights, home-based resistance programmes have been increasing in popularity. Home-based resistance training that uses bodyweight exercises, or a weighted belt, to increase bodyweight resistance, limb weights, elastic resistance bands, and dumbbells have been reported to increase strength and bone mineral density (BMD) (Judge et al 2005). After a year-long home-based strength and balance programme using bodyweight and ankle weights, the risk of falls is reduced in older people (Robertson et al 2001). However, whilst home-based training may have advantages in terms of convenience, potential disadvantages include suboptimal loading and a lack of supervision that may reduce motivation and adherence. Supervision has been found to increase the rate of improvement in muscular strength in response to training (Mazzetti et al 2000).

Because functional ability is highly related to strength, it might be reasonable to assume that an increase in muscle strength would lead to an improvement in function (Hyatt et al 1990). However, improvements in strength do not always translate into improvements in daily functioning (Skelton et al 1995). Combining strength training with more functional training has resulted in more functional gains both in non-frail elderly (Skelton et al 1996) and in frail elderly (Fiatarone et al 1990, Jette et al 1999) and this combination should, therefore, be integrated into the programme.

Resistance training is highly effective at countering the decline in muscle strength and power, with significant increases in strength and power after only a few weeks of training, even in very elderly participants (Fiatarone et al 1990, Skelton et al 1995). Increases in strength and power are attributed to improvements in the nervous system (muscle activation, overall coordination) and morphological changes within the trained muscles (primarily muscle fibre hypertrophy). Resistance training can improve everyday function and mobility including factors such as walking speed and time to stand up from a chair (Skelton & McLaughlin 1996).

Some studies of low-intensity strength training have shown that it increases muscle strength in nursing home residents, frail elderly and elderly people with co-morbidity (Fiatarone et al 1990, McMurdo & Rennie 1994) but has very little effect in healthy elderly people (Jette et al 1996). Traditional resistance training with a relatively slow movement velocity and use of resistance exercise weight stack machines has been criticized for having a lack of specificity for the mobility requirements of older people. Older individuals may benefit more from improvements in power than strength (Skelton et al 1995). Performing mobility-specific exercises appears to produce greater improvements in functional outcomes than traditional resistance exercise (Skelton & McLaughlin 1996). The duration of training is important. In the first 8–12 weeks of resistance training in nonagenarians, just as at earlier ages, there are huge improvements in strength but little change in muscle mass (Fiatarone et al 1990). In the first 8–12 weeks, all improvements in strength are neurally mediated, so for changes to muscle bulk, longer training periods must be considered (Itoi & Sinaki 1994). Finally, the importance of duration of training is highlighted by evidence suggesting that the preservation of muscle mass and/or reversal of sarcopenia through exercise could be a useful anabolic method to provide a protein reservoir for later use when the older person is exposed to infection, inflammation and/or severe trauma (Spirduso et al 2005) and as padding if they fall (Rutherford 1999).

Bone

Much of the initial work aimed at improving bone mineral density (BMD) concentrated on the types of endurance activity that had been shown to be beneficial for cardiovascular health (Rutherford 1999). There is increasing acknowledgement that the same type of exercise may not be optimal for bone health or for reduction of falls risk. Bone loading is necessary, but bodyweight by itself is not sufficient to create the loading levels necessary for an osteogenic response (Kohrt et al 2004, Rutherford 1999). Bone health requires the following basic principles of training (Kohrt et al 2004):

- Principle of specificity: only sites loaded by the exercise will respond as the effects are localized.
- Principle of overload: the training stimulus must exceed the normal loading experienced by the skeleton in everyday activities and, as the bone responds, the stimulus must be increased progressively.
- Principle of reversibility: any positive effects of training on BMD will only be maintained as long as the exercise is continued.
- Principle of initial values: the most benefit is likely to be achieved in those with the lowest initial BMD.

The forms of exercise shown to be beneficial for slowing or reversing the age-related loss of bone include brief bouts of weight-bearing exercise such as intermittent jogging (Kohrt et al 2004), exercise classes (Welsh & Rutherford 1996) and also weight training using weights in excess of 80% of personal maximum (1-RM) (Kerr et al 1996). However, walking alone does not increase bone density, it merely helps maintain it (Cavanaugh & Cann 1988). Regular exercise could delay the point at which osteopenia progresses to clinically significant osteoporosis (Nelson et al 1994, Welsh & Rutherford 1996). Indeed, home-based resistance training improves BMD in women on treatment (Judge et al 2005).

The ACSM suggests that weight-bearing exercises (e.g. weight training, stair climbing, walking, running, jogging, dancing, aerobics, racquet sports, court sports and field sports), three times per week, for 20–30 minutes are required to help maintain a healthy bone mass (Kohrt et al 2004). In all activities, it is important to consider the basic principles of training for bone health (Kohrt et al 2004).

In postmenopausal women, simple daily squeezing of a tennis ball for 30 seconds has significant benefits in the non-injured forearm of women who had already sustained a Colles' fracture (Beverly et al 1989). In addition, a set of dynamic bone loading exercises for the distal forearm results in increased bone strength at the wrist (Ayalon et al 1987). Total body calcium is improved in postmenopausal women training at a repetitive low force, as well as in those who train at a similar level with the addition of light weights attached to their wrists and ankles during the exercise classes (Chow et al 1987). In postmenopausal women, Tai Chi Chun exercise has been linked with a three- to fourfold slowing down in the rate of bone loss in both trabecular and cortical compartments of the distal tibia compared with a sedentary lifestyle (Chan et al 2004). Interventions to reduce the effects of immobilization or bed rest have found that quiet standing for a daily total of 3 hours (as opposed to an exercise intervention) prevents the changes in mineral metabolism (Issekutz et al 1966). Whether shorter total periods of standing would be equally effective is unknown.

Whole body vibration (WBV) has recently been considered as a possible modality for skeletal loading. In older adults, WBV at 35–40 Hz three times weekly for 24 weeks (Verschueren et al 2004) has been linked with increased bone strength. However, at 20 Hz for 4 minutes once a week for 12 months, microvibrations appeared to have no additional positive bone strength effect (compared with a course of 5 mg daily of alendronate), in postmenopausal women (Iwamoto et al 2005). More work is needed on this type of bone loading, not least on the potential side effects that may occur from the vibration to the head and neck region.

For postmenopausal women with substantial thoracic kyphosis, progressive back strengthening exercises for 2 years have been found to decrease kyphosis and improve posture (Itoi & Sinaki 1994). In a follow-up study, women who had participated in back strengthening exercises for 2 years, but none thereafter, were found 8 years later to have greater back extension strength and bone mineral density of the lumbar spine, and less than half the incidence of vertebral fractures, compared to a control group of comparable women who had not performed back strengthening exercises (Sinaki et al 2002). This suggests that a prolonged period of resistance training can provide musculoskeletal health benefits for a considerable period even after cessation of the exercise. Even frail older patients with osteoporosis gain benefit from exercise. However, when working with these patients, exercise must be low risk and low impact for safety. For example, those with a previous history of vertebral fractures should avoid unsupported spinal flexion, such as abdominal curls (Sinaki 1982). These patients are likely to have weak back extensor muscle strength and must focus on back extensor strengthening and start with the lowest workload and progress slowly (Sinaki 1982).

Flexibility

There is plenty of evidence that older adults can increase their range of motion and flexibility. It does not seem to matter what type of exercise is used as long as it works the joint through its full range of movement. Improvements have been found with traditional range of movement and static stretches, aerobic sessions, resistance training, yoga, dance, tai chi and aquatic exercise (Jones & Rose 2005).

Effects on the nervous system

Despite the paucity of human research, basic animal models and clinical data overwhelmingly support the notion that exercise treatment is a major protective factor against neurodegeneration (Kiraly & Kiraly 2005). Unfortunately this is an under-researched area and there are no clinical guidelines on exercise modes or intensities for retaining neuron integrity in older adults. However, significant increases in brain volume, in both grey and white matter regions, were found for aerobic fitness training group but not for the older adults who participated in the stretching and toning (non-aerobic) control group (Colcombe et al 2006). Improvements in muscle steadiness, decreases in muscle relaxation time and reaction times and generally improved neural control of movement have been found with a variety of exercise modalities including tai chi, functional strength training, aerobic classes and balance training (Skelton 2001, Spirduso et al 2005). Exercise may help protect older people from depression, not only by increasing blood flow to the brain but by directly enhancing neurotransmitters and neuronal growth factors (Cotman & Berchtold 2002).

To help prevent, slow or even reverse the effects of cognitive decline, activities must specifically target the cause (Verghese et al 2003).

- To combat disuse, activities must repeatedly and progressively engage the brain in new and demanding tasks.
- To improve input, activities must require careful attention and focus.

- To improve regulation and production of neuromodulators, activities must include rewarding, surprising and focusing.
- To re-pattern maladaptive compensatory behaviours, activities must require confrontation rather than avoidance of challenges.

Learning to play an instrument or sing, learning a foreign language, juggling, dancing, jigsaw puzzles and table tennis and aerobic exercise have all been effective (Colcombe et al 2006, Kramer et al 2002, Verghese et al 2003).

Effects on the endocrine system

Every bout of resistance exercise helps endocrine function. Men and women over the age of 65 have increased circulating levels of IGF-1 and decreased cortisol levels after only two sets of leg extensions, thereby increasing serum anabolic/catabolic hormone ratios (Kostka et al 2003). Aerobic exercise initiates a release of circulating growth hormone that varies by intensity of exercise but is measurable even in older adults at low intensities (Weltman et al 2006). Moderate exercise can help to reverse the adverse effects of ageing on the immune system by increasing the production of anabolic endocrine hormones and reducing the effects of catabolic hormones (Venjatraman & Fernandes 1997). Aerobic exercise can enhance immune function of healthy older people, potentially increasing resistance to viral infections and preventing the formation of malignant cells. It can also reduce the age-related decline in certain aspects of circulating T-cell function and related cytokine production (Venjatraman & Fernandes 1997).

Effects on falls and fall-related injuries

Recent reviews and guidelines suggest multidisciplinary falls assessment and intervention, including exercise, should be considered alongside osteoporosis diagnosis and management to reduce the number of falls and fall-related injuries (Gardner et al 2000, Gillespie et al 2005).

Falls in the home-dwelling elderly take place during periods of maximal activity (Luukinen et al 1995), so there may be a U-shaped relationship between the amount of physical activity and the number of falls, with a higher incidence of falls in the least active and the most active as suggested in one study (Gregg et al 2000). Care must be taken over which activities are suggested to those with poor balance and mobility (Dinan 2001, Skelton 2001, Skelton & Dinan 1999). Indeed, one walking intervention in patients with a previous Colles' fracture actually increased the risk of fractures compared to not walking (Ebrahim et al 1997).

Some exercise-only interventions have shown little or no effect on falls risk despite improvements in known risk factors (e.g. strength). It appears that individualized exercise interventions with balance training at the core of the programme are most effective for those at risk of falls (Robertson et al 2001, Skelton et al 2005, Wolf et al 1996).

In New Zealand, a targeted home exercise programme, for women aged over 80 years, a population at high risk of falls, was taught to participants in their own homes by a physiotherapist (and then repeated with specially trained nurses) and compared to social visits only as a control (Robertson et al 2001). Exercises were individually prescribed from a set number of warm-up, muscle strength and balance training exercises to perform three times a week for a year. The subjects were also encouraged to walk outdoors at their desired pace, building up to 30 minutes two to three times a week. The physiotherapist visited each intervention participant four times over the first 2 months, following on with regular telephone contact. The exercise group had a significantly lower rate of falls and the intervention was cost-effective in the group concerned (Robertson et al 2001).

In those aged over 65 years, with poor strength and balance, modified Tai Chi appears effective as a group exercise programme to reduce the risk of the first fall (Wolf et al 1996). A modified programme of Tai Chi (which took account of poor balance in the subjects) over a 48-week period, however, was not beneficial in reducing falls in an older (aged 70 years and over) group with signs of frailty (Wolf et al 2003).

In the UK, independent-living frequent fallers halved their risk of falls (incidence rate ratio (IRR) 0.46, 95% CI 0.34 to 0.63) with 9 months of weekly group balance and strength exercises, led by a postural stability exercise instructor, combined with twice weekly home exercises (Skelton et al 2005) (Fig. 6.3). The women undertaking this falls management exercise (FaME) had significantly lower mortality and morbidity at 3-year follow-up than the randomized control group (Skelton et al 2005). The exercise intervention consisted of progressive resistance, gait, balance, functional activity, floor work, endurance and flexibility training. The exercise was individually tailored in both type and intensity, with most exercises in weight-bearing positions, reducing upper limb support. There were also significant improvements in strength, power and bone mineral density at the lumbar spine and one area of the hip (Fig. 6.3).

On a population/public health basis, encouraging physical activity and the provision of exercise sessions as part of a wider campaign including literature, medication reviews and environmental changes has been shown to decrease fall-related injuries (McClure et al 2005). One large population approach trial, over 10 years, has seen a reduction in fracture rate by advocating increased physical activity and other lifestyle changes (Grahn Kronhed et al 2005).

Effects on psychological function

Physically active and fit older adults have been found to process cognitive information more efficiently than less fit individuals of the same age (Kramer et al 2002). The results were independent of sex, self-rated health and level of social activity. Both aerobic exercise and combined aerobic and strength exercise are associated with improvements in cognitive function, with the combined aerobic and strength exercises being most effective (Kramer et al 2002).

There is a strong association between self-esteem, self-efficacy and long-term exercise; it is strongest in cross-sectional studies; it is less clear whether short-term exercise training causes changes in global aspects of self-esteem. A number of comprehensive reviews (Biddle & Faulkner 2001, Boutcher 2000, McAuley & Rudolph 1995) have covered the literature on research studies on exercise and psychological well-being in people over the age of 45. Moderate-intensity has been shown to be more effective than high- or low-intensity training (King et al 1993) and training programmes of more than 10 weeks have greater effect than shorter programmes (McAuley & Katula 1998, McAuley & Rudolph 1995). There is a very clear positive effect for physical activity on psychological well-being (Table 6.3) in older adults, with 86.7% of studies reporting positive results, only 13.3% showing no effects and, of particular note, no studies showing negative effects.

The studies have diverse measurements of psychological well-being (46.7% assess stress, 50% assess positive well-being, 23.3% mood, 36.7% life satisfaction and 23.3% other variables) as well as diverse age ranges (86.6% of studies investigating the

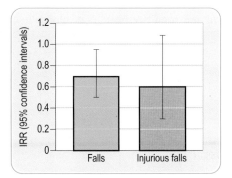

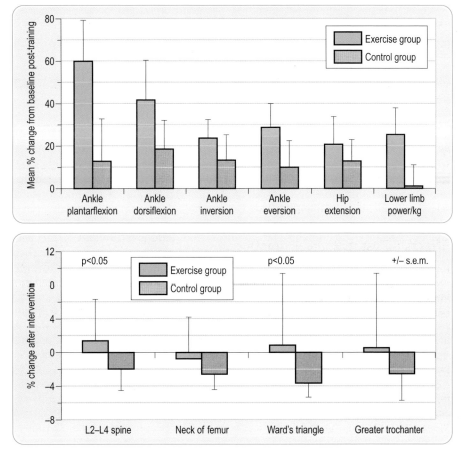

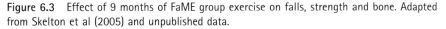

Figure 6.3 Effect of 9 months of FaME group exercise on falls, strength and bone. Adapted from Skelton et al (2005) and unpublished data.

'young old' (60–75 years), 63.3% the 'middle old' (76–85 years) and 36.7% the 'old old' (>85 years)) (Biddle & Faulkner 2001).

A recent trial considered different intensities of resistance training versus normal GP care in clinically depressed older adults and found high-intensity progressive

Table 6.3   Psychological and cognitive benefits of physical activity for older people

Immediate benefits
  Relaxation
  Stress and anxiety reduction
  Enhanced mood state
  Regular physical activity
Long-term benefits
  General well-being
  Regularly active individuals have stronger self-esteem and self-efficacy
  Greater sense of control
  Improved mental health: regular activity can help in treatment of depression and anxiety
  Cognitive improvements: can help to postpone age-related declines in cognitive performance
Motor control
  Prevent or postpone age-associated decline in both fine and gross motor control
Skill acquisition
  New skills can be learned and existing skills refined through physical activity

Adapted from AARP (2001), Chodzko-Zajko & Moore (1994), WHO (1997).

resistance training (PRT) more effective than GP care or low-intensity PRT (Singh et al 2005).

Self-efficacy is defined as situation-specific self-confidence and is typically studied as a determinant of exercise. However, more recently it has been suggested that self-efficacy can be changed as a result of physical activity and therefore can also be seen as an outcome variable (Biddle & Faulker 2001). For example, increasing physical activity confidence in older adults could have a significant impact on physical and psychological functioning and quality of life. Biddle & Faulkner (2001) concluded that positive effects on self-efficacy are evident across all age groups. Their final conclusions were that: physical activity has a significant and large antidepressant effect in depressed older adults (e.g. O'Connor et al 1993); there is evidence linking physical activity with improved cognitive functioning, particularly in older adults who achieve an increase in aerobic fitness (Hill et al 1993, Lavie & Milani 1995). Social factors may influence participation in physical activity as well as mental health and quality of life, but there is no evidence that the positive psychological effects of physical activity are due to social factors alone (Brown et al 1995, Hassmen et al 2000).

Physical activity also helps older people to adjust to their changing roles by providing opportunities to widen their social contacts, stimulate new friendships and acquire positive new roles in a contracting social network (Chodzko-Zajko & Moore 1994, McAuley et al 2000). This can help older people gain a sense of control, especially at a time when major health challenges may otherwise foster a sense of helplessness (Young 2001).

EVIDENCE-BASED GUIDANCE ON THE ROLE AND TYPES OF ASSESSMENT

The prevalence of chronic and degenerative disease and, in particular, the higher rates of underlying coronary artery disease mean that the rationale for exercise testing of the elderly may be even greater than that for the general adult population

(ACSM 2000). Indeed, exercise prescription and dynamic assessment of exercise ability and function for older adults may require subtle differences in protocol, methodology and dosage as compared with younger and middle-aged people (ACSM 2000).

A systematic and multifaceted approach to pre-exercise and health screening and assessment is essential to optimize the older adult's safety during performance testing and exercise and to develop effective exercise prescriptions across the functional continuum (ACSM 2000, Jones & Rikli 2005). The frailer the individual, the more relevant the need for assessment and the greater the importance of safe, functionally relevant and validated assessment tools (Jones & Rikli 2005). An example of this is the use of body mass index (BMI). If there is high muscle mass (veteran athletes) BMI can give the impression that the person is obese. Or if there is very little muscle and more fat mass, characteristic of sedentary, frailer, older adults, BMI can give the false impression that the person is in the correct range (Rogers 2005). However, even correctly calculated BMI can give totally misleading indications of obesity.

Screening and assessment principles

Pre-activity screening has different meanings for different older adults, resulting in potentially different motivational implications for adopting more active lives (Resnick et al 2005). For many, screening increased their sense of confidence and served as a positive motivator whilst for others screening was irrelevant and actually hindered their motivation to join an activity group (Resnick et al 2005). To avoid creating a barrier or over-medicalizing the process, it is important to emphasize that the aim of the assessment is not to exclude those at risk, but rather to ensure inclusion of each individual in an appropriate exercise programme, setting and level of supervision (Dinan 2001).

Initial screening must establish:

- the health and disability status, including current medications
- signs and symptoms associated with certain diseases
- risk factors that predispose to certain diseases (Rogers 2005)
- risk factors that contraindicate performance testing and exercise or adaptation and tailoring to minimize risk during exercise (Table 6.4).

In addition, for older participants, we need to include a range of assessments to establish:

- nature and degree of physical impairment
- specific functional limitations (e.g. restriction in rising from a chair or climbing stairs (Jones & Rikli 2005); inability to get down to and up from the floor (Skelton & Dinan 1999))
- activity history, current interests, preferences and means
- current readiness to exercise (Dinan 2001)
- ability to get to the session (transport/carer) (Dinan 2001).

The specific pre-exercise assessment provides the opportunity to identify (Dinan 2001, Dinan et al 2006, Jones & Rikli 2005):

- who is, or will be, at risk of decreased mobility or disability
- which programme, instructor and setting is appropriate for a particular older person
- what motivates the person (information needed in order to set behavioural goals)

Table 6.4 Contraindications to pre-exercise assessment and exercise participation for older people requiring specific direction from the referring clinician and subsequent programme adaptation by exercise practitioner

---

Absolute contraindications
Severe coronary artery disease/unstable angina pectoris and acute myocardial infarction
Decompensated congestive heart failure
Uncontrolled ventricular arrhythmias
Uncontrolled cardiac arrhythmias (compromising cardiac function)
Severe valvular heart disease including aortic, pulmonic and mitral stenosis
Uncontrolled systemic hypertension (e.g. >200 mmHg/105 mmHg)
Pulmonary hypertension
Suspected or known dissecting aneurysm
Acute myocarditis
Acute pulmonary embolus
Acute infections
Uncontrolled acute systemic illness
Significant drop in blood pressure during exercise
Recent injurious fall without medical attention
Uncontrolled vestibular or visual disturbances
People with proven inability to comply with the recommended adaptations to the exercise
  programme
Relative contraindications
Coronary artery disease
Congestive heart failure
Significant valvular heart disease
Cardiac arrhythmias including ventricular and atrial arrhythmias and complete heart block
Severe arterial hypertension (>200 mmHg/>105 mmHg)
Fixed-rate, permanent pacemaker
Cyanotic congenital heart disease
Congenital anomalies of coronary arteries
Cardiomyopathy including hypertrophic cardiomyopathy and dilated cardiomyopathy
Marfan's syndrome
High-degree atrioventricular heart block
Ventricular aneurysm
Peripheral vascular disease
Severe obstructive or restrictive lung disease
Electrolyte abnormalities, especially hypokalaemia
Uncontrolled metabolic disease (e.g. diabetes, thyrotoxicosis, myxoedema)
Any serious systemic disorder (e.g. mononucleosis, hepatitis)
Neuromuscular, musculoskeletal or rheumatoid disorders exacerbated by exercise
Marked (gross) obesity
Idiopathic long-QT syndrome

Adapted from ACSM (2000), Dinan (2001), Rogers (2005).

- which goals are realistic/achievable for that individual
- the selection and combination of exercises that address their needs
- the most meaningful feedback approach for that individual if an onward referral to a medical or therapy professional is necessary.

Assessment also provides the opportunity to promote and document the benefits of the physical activity programme and the expertise available and to introduce a few of the key exercises to assist safety and familiarization (Dinan et al 2006, Jones & Rikli 2005). Unfortunately, this assessment session is often little more than an unsupervised completion of a health screening tool, which fails to collect the functional, motivational, social and personal information essential to tailoring the prescription.

Written informed consent must be obtained from each participant to take part in the pre-exercise screening and assessment as well as in the exercise programme (ACSM 2000, Rogers 2005). All information must be stored securely.

Being able to select, administer and interpret appropriate tests/assessment is a necessary skill for all physical instructors of older adults (Cress et al 2005, Jones & Rikli 2005, Zhu & Chodzko-Zajko 2006).

No single assessment tool can measure all factors related to disease and disabilities, physical limitations, balance and mobility problems and falls risks (Close et al 2005, Jones & Rikli 2005).

Assessment of ability to exercise

A common concern when assessing older people for participation in a physical activity or exercise programme is whether or not a medical evaluation is needed (e.g. exercise treadmill testing to assess for the likelihood of adverse cardiac events) (Jones et al 2005, Ory et al 2005) (Table 6.4). For older people with no active cardiopulmonary symptoms embarking on a moderate-intensity programme (as opposed to a vigorous one that causes the person to breathe hard and sweat profusely), formal testing is generally not necessary and is not supported by the current evidence (ACSM 1998, Buchner & Coleman 1994, Gill et al 2000, Heath 1988, Jones et al 2005, Ory et al 2005). It can also deter participation by portraying exercise as potentially hazardous when the opposite message needs to be conveyed. Formal instruments have been developed to identify if further cardiorespiratory testing and ongoing physician monitoring is advisable. The Physical Activity Readiness Questionnaire (PAR-Q) has been adapted for older people (Thomas et al 1992).

The ACSM guidelines on 'Contraindications to exercise testing' and 'Exercise participation without medical clearance from the person's physician' have both been extended to include medical considerations specific to older people (Table 6.4).

If further cardiorespiratory testing is advised, the following special considerations should be taken into account (ACSM 2000):

- For those with expected low work capacities, the initial workload should be low (2–3 METs) and increments should be small (0.5–1 METs) – the Naughton protocol.
- A cycle ergometer may be preferable to a treadmill for those with poor balance, coordination, vision, gait patterns, weight-bearing ability or foot problems. If there is no cycle ergometer, it may be necessary to add handrail support to the treadmill handrail support, but this will impact on accuracy of measurement of peak workload.
- For those who have difficulty adjusting to the exercise equipment, the initial stage may need to be extended, the test restarted or the test repeated.
- Exercise-induced arrhythmias are more frequent in older people than in other age groups.
- Prescribed medications may impact on exercise electrocardiographic and haemodynamic responses.

Despite this long list of special considerations, the criteria for exercise test termination in older people are no different to those in the younger age groups (ACSM 2000, Heath 1988).

Older people with impaired balance or mobility at high risk for falls, but no specific cardiorespiratory risk factors, will benefit from an evaluation by a physiotherapist or occupational therapist prior to initiating a programme of regular physical activity.

Assessment of physical activity

Physically inactive older adults can be identified in many ways (Jørstad-Stein et al 2005). Indeed, the assessment of physical activity can be considered an additional vital sign for all older people, irrespective of health or functional status. For example, PASE, or the Physical Activity Scale for the Elderly, measures total leisure and work activity through a weighted scoring of hours per activity in the previous 7 days (Washburn et al 1993). PACE, or Physician-based Assessment and Counseling for Exercise, measures attitudes and behaviours related to physical activity (Norris et al 2000). The 7-day recall physical activity questionnaire is considered more appropriate for older people (Hayden-Wade et al 2003).

Although no questionnaire on physical activity is going to be as accurate as the use of body-fixed sensors (Jørstad-Stein et al 2005), it is highly unlikely that you will have access to or be able to fund these kinds of objective physical activity measures. The minimum assessment of physical activity should be a history of participation in sport or recreational activities and current activity preferences and dislikes.

Assessment of functional ability

There are literally hundreds of possible functional tests that can be administered with older people (Jones & Rikli 2005). The choice of test depends on the fitness and functional ability of the individual (e.g. a shuttle test is not appropriate for a frail person living in a nursing setting) and whether that test is appropriate to the outcomes of the exercise programme (e.g. a single sit-to-stand is not appropriate if you are interested in seeing the effects of the programme on endurance). It is also important to choose a test that has been validated and has normative values available in the same population group and age (Jarnlo 2003, Jones & Rikli 2005) and to remember that older people are not a homogeneous group so it is unwise to assume that a person of a certain age will always have certain abilities (ACSM 2000).

The Functional Fitness Framework (Jones & Rikli 2005) identifies the physical fitness parameters associated with functional mobility and can be used as a guide in selecting appropriate assessment tools. The Senior Fitness Test (SFT) has seven functional tests and is practical and relevant for older people with a wide range of physical abilities (Rikli & Jones 2001). It consists of the following tests: 30-second chair stand, arm curl, 6-minute walk, 2-minute step, chair sit and reach, back scratch and 8 foot up and go (Rikli & Jones 2001). The Fullerton Advanced Balance (FAB) Scale is a newly developed test to measure multiple dimensions of balance in different sensory environments (Jones & Rikli 2005, Rose 2003). Both the SFT and the FAB have normative values for older people aged 60 to 95 years of age.

If you are working with older adults living in nursing settings, it is highly unlikely that they will be able to perform many functional tests without getting unduly fatigued; therefore consideration must be given to picking one or two tests that reflect the outcomes you are working to improve. If the aim of your programme is to reduce falls risk then the timed up and go or the 180° turn are the two recommended tests (Jarnlo 2003).

EVIDENCE–BASED GUIDANCE ON EXERCISE TRAINING FOR OLDER PEOPLE

Programming adaptations for older people have to consider an extreme distribution that ranges from elite athletic masters accomplishments at one end to physical disability and dysfunction at the other. The general principles of exercise prescription apply to adults of all ages; however, as with the assessment process, older adults will require subtle differences or 'adaptations' in protocol and dosage of exercise prescription (ACSM 2000). Special consideration in order to minimize medical problems and meet the range of fitness and functional levels of this diverse continuum (Dinan 2001). The focus here is on health-related exercise rather than sports performance as, at advanced ages, the emphasis shifts to the preservation of physical performance in activities of everyday life and to maintaining functional independence for as long as possible (Table 6.1) (Spirduso et al 1996). To respect the heterogeneity and assist compliance, whilst aiming high and observing the current exercise prescription guidelines, optimal training for older people needs to shift away from the purely physiological parameters appropriate for younger participants and older athletes towards programmes that emphasize functional relevance, minimum levels of effort, choice of modalities and opportunities to socialize (Dinan 2001).

Exercise guidelines for older people

In the last decade, the remarkable growth in the literature on physical activity and exercise prescription in older people has led to the publication of a number of best practice guidelines and expert texts on the programming of exercise both for relatively healthy older people wishing to engage in regular moderate to vigorous physical activity (AARP 2001, ACSM 1998, 2000, Ecclestone & Jones 2004, Evans 1999, Jones & Rose 2005, NIA 1998, Rose 2003) and for vulnerable older people (Dinan 2001, Mazzeo et al 2000). All emphasize the need to conscientiously adapt exercise for all older individuals in line with the evidence and published guidelines or where insufficient evidence exists, with expert best practice recommendations. All also endorse the importance of specialist training for physical activity instructors of older people (AARP 2001, ACSM 1998, 2000, Ecclestone & Jones 2004, Jones & Clark 1998, Jones & Rose 2005, NIA 1998, WHO 1997). The initial ACSM (1998) primarily health-promotion-based guideline focused on the message that regular exercise and physical activity can improve functional capacity and health and lead to greater independence and quality of life for older adults but had little guidance on how best to programme exercise variables such as frequency and duration. Increasing evidence about specificity, progressive overload, monitoring and motivational strategies has informed more prescriptive guidance on exercise testing and programming (ACSM 1998, 2000, NIA 1998) (Table 6.5).

The ACSM guidelines (1998, 2000) include the following:

- older adults should accumulate at least 30 minutes of moderate-intensity exercise (such as brisk walking and heavy gardening) on most, and preferably all, days of the week

Table 6.5 Exercise prescription for the older person

Fitness component	Type	Modality	Frequency	Intensity	Duration (minutes per session)	Special considerations

Flexibility	• Static[A,B,D,F]
	• Passive[D,F]
	• Dynamic (slow controlled)[D,E]
	• Functionally relevant stretching activities[A,D,E]
		• Integrated into endurance/strength training[A,B,D,F]
		• Flexibility programme[A,D,F]
		• Tai chi and yoga[A]
		• Bed/plinth/chair/seated/floor[D,F]
		• Daily active lifestyle activities
		  – reaching up the wall
		  – reaching into a cupboard
		  – stepping onto a high step (bus)
			• Daily[B,D,F]
			• 3–7[B,D,F]
			• 2–3[A]
				• 'Soft exercise'[F]
				• Maintenance 8–10 seconds[D,E,F]
				• Developmental 10–30 seconds[A,B,E,F]
				  10–90 seconds[D]
				• ×4 reps[A]
				• ×1[A,B,D,F] maintenance of all main muscle groups
				• ×1–4 developmental of appropriate muscles (e.g. adductors, hamstring) and/ or targeted joint complexes[A,D,E,F]
					• Approx 10–15 minutes (i.e. long enough to exercise the major muscle/tendon groups)[A,D,F]
					• An entire session may be appropriate for older beginners[A,D,F]
						• After endurance and strength training[B,D,F] or warm-up[A,B,D,F]
						• Include as part of warm-up (maintenance only) and as part of a cool-down[A,B,D,F] (maintenance and developmental)
						• If time limited ensure stretch all major muscles 8–10 seconds once; if flexibility training then multiple reps etc.[D,F]
						• Use chair or wall for support to reduce balance problems that compromise stretch[F]
						• Tailor type, repetitions, limb angle to individual[D,F]
						• Ensure alignment before and during stretch[D,F]
						• Ease slowly and gradually into and out of stretch[A,D,E]
						• Stretch to point of mild tension but not pain[D,F]
						• Do not bounce or force stretch[D,F]
						• Inhale at start, exhale as move into and breathe regularly on hold[D,F]
						• Include slow controlled moving/ dynamic stretches in warm-up and especially for people with poor body awareness[D,F]
						• Static only: in people with arthritis or severe adaptive shortening around joint[D,F]
						• For comfort, ensure long thick, light mats and pillows for neck support[F]

Muscular strength						

• Isotonic[A-H]
• Controlled (5-6 seconds) Isometric[A,C,E]
• Closed (and open) chain[A,D,E,F]
• Functionally relevant strength activities[D,E,F]
	• Resistance bands[D,E,F]
	• Velcro ankle/wrist weights[D,E,F]
	• Free weights[D,E,F]
	• Fixed machines[D,E,F]
	• Floor work/standing/sitting[D,E,F]
	• Resistance balls/tennis balls[D,F]/Parachutes etc.[F]
	• Sit-to-stand, lifting, carrying[D,F]
		• 2-3[A-H]
		• 48 hours between sessions (48-72 hours for beginners,[A,B,D,E,F] for advanced 24 hours recovery between some muscle groups or 'split' workout where schedule different muscle groups on different consecutive days[B,D,E,F])
			• ×8-10 exercises using all major muscle groups[A,B,D,E,F]
			• ×10-15 reps[A,D,E,F] @ 45/50% of 1-RM[D,F]
			• RPE 12-13 (somewhat hard; 3-4 (moderate)- Borg CEtCR scales)[A,B,D,F] (Advanced only: ×6-8 reps @60%/80% of 1-RM = RPE 14-15 (hard); 4-5 (strong))
			• ×1 set training; build to 2 and maximum of 3 sets[A,E,F]
			• To fatigue not to failure[A,D,E,F]
			• Progressive
			  %1-RM Reps
			  65% 14-15
			  70% 12-13
			  75% 10-11
			  80% 8-9[D,E,F]
			• Speed: 6-9 seconds per rep; rest: 1-3 seconds between reps (hard)[D,E,F]
			• Peak strain to target hold at peak of contraction to target bone[F]
				• 20-30[A,B,D-F]
				• NB sessions lasting longer than 60 minutes may have a detrimental effect on exercise adherence
					• Major goal = life related = strength, endurance/power[A-H]
					• Individualization of prescription is essential[A,D,E,F]
					• Increase repetitions before increase resistance (i.e. when 15 reps or more)[A,E,F]
					• When returning from a lay-off start with 50% or less of previous prescription and progress gradually[A,E,F]
					• Close supervision by trained specialist older person instructors[A,B,D,E,F]
					• Exercise order – exercises using larger muscle groups at beginning; (multi-joint) single joint or isolated muscle action (e.g. biceps) at end[A]
					• Multi-joint versus single joint exercises the priority[A,D,E,F]
					• Do not exercise same muscle groups on two consecutive days[A,B,D,E,F]
					• One set training initially reduces fatigue and likelihood of muscle soreness[A,E,F]
					• First 8 weeks minimal resistance to allow for connective tissue adaptation[A,D,E,F]
					• Bone load by targeting fracture sites, wrist, spine, hip
					• Utilize controlled isometric work and peak strain (limit hold to 5-6 seconds)[A,F]
					• Emphasize normal, even breathing pattern
					• Teach 'strict form' and programming and progression techniques so all major muscle exercises are included[D,E,F]
					• Emphasize controlled speed on lifting and lowering phase[D,E,F]

(Continued)

Table 6.5 Exercise prescription for the older person—Cont'd

Fitness component	Type	Modality	Frequency	Intensity	Duration (minutes per session)	Special considerations
Muscular strength—Cont'd						• Do not do ballistic movements[D,E,F] • Perform in a 'pain-free arc' or maximum natural range of motion[D,E,F] • Whenever possible, use fixed machines as less skill needed, greater back stability, lower baseline, smaller increments of progression, increased range of movement control[A,D,E,F] • Arthritic patients should begin with isometric work to minimize joint tension[A,F] • Contraindications to resistance training (at any age): uncontrolled angina, uncontrolled hypertension or arrhythmia, abnormal haemodynamic responses during exercise, acute orthopaedic condition, acute systemic condition[A,D,E,F] • For frailer or osteoporotic patients avoid any resisted retraction of shoulder girdle and resisted spinal flexion[A,E,F] • Emphasize benefits of all-year-round resistance training[A-G]
Cardiorespiratory fitness	• Aerobic endurance exercise[A,B,C,D,F,G,H] • Continuous rhythmic large muscle group activity that can be maintained for a prolonged period[F,G]	• Brisk walking, swimming, aqua exercise, cycling, jogging ergometers, rowing etc., continuous dancing[A,F,G] • Active lifestyle options: gardening/yard work (raking leaves), housework, climbing	• 5–7 most days[*A,B,C,G,F] • 3 (alternating no exercise and exercise days)[A,B]	• Moderate 40–75% $\dot{V}O_2$max (initially 40–50% building to 75% and advanced vigorous to 85%) RPE 12–14 (Borg 6–20) 3–4 (Borg 0–10) (initially 9–11 building to 11–12 and advanced 12–14)[A,G] • Initial workload should be low (2–3 METs) and	• 30 (×3 of 10 minutes) for health benefits[A,B,G] • longer duration (up to 60 minutes) offers additional health and fitness benefits[A,B,G]	Ensure • Start low and progress duration before intensity (for safety and injury prevention)[A,B,C,G,H] • Progress in small increments of duration and intensity[A,B,G,H] • Low to medium impact[A,B,G,H] • Utilize interval conditioning prior to continuous[G,F] • Avoid moves with high falls risks[D,F]

- Interval conditioning (a higher-intensity cardiorespiratory interval followed by a lower active recovery interval)[F,G]
- Continuous conditioning
- Functionally relevant active lifestyle activities[A,B,C,F,G,I]
- Low-medium impact to avoid orthopaedic problems[A,F,G,I]

stairs and active recreational pursuits (e.g. bowling)[A,F,G]

increments small (0.5-1.0 METs)
- METs – age categorization 'rough' guide:
  - 'Athletic old' 55+ = VO_2max = 10 METs
  - 'Young old' 55-75 = VO_2max = 6-7 METs
  - 'Old old' 75+ = 2-3 METs[H]

- Transitions between activities should be active low intensity, and longer than with younger people[F]
- Longer, more gradual aerobic curve build-up and endurance cool-down[A,B,F]
- Longer duration can increase cardiovascular/musculoskeletal risks and reduce compliance[A,B,H]
- Shorter duration 10-minute periods can increase compliance and exercise tolerance[F]
- Many older people have one or more medical conditions and are more likely to be on medications that can influence peak heart rate response[A-H]
- Progress according to individual tolerance and preference to minimize medical problems and promote compliance[A-H]
- Including controlled changes of pace, level, direction, e.g. side steps, forward movements and arm movements, can also increase endurance, intensity and balance gains[F]
- Simple, few repetitive moves[F]
- NB: A measured peak heart rate (HR) is preferable to an age-predicted peak HR when prescribing aerobic exercise for 65+ because of the variability in peak HR and increased risk of coronary artery disease – % of peak HR may provide more accurate estimate of % of peak VO_2 than the HR reserve method when calculating a target HR range[A,F,G,H]

(Continued)

Table 6.5 Exercise prescription for the older person—Cont'd

Fitness component	Type	Modality	Frequency	Intensity	Duration (minutes per session)	Special considerations
Balance and agility training	• Dynamic balance – prescriptive ways of transferring bodyweight between different points of support[D,F] • Integrated dynamic balance[A,B,F] • Functional, relevant 'applied', integrated dynamic balance[D,F] • Sensory integration and organization activities[D] • Proprioceptive visual, aural tasks[D,F]	• Falls prevention = – general exercise for the older person session – adapted tai chi[D,F] – Falls management = – specific balance (and strength) exercises[D,F] – Integrated balance training – endurance session with walking and stepping patterns[D,F] – dance, adapted tai chi[D,F] – floor work, functional floor activities[F] – balance circuits/obstacle course[D,F] – ball games etc.[D,F]	• 3[B,D,F]	• Degree of support (two hands, one, one finger, no hands etc.)[D,F] • No of steps (reps) and sets[D,F] • Different paces, levels, surfaces, obstacles[D,F] • Carrying different objects[D,F] • Catching and throwing etc. • Increased multi-tasking – number and complexity of tasks[D,F] • Floor work – transfer down to and up from the floor, rolling, crawling[F] • Balancing on uneven, unfamiliar surface, e.g. foam blocks etc.[D,F]	• 30 (i.e. integrated strength and balance)[D,F]	Considerations • In 'static' dynamic balance exercises increase the duration before decreasing the support[F] • In travelling dynamic balance exercises increase the number of steps before decreasing the support[F] • Add balance training as part of lower body strengthening (e.g. toe walks/heel walks)[B,D,F] • Introduce all sensory-specific tasks as single stimulus tasks[D] • Introduce all complex movement skills (e.g. getting down to and up from floor) as single step-by-step links in the movement chain[D,F] • Ensure each link in the chain is mastered competently and confidently before moving on to the next stage or link (backward chaining approach)[D,F] • Poor balance is closely associated with fear of falling and loss of confidence. Ensuring a step-by-step approach, close observation, praise and encouragement is essential[D,F] • Improved balance and strength can result in over-confidence and increased risk taking and increase risk. Therefore ensure postural stability is sufficient before the sensory and social tasks, e.g. ball games[F]

Key: A, ACSM (1998, 2000); B, IIA (1998); C, WHO (1997); D, Rose (2003); E, Kraemer & French (2005); F, Skelton & Dinan (1999), Dinan et al (2004), Dinan & Skelton 2007; G, Brooks (1997); H, Smith (1984).

- additional benefits can be obtained by performing higher-intensity exercise (after discussing this with a physician)
- for strength and muscular endurance gains, older adults need to do resistance training at least twice per week (with at least 48 hours of rest between sessions)
- to maintain flexibility and improve balance and agility older adults need to ensure they have a well-rounded programme that includes stretching at least two to three days of the week; tai chi and yoga are suggested as useful ways of obtaining these particular benefits.

Today, with the benefit of further evidence we can be more specific in relation to balance and tai chi. These have been included in the best practice guidelines summary, Table 6.5.

The NIA (National Institute on Ageing) guidelines (1998) included more specific detail for practitioners, especially on balance training. Illustrations and instruction for specific exercises were also included. It recommended:

- gradually progressing to at least 30 minutes of endurance exercise on most, or preferably all, days of the week and that the 30-minute goal can be accomplished by accumulating time in shorter 10-minute sessions or 'activity snacks'
- for advanced exercisers, 24 hours between sessions was sufficient provided that the same muscle groups are not exercised on two consecutive days
- balance training components should be added progressively as part of the lower body strengthening programme and additional balance exercises (e.g. standing on one leg) can be done any time
- stretching exercises should only be done after endurance and strength training, or after warming up – 3 to 7 days per week for those not participating in other types of exercise.

Importantly, both these guidelines emphasize the need for individualization in relation to cardiorespiratory endurance and resistance training programmes and for pre-exercise and ongoing health and risk assessment and exercise prescription. Both also promote the benefits of additional information on clinical status and functional capacity (ACSM 1998, 2000, NIA 1998).

Best practice begins with the conscientious observance of these guidelines for all older participants, with further specific adaptations being made to session aims, structure, content, programming and teaching methods (Dinan 2001).

Injury prevention

Injury prevention is a high priority. Even stiffness and minor overuse injuries reduce enjoyment, may affect compliance and everyday function, and can be avoided. The design of the session, supervision and monitoring of performance, together with education and guidance of participants can substantially reduce hazards. Overuse or 'too much too soon' injuries are not uncommon in older participants (Carroll et al 1992, Pollock et al 1991, 1997). The risk of an event, an accident or an exacerbation of an existing joint condition can be controlled by ensuring biomechanically sound positions, cautious training loads and by introducing exercises one by one around affected joint(s). All activities must avoid undue spinal stress or disc compression (e.g. sit ups or other exercises that cause spinal loading in flexion (Dinan 2001, Sinaki 1982)); moves with high falls risk (turns of more than 90° or exercises involving lateral movement of one leg across the other (Skelton & Dinan 1999)); and uncontrolled isometric contraction (Bell 2001). Older people with muscular weakness, particularly those with a history of joint, muscular or connective tissue damage caused by overuse injury or disease, should use an especially conservative training load initially with predominantly controlled isometric work at first and then progression to light isotonic work loads (Ettinger et al 1997). Wearing hip protectors during exercise reduces the risk of a hip fracture if a fall does occur and improves both self-efficacy in the participant and confidence in the instructor (Skelton & Dinan 1999). Balance training should be progressed cautiously in frailer older adults, first by increasing the number of repetitions, then decreasing the support (e.g. chair support to no support, bipedal to unipedal base of support, increasing the difficulty of the surface etc.) (Rose 2003, Skelton & Dinan 1999), whilst being aware of potential hazards of asymmetry in lower limb strength and power (Skelton et al 2002) (Table 6.5). Particular care during transitions between exercises and components, particularly floor work transfers, is also necessary (Dinan 2001, Skelton & Dinan 1999).

Specificity

In defining cardiorespiratory overload, the first step is to identify the right type of activity. For a significant training effect, it is essential to select activities that sustain a large volume of venous return. When designing for senior participants, endurance training should be multipurpose. It must have energy-source specificity (aerobic and anaerobic) and everyday life specificity. A combination of walking, stationary cycling, swimming and/or water-fitness will meet most of the criteria for most seniors (Dinan et al 2004, Young & Dinan 2005) (Table 6.5). The combination of activities is as important as the selection in terms of safety, function and adherence.

The type of training approach is also important for successful energy source outcomes for older people. Cardiovascular training can be continuous or it can utilize an adapted interval training approach (i.e. interval conditioning) (Bompa 1999). Although both types have a role to play in long-term cardiorespiratory programming, interval conditioning is recommended as the initial and core approach, because it is the most effective way of achieving overload and meeting functional fitness needs. Everyday tasks such as quickening our pace to catch a bus or climbing a hill during a walk to the shops, and leisure activities such as timed swimming, are examples of 'interval' demands placed on the body during any given day or exercise session. They all involve an effort interval where the work rate is a little harder than 'steady state' or what is comfortable, followed by a moderate recovery interval or time period where activity returns to this comfortable, easily sustained level of effort (Brooks 1997). The physiological benefits of interval conditioning (1–6 minutes) and continuous training (6 minutes or longer of uninterrupted activity, usually performed at a constant submaximal intensity) are similar (Ahmaidi et al 1998, Brooks 1997, Haskell 1997, Shephard, 1991). However, the advantage of interval conditioning is that at any age, the stimulus to physiological change is greater, as the total *volume* of work is greater than when the same intensity of exercise is continuous (Brooks 1997, De Busk et al 1990). This enables the older person to meet the generally lower anaerobic thresholds and to work harder with greater comfort for up to three times longer (Bompa 1999, Dinan et al 2004, Malbut et al 2002, Vogiatzis et al 2002).

In strength training, a wide range of types of activity and equipment is needed to ensure that specificity is met and there are improvements in strength, power, size of muscle, functional strength and quality of life (Dinan 2001, Kraemer & French 2005, Pollock et al 2000). An eclectic mix of resistance bands, free weights, Velcro ankle and wrist weights, fixed resistance machines and bodyweight, cans of food or even parachutes can be utilized to ensure both progression of resistance and functional specificity (e.g. sit-to-stands) that will enable better function in everyday life (Table 6.5).

As noted earlier, resistance training alone, without functional training, does not improve everyday function (Skelton et al 1995, Skelton & McLaughlin 1996). The linear movements of traditional weight training machines are not sufficient to address the more three-dimensional, functional everyday movement patterns that involve acceleration, deceleration and stabilization of joint structures and it is the stabilizer muscles, not the mobilizers, that limit functional strength. In order to improve transfer from and to the floor, this must be practised in the training session in order to retrain the movement pattern and also must be combined with strengthening exercises for the core muscles of the spine, pelvis and scapula (Dinan 2001, Kraemer & French 2005, Skelton & Dinan 1999). For power training, current research suggests including some higher velocity but non-ballistic movements with multiple and single joint exercises (Table 6.5). The recommended type of strength training approach for older people is periodization (the systematic alteration of the training variables of volume and intensity over time to create variation in the physiological stresses, to optimize the training stimulus). Periodization closely mimics the demands of everyday life and is the most functionally relevant approach to strength training (Dinan & Skelton 2007, Fleck & Kraemer 2004, Kraemer & French 2005).

Effective balance training needs to target the multiple sensory dimensions of balance, altering task demands for motor system improvements and environmental demands for sensory improvements (Rose 2003, Skelton & Dinan 1999). Guidelines on the types of exercise and approach for the specificity and overload for balance and flexibility training are given in Table 6.5.

Progressive overload

Overload is influenced most strongly by the type of exercise and then further defined by frequency, intensity and duration, modes of exercise and approaches to training.

Everyday tasks, such as dressing, require as much as 50–75% of a frail 80-year-old woman's VO_2max (Fig. 6.2A) (Malbut et al 2002, Saltin 1980, Young 1986); therefore, endurance overload may initially be as little as a 3-minute walk. To maintain improvements, overload must be progressive in nature but, for safety with older participants, must be progressed gradually and cautiously. Recommendations include always allowing a minimum of 3 weeks for adaptation before progressing the overload, progressing duration first and always in 1-minute increments as tolerated (Bell 2001) and progressing intensity by increasing resistance (e.g. incline of treadmill, hill, cycle or resistance and skill, e.g. carrying objects) rather than speed (ACSM 2000).

In practice, with beginners of all ages, most particularly with frailer older participants, it is recommended that resistance training begins with local muscular endurance training to allow time to master the technique of each exercise and feel confident and competent in performing it and then progresses steadily and cautiously up through the recommended strength training ranges. It is important to remember that strength training will maintain local muscular endurance gains but local muscular endurance training alone will not bring the crucial muscle mass, strength and force changes of strength training (Table 6.5) (Fleck & Kramer 2004, Kraemer & French 2005). In people with clinically significant arthritis and those with osteoporosis, progression of resistance training must be slow and cautious (Dinan 2001, Ettinger et al 1997). Where resistance training with vulnerable, older patients is concerned, avoidance of isometric work held for over 5 seconds is preferred (Haskell 1997). Recent studies have reported similar cardiovascular and haemodynamic responses to resistance training in patients both with and without coronary artery disease and indicate that myocardial perfusion may even be enhanced due to the increase in diastolic pressure (Squires et al 1991). Caution must be taken, how-ever, to avoid the risk of rapid rises in systolic and diastolic blood pressure associated with prolonged high-intensity isometric work (Bell et al 1995, Bell 2001, Fleck & Kramer 2004, Kraemer & French 2005). When utilizing isometric (static) work, to achieve a targeted strength gain in specific muscle groups, a moderate workload should be used and each contraction should be held for a maximum of 3–4 seconds (Bell 2001). For patients with hypertension, coronary artery disease or peripheral vascular disease, this would be adapted even further. There is, however, no evidence that brief bouts of moderate-intensity static exercise of 5–10 seconds duration significantly increases the risk of a clinical event in older people (Haskell 1997).

Whatever the type of resistance training or mode selected, the criteria must be that the exerciser can control the movement through the fullest possible range. On some fixed-weight machines, even the lightest resistance is too great and some participants are unable to produce the initial forces to start the movement and the incremental progressions are too large to allow smooth, safe progression. Resistance bands can overcome some of the initial problems, provide easier initiation of movement and, for frailer adults unwilling to travel, may be the only practical and acceptable starting point in some settings (Skelton et al 1996).

Adaptations to session structure

Warm-up and cool-down

For all older participants, sessions should start and finish gradually, providing safe transition to, and adequate recovery from, more vigorous exercise. The warm-up period should be longer than for younger adults (15–20 minutes), gradually pro-gressed in intensity, to safely improve the efficiency of the cardiovascular response and help to prevent ischaemic ST segment changes, arrhythmias, a reduction in left ventricular ejection function and other cardiovascular irregularities commonly brought on by sudden strenuous exercise (ACSM 2000, Bell 2001, Haskell 1997, Malbut et al 2002). Additional advantages of extended warm-up are that it improves blood saturation to, and elasticity in, the muscles, tendons and ligaments, decreases viscosity of the muscles, improves mechanical efficiency and helps prevent musculo-skeletal injuries – all considerations which are more important with age (Haskell 1997).

The long, gradual continuous cool-down (a warm-up in reverse) is recommended to preserve venous return and safely decrease heart rate, respiration and catechol-amine levels (Shephard 1997), allow muscle and skin vasodilatation to return to rest-ing levels (Dinan 2001) and help prevent the dizziness and cardiac-related irregularities which are more common in older people (Haskell 1997) and other high risk populations (Bell 2001).

Monitoring exercise intensity

The most common method of prescribing and monitoring exercise intensity is by target-ing a training heart rate, established as a percentage of either maximal heart rate (HRmax) or heart rate reserve (HRR, defined as maximal heart rate minus resting heart rate). Both of these methods have certain disadvantages, unless a true measure of HRmax has been obtained. Estimates of HRmax and HRR are particularly unreliable in older people (Cooper et al 1977). But maximal tests on older individuals, and/or indi-viduals with risk factors, should only be performed with medical supervision and are, therefore, inappropriate for older people (Kallinen et al 2006). During exercise, the majority older people must slow down or stop exercising in order to take their heart rate and, even then, heart rates self measured by palpitation are inaccurate (Bell 2001). Also HRR may represent a higher percentage of $\dot{V}O_2$max than expected, so using HRR may result in the older person working at a higher intensity than desired (Dinan et al 2004). The use of medications that may affect heart rate response is common and use of heart rate measures can cause concern and even reinforce ideas that exercise is high risk.

An alternative to using target heart rate to obtain the desired training intensity is the use of Borg's rating of perceived exertion (RPE) scale (Borg 1998), effective in both young and older people (Dinan et al 2004, Malbut et al 2002). This scale of self-perceived effort takes into account both central (e.g. heart rate and breathing) and local (e.g. muscle fatigue) sensations. It also does not require a slowing down or stopping of exercise.

A training intensity between 13 and 15 on the 6–20 RPE scale is approximately equivalent to working at 70–80% of $\dot{V}O_2$max and an RPE of 11–13 approximates to working at 49–70% of $\dot{V}O_2$max (ACSM 2000, Malbut et al 2002, Pollock et al 2000). According to the ACSM (1998, 2000) starting with an exercise intensity of 11–13 on the RPE scale and never exceeding a hard intensity (15 on the scale) appears to be most appropriate for sedentary older people. For a frailer older adult, a starting intensity of 9–11 may be preferable (Dinan 2001, Dinan et al 2004). It is essential that the instructor and participant understand what they are assessing and there is clear instruction in the use of the scales (Borg 1998).

The intensity of exercise can also be regulated by selecting activities based on known metabolic equivalent (MET) values. Some activities have a wide range of MET values (e.g. ballroom dancing 4–8 METs, aerobic dance 6–9 METs and skipping 8–12 METs), while others vary little (e.g. walking at normal pace 3–4 METs, cycling 5–6 METs). Ideally for the first 8–10 weeks of a programme, endurance activities should be of a type that is easy to perform and to monitor and can be maintained at a moderate intensity (Bell 2001). Smith's age classification guide raises awareness of the key real need for adaptation: athletic old 55+, $\dot{V}O_2$max = 10 METs; young old 55–75, $\dot{V}O_2$max = 6–7 METs; old old 75+, $\dot{V}O_2$max = 2–3 METs (Smith 1984).

Rest and recovery

It is crucial when planning an endurance programme for older people to systematically plan recovery periods between and within each component and between sessions (ACSM 1998, 2000). The use of interval training (Ahmaidi et al 1998, Brooks 1997) and alternating muscle groups is also recommended (Dinan 2001). A fartlek training approach (speed play) is utilized to accommodate the lower anaerobic thresholds found in older people. This allows participants to continue for longer without undue fatigue. Adequate recovery enhances the cardiorespiratory stimulus, improves performance, improves long-term commitment and, above all, prevents overuse injuries, fatigue (Bompa 1999, Fleck & Kramer 2004) and fatigue-related events such as falls (Dinan 2001). Strength training rests and recovery desirable in an older population are quite different to recommendations for a younger population (see Table 6.5).

Observation and interpretation

At any age, it is important not to rely on any single indicator of exertion levels during exercise. The instructor should be alert to the physical signs or symptoms that indicate deterioration in health, or the onset of a new condition and other 'triggers' that signal to the need to refer back to the medical setting for further investigation. It is important to be aware that the frailer the individual, the greater the fluctuation in day-to-day health, energy, mood and anxiety levels, and these may have an effect on general performance, postural stability and, therefore, safety and comfort during the session (Dinan & Skelton 2007).

Group versus home-based exercise programmes

Participation in a structured group exercise programme (e.g. at a healthcare facility or in a community senior centre) versus a home-based programme is a matter of personal preference. Comparable results can be achieved in either setting (Judge et al 2005, King et al 1991, Robertson et al 2001, Skelton et al 2005, Wallace et al 1998). The group setting, however, affords additional benefits by creating an environment for peer support, self-efficacy and increased socialization that can counteract the negative effects of social isolation and associated depression (Leveille et al 1998, Lorig et al 1999). Also, older people who exercise in a group setting may feel a greater sense of personal safety that may reduce fear of injury as a potential barrier to exercise. For those who prefer the convenience or privacy of a home-based programme, specific protocols have been developed that use resistance bands, light weights, stationary bicycles or common household objects such as a chair or a towel (Jette et al 1996, King et al 1991, Robertson et al 2001).

Motivation and adherence to exercise

Multiple studies have shown that physicians are an important source of motivation for people contemplating the initiation of a physical activity programme (Andersen et al 1997, Christmas & Andersen 2000, Damush et al 1999). Also there is increasing evidence that positive images of ageing can reverse the age-related declines in gait, with one trial showing that positive stereotypes of ageing have a powerful positive impact on the gait speed (9%) of older people (Hausdorff et al 1999).

There are multiple barriers to improving physical activity levels in older people (Finch 1997) (Table 6.6). These include intrinsic barriers such as: lack of knowledge or misperceptions about community physical activity programmes; fear of crime (mugging); fear of falling (Yardley & Smith 2003); fear of overexertion; not having someone to exercise with (spouse or friends may have died) (Finch 1997). Extrinsic barriers include weather that is not conducive to physical activity (e.g. excessive cold or heat); influence of significant others (Yardley et al 2006) such as a partner, family, peers, carer or health professional; ease of access to activities, safe streets and neighbourhoods (Finch 1997) (Table 6.6). Finally, myths and stereotypes about exercising in older age (no pain, no gain, etc.) are often cited (Finch 1997).

No single factor will predict whether or not an older person will start and sustain an exercise programme. Participation is determined and regulated by a range of factors, unique to the individual. For many older people this will be a significant change in lifestyle or an unfamiliar experience, and those with the poorest health and the most likely to visit their GP may be the most resistant to change (Chodzko-Zajko & Resnick 2004, Marcus & Forsyth 2003). Readiness to change may be significantly influenced by a referral from a health professional, often following the diagnosis of a chronic disease or following a significant life event such as a fall or heart attack or by individuals recognizing for themselves the tell-tale signs that they are losing function (e.g. having difficulty using the stairs or crossing the road). Exploring the individual's readiness

Table 6.6   Exercise barriers and motivators for older adults

Barriers to exercise	Motivators for exercise
Health and medical	**Health and medical**
○ Illness or injury	○ To feel good physically
○ Pain or discomfort	○ To improve overall health
○ Lack of strength or stamina	○ To reduce risk of disease
○ Fear of a medical event during exercise	○ To maintain or improve mobility
	○ To maintain activities of daily living
Knowledge	○ To reduce risk of falls
○ Lack of knowledge or ability	○ To improve fitness
Motivational or psychological	○ To improve strength
○ Lack of time	○ To reduce/manage bodyweight
○ Lack of self-motivation, low self-efficacy or confidence	○ For rehabilitation
	Mental health
○ Not a priority	○ To have more energy
○ Fear of injury	○ To reduce stress or anxiety
○ Exercise perceived as inappropriate, unnecessary or 'not for me'	○ To reduce depression
	○ To enjoy life more fully
○ Poor body image	○ To feel more confidence
○ Depression or anxiety	**Appearance–related**
○ Lack of support from family, peers, health professionals	○ To maintain/improve appearance
	○ To reduce/manage bodyweight
Programme–related	**Social**
○ Lack of appropriate classes/activities	○ For social contact/interaction
○ Intensity too high/too low	○ Encouragement by family/friends
○ Inconvenient times of sessions	**Other**
○ Programme cost	○ For enjoyment of activity
○ Travel to session (availability, cost and fear of travelling alone)	○ For competition/personal challenge
	○ Recommendation of health professional
Environmental	○ Feel it is appropriate for them
○ Poor weather conditions	

Adapted from Finch (1997), Jones & Rose (2005), Yardley et al (2006).

to change will reveal positive and negative behaviour attitudes towards participation and will determine the strategies to use when setting and agreeing realistic and meaningful goals (Chodzko-Zajko & Resnick 2004, King et al 1998).

Exercise self-efficacy, or confidence in one's ability to undertake regular exercise successfully (even when faced with difficulties), is a strong predictor of exercise adoption among older people (King et al 1998, Marcus & Forsyth 2003, Yardley et al 2006).

Dispelling myths and stereotypes

There are five common myths and stereotypes about physical activity and ageing that need to be dispelled (Jones & Rose 2005). These are described below with reminders on how to assist older people dispel them.

- You have to be healthy to exercise – find appropriate role models of people with chronic disease who have had improvements to their quality of life with exercise.
- I'm too old to start exercising – use appropriate images to show that age is not a barrier to physical activity.
- You need special equipment and clothing – apart from comfortable shoes and loose-fitting clothing there is no special clothing or equipment. However, cultural and generational factors have to be taken into consideration.
- No pain, no gain – reinforce the notion that vigorous exercise is no longer recommended and that moderate physical activity can be easily incorporated into daily life.
- I'm too busy to exercise – help identify opportunities within their schedule.

Induction

An appropriately designed induction session which provides information and reassurance about the level of physical activity, clothing, safety and how the programme is designed to meet individual needs and goals will assist in overcoming many of the concerns a new participant may have. Programme factors (Jones & Rose 2005) cited as motivating amongst older people taking part in group activities include: the mode of exercise, the interpersonal skills and expertise of the instructor and social support from peers (King et al 1998, Stewart et al 2006).

Support strategies

There needs to be a greater emphasis on scheduling, funding and training. Support strategies (e.g. social support from family, peers and other exercisers within a group and professional instructor support), including regular telephone contact to monitor progress, together with regular review of programme goals, are known to improve adherence (Hillsdon et al 2005). A 'relapse' to sedentary behaviour can be avoided by prevention strategies that anticipate high risk of drop-out situations and the understanding that short lapses are normal behaviour (Chodzko-Zajko & Resnick 2004). The importance of involvement of peer mentors in the adoption and maintenance of exercise amongst other older adults and of professional support in adherence to a home exercise programme cannot be underestimated (Robertson et al 2001, Stewart et al 2006).

A recent trial of primary care exercise referral for older adults showed that, with structured support strategies, including transport, it is possible to get high rates of uptake and adherence to exercise programmes even amongst frail older adults (Dinan et al 2006). In people aged 75 and over, 89% took up the exercise programme; 73% completed stage I and 63% made the transition to the community stage II programme (Dinan et al 2006).

Finally and importantly, designing and delivering exercise for older people requires specialist skills and training. Shephard (1991) emphasized that programming physical activity for older people requires more care and more expertise than for any other age group, with only a fine line separating effective from dangerous procedures. The recognition of the importance of specialist skills culminated in the publication and current implementation of the International Curriculum Guidelines for Physical Activity Instructors of Older People (Ecclestone & Jones 2004).

KEY POINTS

Man does not cease to play because he grows old.
Man grows old because he ceases to play.
(George Bernard Shaw)

1. Disease and sedentary behaviour accelerate the rate of ageing.
2. The only three interventions that have slowed the rate of ageing are calorie restriction, genetic manipulation and regular physical activity involving moderate amounts of physical exercise.
3. Life expectancy for both sexes and most countries has almost doubled from 40 to 80 years of age since the beginning of the 20th century. In contrast, lifespan has remained relatively stable and is limited to 85 years, with only 12% of the population exceeding that age.
4. This demographic shift to an older age structure is mainly a consequence of long-term downward trends in fertility.
5. Increased longevity has been accompanied by an increase in unhealthy, sedentary lifestyles, disease and morbidity.
6. There are three main theories of ageing: biological (genetic, damage and gradual imbalance), psychological (Maslow's hierarchy of needs, Erickson's stages of psychosocial development of personality and Baltes' optimization and selective compensation), and sociological (activity and continuity).
7. Active life expectancy is the number of years an individual may expect to maintain ADLs and IADLs.
8. Morbidity can be compressed by adopting a healthy lifestyle early in life.
9. The predictors of successful ageing include: physical and mental health, functional and social competence, productivity, personal control and life satisfaction; these are influenced by the interplay of: genetics, personal and social environment and support, and behaviour, attitudes and personality.
10. In all body systems it is difficult to distinguish between normal body ageing, the effects of age-related decreases in habitual physical activity and the pathology that develops with advancing years and chronic inactivity.
11. Age-related structural changes and effects in the cardiorespiratory system include: increased thickening of the blood vessel and left ventricular walls, increased arterial stiffness, reduced elasticity (greater cross-linkage between the collagen molecules), increased systolic and diastolic blood pressures (aorta thickening and hardening, increased total peripheral resistance), increased hypertrophy and hyporesponsiveness of the heart and vasculature to sympathetic stimulation. Heart rates remain higher and recover more slowly after maximal exertion; postural hypotension increases and appears to be related most closely to high systolic blood pressure.
12. Although cardiac function in most older adults is adequate at rest and for submaximal activities: heart rate, stroke volume and therefore, cardiac output, is reduced. $\dot{V}O_2$max declines at about 10–15% per year after age 25, but the decline is much less in active individuals with many older exercisers having a higher $\dot{V}O_2$max than sedentary 20-year-olds.
13. Age-related structural changes in the respiratory system include: a reduction in elastic tissue content (and hence elastic recoil) of the lungs, a decrease in some volumes and capacities (particularly FEV), increased chest wall stiffness,

decreased strength of the respiratory muscles and decreased sensitivity of the respiratory centres in the nervous system.

14. Pulmonary function is satisfactory in healthy older individuals under resting and moderate exercise conditions. The limiting factor in maximal work is the decreased cardiac output.

15. Structural and functional deterioration in the cardiorespiratory systems is attributable to disease rather than the ageing process. Habitual exercise both prevents and remediates cardiovascular disease, hypertension and diabetes and postpones many characteristics of ageing in the cardiovascular and respiratory systems.

16. The capacity of the cardiorespiratory system to adapt to an endurance training load is not affected by age, with similar percentage increases in $\dot{V}O_2$max being reported for young and old adults.

17. Combined strength and aerobic training, and strength training alone, are as effective as aerobic training alone at improving $\dot{V}O_2$max in older participants.

18. The age-related structural changes to the muscular system include: reduction in muscle mass; size and number of muscle fibres (with greater atrophy and greater mitochondrial dysfunction in type II fibres); changes in muscle architecture and tendon mechanical properties; strength losses are also due to loss of total number of motor units and a larger innervation ratio (number of muscle cells per motor neuron) in the remaining units.

19. Strength and power declines from 30 years by 10–15% per decade and accelerates after 60 years with power declining more rapidly than strength due to the selective type II fibre loss. Isometric and eccentric strength declines less than concentric. Men and women experience similar losses though women show fewer age-related declines in upper body strength.

20. Older muscle shows a normal response to training with improvements equivalent to 10–20 years' 'rejuvenation'; 8–12 weeks of training can reverse sarcopenia.

21. Functional ability and mobility is highly related to strength; however, strength improvements will only translate into improvements in daily function if functional training is combined with strength training.

22. Bone mass peaks between 20 and 40 years, and then declines at 0.5–1% per year, with an accelerated period of loss in women for 5–10 years after the start of the menopause (leading to a total loss of 25–30% cortical and 35–50% trabecular bone over this period); men lose at about two-thirds this rate. Bone strength depends not only on bone mass but also on bone quality (bone architecture, fatigue damage, bulk material properties).

23. Bone remains responsive to site- and load-specific training throughout the lifespan though the exercise modality needs to be more specific as we age, i.e. high-intensity weight training through intermittent jogging, exercise classes and WBV are effective even in postmenopausal women, but jumping is not.

24. The age-related structural changes in joints include: increased inter- and intramuscular connective tissue, less extensible connective tissue due to a change in chemical composition, and a breakdown of articular cartilage; the combined effect is stiffness and loss of ROM in all joints.

25. ROM and flexibility can be improved in older adults by a wide range of physical activities; frequency rather than type is key.

26. The age-related structural changes in the nervous system include: decline in number of nerve cells, connective networks in, and weight of, the brain, preferential loss of distal, large, myelinated sensory fibres, receptors, enzymes, neurotransmitters and cerebral blood flow.

27. In addition to reduction of volume and strength, the functional changes in muscle include abnormalities in somatosensory (temperature, pressure, pain and muscle/joint position sensation) and vestibular and visual responses together with musculoskeletal changes which increase the risk of falls and fracture.

28. Major disturbances of the vestibular system and eye infections and structural eye disease are more common as we age.

29. Aerobic exercise increases brain volume, in both grey and white matter regions, and, along with functional strength training, tai chi and balance training, improves reaction time and movement control and may protect older people from depression.

30. The endocrine system becomes more catabolic with age as cortisol is produced more readily in response to stress and inflammation, and the target tissues become less responsive, impairing muscle, bone and cognitive function.

31. Regular moderate activity and resistance exercise is associated with higher levels of circulating IGF-1, improved thyroid and immune function and decreased cortisol.

32. Cognitive performance is impaired by poor health, disease and decreased quality of life; keeping the brain active (dancing, playing an instrument, learning a foreign language) has been shown to maintain cognitive fitness.

33. Falls increase with age due to: impaired integration of body systems involved in maintaining postural stability; increased, slower body sway; wider base of support in standing, decreased trunk rotation, stride length and time in single leg support; less sensory sensitivity; poor coordination and reaction times; poor eye sight and vestibular function.

34. Individualized dynamic, balance and strength, group and home-based training can reduce the risk and number of falls, and the severity of fall-related injury and fear of falling.

35. Pre-exercise screening and additional health and functional assessment is crucial to the individual tailoring of exercise prescription for older adults; because of the prevalence of chronic and degenerative disease and chronic inactivity it will require subtle differences in protocol, methodology interpretation and dosage.

36. Pre-exercise screening and assessment should aim to be inclusive, i.e. ensuring each individual is matched to an appropriate programme, setting and level of expertise, undergoes evaluation of functional impairments and risk of injury or disability, and is assessed through utilization of a range of validated outcome measures appropriate for that individual, their setting and level of fitness.

37. No single assessment tool can measure all factors related to disease, disabilities, physical limitations, balance and falls risks.

38. Exercise testing for older adults (embarking on moderate exercise) is generally not necessary, not supported by the current evidence, creates unnecessary and unhelpful anxiety about exercise as a high risk activity. Pre-exercise assessment that includes the ability to perform with equipment, must align with the ACSM's older person specific considerations of METs values, modality, supported balance recommendations and practical guidance on testing those who are unfamiliar with equipment.

39. Exercise prescription for older participants requires adaptation to aims, content, programme and teaching methods, yet to respect the heterogeneity of this group, the prescription must be tailored to individual health, fitness, functional, socio-cultural needs, preferences, interests and means.

40. Injury prevention is the highest priority; warm-up and cool-down must be longer and more gradual; modalities and exercises should be functionally relevant; endurance training should aim to utilize interval conditioning approaches and

walking activities and incorporate changes of direction, level and pace; strength training should aim to incorporate functional movement training, balance and flexibility training and programmes should provide a wide range of choice (modality, levels, scheduling, formats, e.g. indoor, outdoor, group, home options) and be varied, comprehensive, accessible, affordable, all year round, include opportunities to socialize and be accessible and inclusive; instructors should have specialist training, qualifications and competencies.

Acknowledgement

We wish to thank Robert Laventure, British Heart Foundation National Centre for Physical Activity and Health, Loughborough University for his invaluable input on the motivational strategies for increasing uptake and adherence to exercise amongst older people.

References

Ahmaidi S, Masse-Biron J, Adam B et al 1998 Effects of interval training at the ventilatory threshold on clinical and cardiorespiratory responses in elderly humans. European Journal of Applied Physiology and Occupational Physiology 78:170–176

American College of Sports Medicine (ACSM) 1998 Position Stand: exercise and physical activity for older adults. Medicine and Science in Sports and Exercise 30:992–1008

American College of Sports Medicine (ACSM) 2000 ACSM's guidelines for exercise testing and prescription, 6th edn. Lippincott Williams & Wilkins, Philadelphia

American Association of Retired People (AARP), American College of Sports Medicine, American Geriatric Society, Centers for Disease Control and Prevention, National Institute on Ageing, Robert Wood Foundation 2001 National blueprint: increasing physical activity among adults 50 and older. Robert Wood Foundation, Princetown, NJ

Andersen R E, Blair S N, Cheskin L J, Barlett S J 1997 Encouraging patients to become more physically active; the physician's role. Annals of Internal Medicine 127:395–400

Aniansson A, Gustafsson E 1981 Physical training in elderly men with special reference to quadriceps muscle strength and morphology. Clinical Physiology 1:87–98

Atchley R C 1972 The social forces in later life. An introduction to social gerontology. Wadsworth, Belmont, CA

Ayalon J, Simkin A, Leichter I et al 1987 Dynamic bone loading exercises for postmenopausal women: effect on the density of the distal radius. Archives of Physical Medicine and Rehabilitation 68:280–283

Bandura A 1997 Self-efficacy; the exercise of control. Freeman, New York

Bao S, Chang E F, Davis J D et al 2003 Progressive degradation and subsequent refinement of acoustic representations in the adult auditory cortex. Journal of Neuroscience 23:10765–10775

Bell J 2001 Delivering an exercise prescription for patients with coronary artery disease. In: Young A, Harries M (eds) Physical activity for patients. An exercise prescription. Royal College of Physicians, London

Bell R, Hoshizaki T 1981 Relationships of age and sex with joint range of motion of seventeen joint actions in humans. Canadian Journal of Applied Sport Sciences 6:202–206

Bell J, Coats A J, Hardman A E 1995 Exercise testing and prescription. In: Coats A J (ed) BACR guidelines for cardiac rehabilitation. Blackwell Science, Oxford

Beverly M C, Rider T A, Evans M J et al 1989 Local bone mineral response to brief exercise that stresses the skeleton. British Medical Journal 299:233–235

Biddle S, Faulkner G 2001 Benefits of physical activity on psychological well-being for older adults. British Heart Foundation National Centre for Physical Activity and Health, Loughborough

Bloomfield S A 1997 Changes in musculoskeletal structure and function with prolonged bed rest. Medicine and Science in Sports and Exercise 29:197–206

Bompa T O 1999 Periodization: theory and methodology of training. Human Kinetics, Champaign, IL

Borg G 1998 Borg's perceived exertion and pain scales. Human Kinetics, Champaign, IL

Bosco C, Komi P V 1980 Influence of aging on the mechanical behavior of leg extensor muscles. European Journal of Applied Physiology 45:209–219

Boutcher S H 2000 Cognitive performance, fitness and ageing. In: Biddle S J H, Fox K R, Boutcher S H (eds) Physical activity and psychological well-being. Routledge, London

Brach J S, Simonsick E M, Kritchevsky S et al 2004 The association between physical function and lifestyle activity and exercise in the health, aging and body composition study. Journal of the American Geriatrics Society 52(4):502–509

Brill P A, Macera C A, Davis D R et al 2000 Muscular strength and physical function. Medicine and Science in Sports and Exercise 32:412–416

Brooks D S 1997 Program design for personal trainers. Human Kinetics, Champaign, IL

Brooks S V, Faulkner J A 1994 Skeletal muscle weakness in old age: underlying mechanisms. Medicine and Science in Sports and Exercise 26:432–439

Brown D R, Wang Y, Ward A et al 1995 Chronic psychological effects of exercise and exercise plus cognitive strategies. Medicine and Science in Sports and Exercise 27 (5):765–775

Buchner D M 1997 Preserving mobility in older adults. Western Journal of Medicine 167:258–264

Buchner D M, Coleman E A 1994 Exercise considerations for older adults. Physical Medicine and Rehabilitation Clinics of North America 5:5–9

Buchner D M, Cress M E, de Lateur B J et al 1997 The effect of strength and endurance training on gait, balance, fall risk, and health services use in community-living older adults. Journal of Gerontology 52A:M218–M224

Campbell M J, McComas A J, Petito F 1973 Physiological changes in ageing muscles. Journal of Neurology, Neurosurgery and Psychiatry 36:71–182

Carroll J F, Pollock M L, Graves J E et al 1992 Incidence of injury during moderate- and high-intensity walking training in the elderly. Journal of Gerontology 47(3):M61–M66

Cavanaugh D J, Cann C E 1988 Brisk walking does not stop bone loss in postmenopausal women. Bone 9:201–204

Centers for Disease Control and Prevention (CDC) 1996 Physical activity and health: a report of the surgeon general executive summary. US Department of Health and Human Services, p 9–14

Centers for Disease Control and Prevention (CDC) 2002 Promoting active lifestyles among older adults. US Department of Health and Human Services. Online. Available: http://www.cdc.gov/nccdphp/dnpa/physical/pdf/lifestyles.pdf

Chan K M, Qin L, Lau M C et al 2004 A randomized, prospective study of the effects of Tai Chi Chun exercise on bone mineral density in postmenopausal women. Archives of Physical Medicine and Rehabilitation 85:717–722

Chaput S, Proteau L 1996 Modification with ageing and the role played by vision and proprioception for movement control. Experimental Aging Research 22:1–21

Chasens E R, Sereika S M, Weaver T E, Umlauf M G 2007 Daytime sleepiness, exercise, and physical function in older adults. Journal of Sleep Research 16(1):60–65

Chaunchaiyakul R, Groeller H, Clarke J R, Taylor N A 2004 The impact of aging and habitual physical activity on static respiratory work at rest and during exercise.

American Journal of Physiology. Lung Cellular and Molecular Physiology 287:1098–1106

Chodzko-Zajko W J, Moore R A 1994 Physical fitness and cognitive function in aging. Exercise and Sport Sciences Reviews 22:1995–2020

Chodzko-Zajko W J, Resnick B 2004 Beyond screening: the need for new pre-activity counseling protocols to assist older adults transition from sedentary living to physically active lifestyles. Journal of Active Aging 3:26–30

Chow R, Harrison J E, Notarius C 1987 Effect of two randomised exercise programmes on bone mass of healthy postmenopausal women. British Medical Journal (Clin Res Ed) 295:1441–1444

Christmas C, Andersen R A 2000 Exercise and older patients: guidelines for the clinician. Journal of the American Geriatrics Society 48:318–324

Close J C T, Lord S R, Menz H B, Sherrington C 2005 What is the role of falls? Best Practice and Research. Clinical Rheumatology 19(6):913–935

Colcombe S J, Erickson K I, Scalf P E et al 2006 Aerobic exercise training increases brain volume in aging humans. Journal of Gerontology A. Biological Sciences and Medical Sciences 61:1166–1170

Coleman E, Buchner D M, Cress M E et al 1996 The relationship of joint symptoms with exercise performance in older adults. Journal of the American Geriatrics Society 44:14–21

Conley K, Amara C, Jubrias S, Marcinek D 2007 Mitochondrial function, fibre types and aging: new insights from human muscle In Vivo. Experimental Physiology 92(2):333–339

Cooper C 1993 The epidemiology of fragility fractures: is there a role for bone quality? Calcified Tissue International 53(Suppl 1):S23–S26

Cooper K H, Purdy J G, White S R, Pollock M L 1977 Age fitness adjusted maximal heart rates. Medicine and Sport 10:78–88

Copeland J L, Chu S Y, Tremblay M S 2004 Aging, physical activity, and hormones in women – a review. Journal of Aging and Physical Activity 12:101–116

Cotman C W, Berchtold N C 2002 Exercise: a behavioral intervention to enhance brain health and plasticity. Trends in Neuroscience 25(6):295–301

Cress M E, Thomas D P, Johnson J et al 1991 Effect of training on VO2max, thigh strength, and muscle morphology in septuagenarian women. Medicine and Science in Sports and Exercise 23:752–758

Cress M E, Prohaska T, Rimmer J et al 2005 Best practices for physical activity programs and behavior counseling in older adult populations. Journal of Aging and Physical Activity 13:61–74

Damush T M, Stewart A L, Mills K M et al 1999 Prevalence and correlates of physician recommendations to exercise among older adults. Journal of Gerontology A. Biological Sciences and Medical Sciences 54(8):M423–M427

De Busk R F, Stenstrand U, Sheehan M, Haskell W L 1990 Training effects of long versus short bouts of exercise in healthy subjects. American Journal of Cardiology 65:1010–1013

Department of Health 2001 National Service Framework for Older People: modern standards and service models. Her Majesty's Stationery Office, London

De Vito G, Hernandez R, Gonzalez V et al 1997 Low intensity physical training in older subjects. Journal of Sports Medicine and Physical Fitness 37(1):72–77

Dinan S M 2001 Exercise for vulnerable older patients. In: Young A, Harries M (eds) Exercise prescription for patients. Royal College of Physicians, London

Dinan S M, Skelton D A 2007 Exercise for the prevention of falls and injuries in frailer older people: a manual for the postural stability instructor, 3rd edn. Later Life Training, London

Dinan S M, Skelton D, Malbut K 2004 Aerobic endurance training. In: Jones J, Rose D (eds) Physical activity instruction of older adults. Human Kinetics, Champaign, IL

Dinan S M, Lenihan P, Tenn T, Iliffe S 2006 Is the promotion of physical activity in vulnerable, older people feasible and effective in general practice? British Journal of General Practice 56(531):791–793

Eastell R, Riggs B L 1988 Diagnostic evaluation of osteoporosis. Endocrinology and Metabolism Clinics of North America 17(3):547–571

Ebrahim S, Thompson P W, Baskaran V et al 1997 Randomized placebo-controlled trial of brisk walking in the prevention of postmenopausal osteoporosis. Age and Ageing 26:253–260

Ecclestone N A, Jones C J 2004 International curriculum guidelines for preparing physical activity instructors of older adults. Journal of Aging and Physical Activity 12:5–21

Ehsani A A, Ogawa T, Miller T R et al 1991 Exercise training improves left ventricular systolic function in older men. Circulation 89:2545–2551

Einkauf D K, Gohdes M L, Jensen G M, Jewell M J 1987 Changes in spinal mobility with increasing age in women. Physical Therapy 67:370–375

Ekonomov A L, Rudd C L, Lomakin A J 1989 Actuarial ageing rate is not constant within the human life span. Gerontology 35:113–120

Ettinger W H Jr, Burns R, Messier S P et al 1997 A randomized trial comparing aerobic exercise and resistance exercise with a health education program in older adults with knee osteoarthritis. The Fitness Arthritis and Seniors Trial (FAST). JAMA 277 (1):25–31

Evans W J 1999 Exercise training guidelines for the elderly. Medicine and Science in Sports and Exercise 31(1):12–17

Ferrari A U, Radaelli A, Centola M 2003 Invited review: aging and the cardiovascular system. Journal of Applied Physiology 95:2591–2597

Fiatarone M A, Marks E C, Ryan N D et al 1990 High-intensity strength training in nonagenarians. Effects on skeletal muscle. JAMA 263:3029–3034

Finch C E 1976 The regulation of physiological changes during mammalian ageing. Quarterly Review of Biology 51:49–83

Finch H 1997 Physical activity – at our age. Qualitative research among people over the age of 50. Health Education Authority, London

Fisher B J 1995 Successful aging, life satisfaction, and generativity in later life. International Journal of Aging and Human Development 41:239–250

Fleck S J, Kraemer W J 2004 Designing resistance training programs, 3rd edn. Human Kinetics, Champaign, IL

Fleg J, O'Connor F, Gerstenbilth G et al 1995 Impact of age on the cardiovascular response to dynamic upright exercise in healthy men and women. Journal of Applied Physiology 78:890–900

Fries J F 1980 Ageing, natural death and the compression of morbidity. New England Journal of Medicine 803:130–135

Fries J F, Crapo L M 1981 Vitality and ageing. Freeman, San Francisco

Frost H M 1990 Skeletal structural adaptations to mechanical usage (SATMU): 2. Redefining Wolff's law: the remodeling problem. Anatomical Record 226:414–422

Gardner M M, Robinson C M, Campbell J A 2000 Exercise in preventing falls and fall related injuries in older people: a review of randomised controlled trials. British Journal of Sports Medicine 34:7–17

Gill G T 2002 Geriatric medicine: it's more than caring for older people. American Journal of Medicine 113:85–89

Gill T M, DiPietro L, Krumholz H M 2000 Role of exercise stress testing and safety monitoring for older persons starting an exercise program. JAMA 284:342–349

Gillespie L D, Gillespie W J, Robertson M C et al 2005 Interventions for preventing falls in elderly people. The Cochrane Database of Systematic Reviews, 2005 (Issue 5). DOI: 10.1002/14651858.CD000340

Golding L A, Lindsay A 1989 Flexibility and age. Perspective 15:28–30

Grahn Kronhed A C, Blomberg C, Karlsson N 2005 Impact of a community-based osteoporosis and fall prevention program on fracture incidence. Osteoporosis International 16:700–706

Gregg E W, Pereira M A, Caspersen C J 2000 Physical activity, falls, and fractures among older adults: a review of the epidemiologic evidence. Journal of the American Geriatrics Society 48:883–893

Grundy E M D 2003 The epidemiology of ageing. In: Tallis R D, Fillit H M (eds) Brocklehurst's textbook of geriatrics, medicine and gerontology, 6th edn. Churchill Livingstone Elsevier Science, London

Guralnik J M, LaCroix A Z, Abbott R D et al 1993 Maintaining mobility in late life: I. demographic characteristics and chronic conditions. American Journal of Epidemiology 137:845–857

Hagberg J M, Graves J E, Limacher M et al 1989 Cardiovascular responses of 70–79 year old men and women to exercise training. Journal of Applied Physiology 66:2589–2594

Haskell W L 1997 Medical clearance for exercise program participation by older persons: The clinical versus the public health approach. In: Huber G (ed) Healthy aging, activity and sports. Health Promotion, Hamburg

Hassmen P, Koivula N, Uutela A 2000 Physical exercise and psychological well-being: a population study in Finland. Preventive Medicine 30:17–25

Hausdorff J M, Levy B R, Wei J Y 1999 The power of ageism on physical function of older persons: reversibility of age-related gait changes. Journal of the American Geriatrics Society 47(11):1346–1349

Hayden-Wade H A, Coleman K J, Sallis J F, Armstrong C 2003 Validation of the telephone and in-person interview versions of the 7-day PAR. Medicine and Science in Sports and Exercise 35(5):801–809

Hayflick L 1997 The cellular basis for biological ageing. In: Eirch C E, Hayfick L (eds). Van Nostrand Reinhold, New York

Haykowsky M, McGavock J, Vonder Muhll I et al 2005 Effect of exercise training on peak aerobic power, left ventricular morphology, and muscle strength in healthy older women. Journal of Gerontology A. Biological Sciences and Medical Sciences 60(3): 307–311

Heath G W 1988 Exercise programming for the older adult. I: Resource manual for the guidelines for exercise testing and prescription. American College of Sports Medicine. Lea and Febiger, Philadelphia

Hill R D, Storandt M, Malley M 1993 The impact of long-term exercise training on psychological function in older adults. Journal of Gerontology 48(1):P12–P17

Hillsdon M, Foster C, Cavill N et al 2005 The effectiveness of public health interventions for increasing physical activity among adults: a review of reviews. Health Development Agency, London

Hirvonen T P, Aalto H, Pyykko I et al 1997 Changes in vestibulo-ocular reflex of elderly people. Acta Otolaryngologica Suppl 529:108–110

Hoenig H, Nusbaum N, Brummel-Smith K 1997 Geriatric rehabilitation: state of the art. Journal of the American Geriatrics Society 45:1371–1381

Hollenberg M, Yang J, Haight T J, Tager I B 2006 Longitudinal changes in aerobic capacity: implications for concepts of aging. Journal of Gerontology A. Biological Sciences and Medical Sciences 61(8):851–858

Horak F B 2006 Postural orientation and equilibrium: what do we need to know about neural control of balance to prevent falls? Age and Ageing 35(Suppl 2):ii7–ii11

Hurley B F 1989 Effects of resistive training on lipoprotein-lipid profiles: a comparison to aerobic exercise training. Medicine and Science in Sports and Exercise 21(6):689–693

Hyatt R, Whitelaw M, Bhat A et al 1990 Association of muscle strength with functional status of elderly people. Age and Ageing 19(5):330–336

Inouye S K, Wagner D R, Acampora D et al 1993 A predictive index for functional decline in hospitalized elderly medical patients. Journal of General Internal Medicine 8:645–652

Issekutz B, Blizzard J J, Birkhead N N, Rodahl K 1966 Effect of prolonged bed rest on urinary calcium output. Journal of Applied Physiology 21:1013–1020

Itoi E, Sinaki M 1994 Effect of back-strengthening exercise on posture in healthy women 49 to 65 years of age. Mayo Clinic Proceedings 69(11):1054–1059

Iwamoto J, Takeda T, Sato Y et al 2005 Effect of whole-body vibration exercise on lumbar bone mineral density, bone turnover, and chronic back pain in post-menopausal osteoporotic women treated with alendronate. Aging Clinical and Experimental Research 17:157–163

Jackson A S, Beard E F, Wier L T et al 1995 Changes in aerobic power of men ages 25–70 yr. Medicine and Science in Sports and Exercise 27:113–120

Jarnlo G 2003 Functional balance tests related to falls among elderly people living in the community. European Journal of Geriatrics 5:7–14

Jette A M, Harris B A, Sleeper L et al 1996 A home-based exercise program for nondisabled older adults. Journal of the American Geriatrics Society 44:644–649

Jette A M, Lachman M, Giorgetti M M et al 1999 Exercise – it's never too late: the strong for life program. American Journal of Public Health 89:66–72

Jones C J, Clark J 1998 National standards for preparing senior fitness instructors. Journal of Aging and Physical Activity 6:207–221

Jones C J, Rikli R E 2005 Field-based physical mobility assessments. In: Jones C J, Rose D (eds) Physical activity instruction of older adults. Human Kinetics, Champaign, IL

Jones C J, Rose D 2005 The field of gerokinesiology. In: Jones C J, Rose D (eds) Physical activity instruction of older adults. Human Kinetics, Champaign, IL

Jones G R, Vandervoort A A, Overend T J 2005 Laboratory-based physiological assessment of older adults. In: Jones C J, Rose D (eds) Physical activity instruction of older adults. Human Kinetics, Champaign, IL

Jørstad-Stein E C, Hauer K, Becker C et al 2005 Suitability of physical activity questionnaires for older adults in fall prevention intervention trials: a systematic review. Journal of Aging and Physical Activity 13(4):461–481

Judge J O, Kleppinger A, Kenny A et al 2005 Home-based resistance training improves femoral bone mineral density in women on hormone therapy. Osteoporosis International 16(9):1096

Kallinen M, Kauppinen M, Era P, Heikkinen E 2006 The predictive value of exercise testing for survival among 75-year-old men and women. Scandinavian Journal of Medicine and Science in Sports 16(4):237–244

Kane R L, Finch M, Blewett L et al 1996 Use of post-hospital care by Medicare patients. Journal of the American Geriatrics Society 44:242–250

Katz S, Branch L G, Branson M H et al 1983 Active life expectancy. New England Journal of Medicine 309:1218–1224

Kennie D C, Dinan S, Young A 2003 Health promotion and physical activity. In: Tallis R D, Fillit H M (eds) Brocklehurst's textbook of geriatrics, medicine and gerontology, 6th edn. Churchill Livingstone Elsevier Science, London

Kerr D, Morton A, Dick I et al 1996 Exercise effects on bone mass in postmenopausal women are site-specific and load-dependent. Journal of Bone and Mineral Research 11:218–225

Kiebzak G M 1991 Age-related bone changes. Experimental Gerontology 26(2–3):171–187

King A C, Haskell W L, Taylor C B et al 1991 Group- vs. home-based exercise training in healthy older men and women: a community-based clinical trial. JAMA 266:1535–1542

King A C, Taylor C B, Haskell W L 1993 Effects of differing intensities and formats of 12 months of exercise training on psychological outcomes in older adults. Health Psychology 12(4):292–300

King A C, Rejeski W J, Buchner D M 1998 Physical activity interventions targeting older adults. A critical review and recommendations. American Journal of Preventive Medicine 15(4):316–333

Kinsella K G 1992 Changes in life expectancy 1900–1990. American Journal of Clinical Nutrition 55(6 Suppl):1196–1202

Kiraly M A, Kiraly S J 2005 The effect of exercise on hippocampal integrity: review of recent research. International Journal of Psychiatry in Medicine 35:75–89

Kirkwood T, Young A 2001 Ageing. In: Blakemore C, Jannet S (eds) The Oxford companion to the body. Oxford University Press, Oxford

Kohrt W, Bloomfield S, Little K et al 2004 Physical activity and bone health. American College of Sports Medicine Position Stand. Medicine and Science in Sports and Exercise 36(11):1985–1996

Kostka T, Patricot M C, Mathian B et al 2003 Anabolic and catabolic hormonal responses to experimental two-set low-volume resistance exercise in sedentary and active elderly people. Aging Clinical and Experimental Research 15(2):123–130

Kramer A F, Colcombe S, Erickson K et al 2002 Effects of aerobic fitness training on human cortical function: a proposal. Journal of Molecular Neuroscience 19:227–231

Kraemer W J, French D N 2005 Resistance training. In: Jones C J, Rose D (eds) Physical activity instruction of older adults. Human Kinetics, Champaign, IL

Krolner B, Toft B 1983 Vertebral bone loss: an unheeded side effect of therapeutic bed rest. Clinical Science (London) 64:537–540

LaCroix A Z, Guralnik J M, Berkman L F et al 1993 Maintaining mobility in late life: II. smoking, alcohol consumption, physical activity, and body mass index. American Journal of Epidemiology 137:858–869

Lakatta E G 1993 Cardiovascular regulatory mechanisms in advanced age. Physiological Reviews 73:413–469

Lamberts S W, van den Beld A W, van der Lely A J 1997 The endocrinology of aging. Science 278(5337):419–424

Lan C, Chou S W, Chen S Y et al 2004 The aerobic capacity and ventilatory efficiency during exercise in Qigong and Tai Chi Chuan practitioners. American Journal Chinese Medicine 32(1):141–150

Lavie C J, Milani R V 1995 Effects of cardiac rehabilitation programs on exercise capacity, coronary risk factors, behavioral characteristics, and quality of life in a large elderly cohort. American Journal of Cardiology 76:177–179

Lemmer J T, Hurlbut D E, Martel G F et al 2000 Age and gender responses to strength training and detraining. Medicine and Science in Sports and Exercise 32:1505–1512

Leveille S G, Wagner E H, Davis C et al 1998 Preventing disability and managing chronic illness in frail older adults: a randomized trial of a community-based partnership with primary care. Journal of the American Geriatrics Society 46:1191–1198

Levy W C, Cerqueira M, Abrass I et al 1993 Endurance exercise training augments diastolic filling at rest and during exercise in older and younger healthy men. Circulation 88:116–126

Lexell J 1995 Human aging, muscle mass, and fiber type composition. Journal of Gerontology. Biological Sciences and Medical Sciences 50(SI UE):11–16

Lexell J 1997 Evidence for nervous system degeneration with advancing age. Journal of Nutrition 127:1011–1013

Lips P 2001 Vitamin D deficiency and secondary hyperparathyroidism in the elderly: consequences for bone loss and fractures and therapeutic implications. Endocrine Reviews 22:477–501

Lord S R, McLean D, Stathers G 1992 Physiological factors associated with injurious falls in older people living in the community. Gerontology 38:338–346

Lord S R, Sambrook P N, Gilbert C et al 1994 Postural stability, falls and fractures in the elderly: results from the Dubbo Osteoporosis Epidemiology Study. Medical Journal of Australia 160:684–685, 688–691

Lord S R, Sherrington C, Menz H B 2001 Falls in older people: risk factors and strategies for prevention. Cambridge University Press, Cambridge

Lorig K, Sobel D S, Stewart A et al 1999 Evidence suggesting that a chronic disease self-management program can improve health status while reducing hospitalization. Medical Care 35:5–14

Lupien S J, Schwartz G, Ng Y K et al 2005 The Douglas Hospital Longitudinal Study of Normal and Pathological Aging: summary of findings. Journal of Psychiatry and Neuroscience 30:328–334

Luukinen H, Koski K, Laippala P et al 1995 Predictors for recurrent falls among the home-dwelling elderly. Scandinavian Journal of Primary Health Care 13:294–299

Lysack J T, Lysack C L, Kvern B L 1998 A severe adverse reaction to mefloquine and chloroquine prophylaxis. Australian Family Physician 27:1119–1120

McAuley E, Rudolph D 1995 Physical activity, aging and psychological well-being. Journal of Aging and Physical Activity 3:67–98

McAuley E, Katula J 1998 Physical activity interventions in the elderly: influence of physical health and psychological function. In: Schultz R, Lawton M P, Maddox G (eds) Annual Review of Gerontology and Geriatrics, Vol 18. Springer, New York, pp 115–154

McAuley E, Blissmer B, Marquez D X et al 2000 Social relations, physical activity, and well-being in older adults. Preventive Medicine 31:608–617

McClure R, Turner C, Peel N et al 2005 Population-based interventions for the prevention of fall-related injuries in older people. The Cochrane Database of Systematic Reviews, Issue 1

McHugh M P, Connolly D A, Eston R G et al 1999 The role of passive muscle stiffness in symptoms of exercise-induced muscle damage. American Journal of Sports Medicine 27:594–599

MacLachlan D 1863 A practical treatise on the diseases and infirmities of advanced life. John Churchill and Sons, London, p 60

MacLennan W J, Hall M R, Timothy J I, Robinson M 1980 Is weakness in old age due to muscle wasting? Age and Ageing 9:188–192

McMurdo M E, Rennie L M 1994 Improvements in quadriceps strength with regular seated exercise in the institutionalized elderly. Archives of Physical Medicine and Rehabilitation 75:600–603

Malbut K E, Dinan S, Young A 2002 Aerobic training in the 'oldest old': the effect of 24 weeks of training. Age and Ageing 31(4):255–260

Manson J E, Greenland P, LaCroix A Z et al 2002 Walking compared with vigorous exercise for the prevention of cardiovascular events in women. New England Journal of Medicine 347:716–725

Marcus B H, Forsyth L H 2003 Motivating people to be physically active. Human Kinetics, Champaign, IL

Mattson M P, Duan W, Lee J, Guo Z 2001 Suppression of brain ageing and neurodegenerative disorders by dietary restriction and environmental enrichment: molecular mechanisms. Mechanisms of Ageing and Development 122(7):757–778

Mazzeo R S, Cavanagh P, Evans W J et al 2000 Exercise and physical activity for older adults. Medicine and Science in Sports and Exercise 30(6):992–1008

Mazzetti S A, Kraemer W J, Volek J S et al 2000 The influence of direct supervision of resistance training on strength performance. Medicine and Science in Sports and Exercise 32:1175–1184

Morey M C, Cowper P A, Feussner J R et al 1989 Evaluation of a supervised exercise program in a geriatric population. Journal of the American Geriatrics Society 37:348–354

Morgenthal A P, Shephard R J 2005 Physiological aspects of ageing. In: Jones C J, Rose D (eds) Physical activity instruction of older adults. Human Kinetics, Champaign, IL

Narici M V, Maganaris C N 2006 Adaptability of elderly human muscles and tendons to increased loading. Journal of Anatomy 208(4):433–443

National Institute on Ageing (NIA) 1998 Exercise: A guide from the National Institute on Ageing (Publication No NIH98-4258). National Institute on Ageing, Washington DC

Need A G, O'Loughlin P D, Morris H A et al 2004 The effects of age and other variables on serum parathyroid hormone in postmenopausal women attending an osteoporosis center. Journal of Clinical Endocrinology and Metabolism 89(4):1646–1649

Nelson M E, Fiatarone M A, Morganti C M et al 1994 Effects of high-intensity strength training on multiple risk factors for osteoporotic fractures. A randomized controlled trial. JAMA 272:1909–1914

Nicholl J P, Coleman P, Brazier J E 1994 Health and healthcare costs and benefits of exercise. Pharmacoeconomics 5(2):109–122

Norris S L, Grothaus L C, Buchner D M, Pratt M 2000 Effectiveness of physician-based assessment and counseling for exercise in a staff model HMO. Preventive Medicine 30:513–523

O'Connor P J, Aenchbacher L E, Dishman R K 1993 Physical activity and depression in the elderly. Journal of Aging and Physical Activity 1:34–58

Office for National Statistics (ONS) 2000 Mortality statistics: cause, England and Wales, 1999 (series DH2, no 26). HMSO, London

Ogawa T, Spina R J, Martin W H 3rd et al 1992 Effects of aging, sex, and physical training on cardiovascular responses to exercise. Circulation 86(2):494–503

Ory M, Resnick B, Jordan P J et al 2005 Screening, safety, and adverse events in physical activity interventions: collaborative experiences from the behavior change consortium. Annals of Behavioral Medicine 29:20–28

Paterson D H, Cunningham D A, Koval J J, St. Croix C 1999 Aerobic fitness in a population of independently living men and women aged 55–86 years. Medicine and Science in Sports and Exercise 31:1813–1820

Pearson S J, Young A, Macaluso A et al 2002 Muscle function in elite master weightlifters. Medicine and Science in Sports and Exercise 34:1199–1206

Phillips S K, Bruce S A, Newton D, Woledge R C 1992 The weakness of old age is not due to failure of muscle activation. Journal of Gerontology. Medical Sciences 47:M45–M49

Pollock M L, Carroll J F, Graves J E et al 1991 Injuries and adherence to walk/jog and resistance training programs in the elderly. Medicine and Science in Sports and Exercise 23(10):1194–1200

Pollock M L, Gettman L R, Milesis C A et al 1977 Effects of frequency and duration of training on attrition and incidence of injury. Medicine and Science in Sports 9(1):31–36

Pollock M L, Franklin B A, Balady G J et al 2000 AHA Science Advisory. Resistance exercise in individuals with and without cardiovascular disease: benefits, rationale, safety, and prescription. Circulation 101(7):828–833

Pride N B 2005 Ageing and changes in lung mechanics. European Respiratory Journal 26(4):563–565

Puggaard L, Larsen J B, Stovring H, Jeune B 2000 Maximal oxygen uptake, muscle strength and walking speed in 85-year-old women: effects of increased physical activity. Aging (Milano) 12(3):180–189

Raric G L 1973 Physical activity, growth and development. Academic Press, New York

Ravaglia G, Forti P, Maioli F et al 2001 Regular moderate intensity physical activity and blood concentrations of endogenous anabolic hormones and thyroid hormones in aging men. Mechanisms of Ageing and Development 122(2):191–203

Resnick B, Ory M, Coday M, Riebe D 2005 Older adults' perspectives on screening prior to initiating an exercise program. Prevention Science 6(3):203–211

Riggs B L, Wahner H W, Dunn W L et al 1981 Differential changes in bone mineral density of the appendicular and axial skeleton with aging. Journal of Clinical Investigation 67:328–335

Rikli R, Jones C J 2001 Senior fitness test manual. Human Kinetics, Champaign, IL

Robertson M C, Devlin N, Scuffham P et al 2001 Economic evaluation of a community based exercise programme to prevent falls. Journal of Epidemiology and Community Health 55:600–606

Rogers M E 2005 Pre-exercise and health screening. In: Jones C J, Rose D (eds) Physical activity instruction of older adults. Human Kinetics, Champaign, IL

Rose D 2003 FallProof: A comprehensive balance and mobility program. Human Kinetics, Champaign, IL

Ross R 1993 The pathogenesis of artherosclerosis: a perspective for the 1990s. Nature 362:801–809

Roubenoff R, Hughes V A 2000 Sarcopenia: current concepts. Journal of Gerontology A. Biological Sciences and Medical Sciences 55:716–724

Rowe J W, Kahn R L 1998 Successful ageing. Pantheon Books, New York

Rutherford O M 1999 Is there a role for exercise in the prevention of osteoporotic fractures? British Journal of Sports Medicine 33:378–386

Rybak L P 1985 Furosemide ototoxicity: clinical and experimental aspects. Laryngoscope 95(9 Pt 2, Suppl 38):1–14

Sager M A, Rudberg M A, Jalajuddin M et al 1996 Hospital admission risk profile (HARP): identifying older patients at risk for functional decline following acute medical illness and hospitalization. Journal of the American Geriatrics Society 44:251–257

Saltin B 1980 Fysisk vedligeholdelse hos aeldre. Manedsskrift for Praktisk Laegegerning 58 (4):198–216

Saltin B 1986 Physiological characteristics of the masters athlete. In: Sutton J R, Brock R M (eds) Sports medicine for the mature athlete. Benchmark Press, Indianapolis

Savine R, Sönksen P 2000 Growth hormone – hormone replacement for the somatopause? Hormone Research 53(Suppl 3):37–41

Sayer A A, Cooper C, Evans J R et al 1998 Are rates of ageing determined in utero? Age and Ageing 27:579–583

Schmidt R A, Lee T D 1999 Motor control and learning: a behavioural emphasis. Human Kinetics, Champaign, IL

Seeman T E, Singer B H, Ryff C D et al 2002 Social relationships, gender and allostatic load across two age cohorts. Psychosomatic Medicine 64:395–406

Sesso H D, Paffenbarger R S Jr, Lee I M 2000 Physical activity and coronary heart disease in men: The Harvard Alumni Health Study. Circulation 102:975–980

Shaffer S W, Harrison A L 2007 Aging of the somatosensory system: a translational perspective. Physical Therapy 87(2):193–207

Shenkin S D, Starr J M, Deary I J 2004 Birth weight and cognitive ability in childhood: a systematic review. Psychological Bulletin 130:989–1013

Shephard R J 1991 Benefits of sport and physical activity for the disabled: implications for individuals and society. Scandinavian Journal of Rehabilitation Medicine 23:51–59

Shephard R J 1994 Aerobic fitness and health. Human Kinetics, Champaign, IL

Shephard R J 1997 Aging, physical activity and health. Human Kinetics, Champaign, IL

Shephard R J, Kavanagh T, Mertens D J 1995 Personal health benefits of Masters athletic competition. British Journal of Sports Medicine 29:35–40

Sinaki M 1982 Postmenopausal spinal osteoporosis: physical therapy and rehabilitation principles. Mayo Clinic Proceedings 57:699–703

Sinaki M, Itoi E, Wahner H W et al 2002 Stronger back muscles reduce the incidence of vertebral fractures: a prospective 10 year follow-up of postmenopausal women. Bone 30 (6):836–841

Singh N A, Clements K M, Fiatarone M A 1997 A randomized controlled trial of progressive resistance training in depressed elders. Journal of Gerontology 52A:M27–M35

Singh N A, Stavrinos T M, Scarbek Y et al 2005 A randomized controlled trial of high versus low intensity weight training versus general practitioner care for clinical depression in older adults. Journal of Gerontology A. Biological Sciences and Medical Sciences 60:768–776

Skelton D A 2001 Effects of physical activity on postural stability. Age and Ageing 30 (S4):33–39

Skelton D A, Dinan S M 1999 Exercise for falls management: rationale for an exercise programme aimed at reducing postural instability. Physiotherapy Theory and Practice 15:105–120

Skelton D A, McLaughlin A W 1996 Training functional ability in old age. Physiotherapy 82:159–167

Skelton D A, Greig C A, Davies J M, Young A 1994 Strength, power and related functional ability of healthy people aged 65–89 years. Age and Ageing 23:371–377

Skelton D A, Young A, Greig C A, Malbut K E 1995 Effects of resistance training on strength, power and selected functional abilities of women aged 75 and over. Journal of the American Geriatrics Society 43:1081–1087

Skelton D A, Young A, Walker A, Hoinville E 1999 Physical activity in later life: further analysis of the ADNFS and the HEASAH. Health Education Authority, London

Skelton D A, Kennedy J, Rutherford O M 2002 Explosive power and asymmetry in leg muscle function in frequent fallers and non-fallers aged over 65. Age and Ageing 31:119–125

Skelton D A, Dinan S M, Campbell M, Rutherford O 2005 Tailored group exercise (Falls Management Exercise – FaME) reduces falls in community-dwelling older frequent fallers (an RCT). Age and Ageing 34(6):636–639

Smith E L 1984 Special considerations in developing exercise programmes for the older adult. In: Matarazzo J D, Miller N E, Weiss S M et al (eds) Behavioural health: a handbook of health enhancement and disease prevention. John Wiley, New York

Spina R J 1999 Cardiovascular adaptations to endurance exercise training in older men and women. Exercise and Sport Sciences Reviews 27:317–332

Spina R J, Ogawa T, Kohrt W M et al 1993 Differences in cardiovascular adaptations to endurance training between older men and women. Journal of Applied Physiology 75:849–855

Spina R J, Turner M J, Ehsani A A 1998 β adrenergic-mediated improvement in left ventricular function by exercise training in older men. American Journal of Physiology 274:H995–H1000

Spirduso W W, Francis K L, MacRae P G 1996 Physical dimensions of aging, 1st edn. Human Kinetics, Champaign, IL

Spirduso W W, Francis K L, MacRae P G 2005 Physical dimensions of aging, 2nd edn. Human Kinetics, Champaign, IL

Squires R W, Muri A J, Anderson L J et al 1991 Weight training during Phase II early outpatient cardiac rehabilitation: Heart rate and blood pressure responses. Journal of Cardiac Rehabilitation 11:360–364

Stearns S, Bernard S L, Fasick S B et al 2001 The economic implications of self-care: The effect of lifestyle, functional adaptations, and medical self-care among a national sample of Medicare beneficiaries. American Journal of Public Health 90:1608–1612

Stewart A L, Gillis D, Grossman M et al 2006 Diffusing a research-based physical activity promotion program for seniors into diverse communities: CHAMPS III. Preventing Chronic Disease 3(2):A51

Stratton J, Levy W, Cerqueira M et al 1994 Cardiovascular response to exercise: effects of aging and exercise training in healthy men. Circulation 89:1648–1655

Taddei S, Virdis A, Ghiadoni L et al 1996 Menopause is associated with endothelial dysfunction in women. Hypertension 28:576–582

Tafaro L, Cicconetti P, Baratta A et al 2007 Sleep quality of centenarians: cognitive and survival implications. Archives of Gerontology and Geriatrics 44S:385–389

Tanaka H, Shirakawa S 2004 Sleep health, lifestyle and mental health in the Japanese elderly: ensuring sleep to promote a healthy brain and mind. Journal of Psychosomatic Research 56:465–477

Taylor A H, Cable N T, Faulkner G et al 2004 Physical activity and older adults: a review of health benefits and the effectiveness of interventions. Journal of Sports Science 22:703–725

Thomas S, Reading J, Shephard R J 1992 Revision of the Physical Activity Readiness Questionnaire (PAR-Q). Canadian Journal of Sport Science 17(4):338–345

Tinetti M E 1994 Prevention of falls and fall injuries in elderly persons: a research agenda. Preventive Medicine 23:756–762

Tinetti M E, Liu W L, Claus E B 1993 Predictors and prognosis of inability to get up after falls among elderly persons. JAMA 269(1):65–70

United Nations 2001 World population prospects: the 2000 revision highlights, Vols I and II. United Nations, New York

US Census Bureau 2001 Population projections of the United States by age, sex, race and Hispanic origin: 1999–2050. Online. Available: http://www.census.gov/prod/www/abs/popula.html

Vallejo A F, Schroeder E T, Zheng L et al 2006 Cardiopulmonary responses to eccentric and concentric resistance exercise in older adults. Age and Ageing 35(3):291–297

Vandervoort A A, Chesworth B M, Cunningham D A et al 1992 Age and sex effects on mobility of the human ankle. Journal of Gerontology: Medical Sciences 47:M17–M21

Venjatraman J T, Fernandes G 1997 Exercise, immunity and aging. Aging (Milano) 9(1–2):42–56

Verghese J, Lipton R B, Katz M et al 2003 Leisure activities and the risk of dementia in the elderly. New England Journal of Medicine 348:2508–2516

Verhaar H J, Samson M M, Jansen P A et al 2000 Muscle strength, functional mobility and vitamin D in older women. Aging (Milano) 12(6):455–460

Verschueren S M P, Roelants M, Delecluse C et al 2004 Effect of 6-month whole body vibration training on hip density, muscle strength, and postural control in postmenopausal women: A randomized controlled pilot study. Journal of Bone and Mineral Research 19:352–359

Vincent K R, Braith R W, Feldman R A et al 2002 Improved cardiorespiratory endurance following 6 months of resistance exercise in elderly men and women. Archives of Internal Medicine 162(6):673–678

Visser M, Deeg D J, Lips P 2003 Low vitamin D and high parathyroid hormone levels as determinants of loss of muscle strength and muscle mass (sarcopenia): the Longitudinal Aging Study Amsterdam. Journal of Clinical Endocrinology and Metabolism 88 (12):5766–5772

Vogiatzis I, Nanas S, Roussos C 2002 Interval training as an alternative modality to continuous exercise in patients with COPD. European Respiratory Journal 20(1):12–19

Wagner E H 1997 Preventing decline in function: evidence from randomized trials around the world. Western Journal of Medicine 167:295–298

Walford R L, Crew M 1989 How dietary restriction retards ageing: an integrative hypothesis. Growth Development, Aging 53:139–140

Wallace J I, Buchner D M, Grothaus L et al 1998 Implementation and effectiveness of a community-based health promotion program for older adults. Journal of Gerontology 53A:M301–M306

Warren B J, Nieman D C, Dotson R G et al 1993 Cardiorespiratory responses to exercise training in septuagenarian women. International Journal of Sports Medicine 14(2):60–65

Washburn R A, Smith K W, Jette A M, Janney C A 1993 The Physical Activity Scale for the Elderly (PASE): development and evaluation. Journal of Clinical Epidemiology 46:153–162

Weindruch R 1995 Diet restriction. In: Maddox G (ed) The encyclopedia of ageing, 2nd edn. Springer, New York

Welsh L, Rutherford O M 1996 Hip bone mineral density is improved by high-impact aerobic exercise in postmenopausal women and men over 50 years. European Journal of Applied Physiology and Occupational Physiology 74:511–517

Weltman A, Weltman J Y, Roy C P et al 2006 Growth hormone response to graded exercise intensities is attenuated and the gender difference abolished in older adults. Journal of Applied Physiology 100(5):1623–1629

Whedon G D 1984 Disuse osteoporosis. Calcified Tissue International 36:S146–S150

Wolf S L, Sattin R W et al 2003 Intense Tai Chi exercise training and fall occurrences in older, transitionally frail adults: A randomized, controlled trial. Journal of the American Geriatrics Society 51:1693–1701

Wolf S L, Barnhart H X, Kutner N G et al 1996 Reducing frailty and falls in older persons: an investigation of tai chi and computerised balance training. Journal of the American Geriatrics Society 44:489–497

World Health Organization (WHO) 1958 Constitution of the World Health Organization. Annexe 1. The first ten years. WHO, Geneva

World Health Organization (WHO) 1997 The Heidleberg Guidelines for promoting physical activity among older persons. Journal of Aging and Physical Activity 5:1–8

World Health Organization (WHO) 2002 Global population profile, international population reports. US Department of Commerce, Economics and Statistics Administration, US Census Bureau

Wright A 1983 The surface structures of the human vestibular apparatus. Clinical Otolaryngology and Allied Sciences 8:53–63

Yardley L, Smith H 2003 A prospective study of the relationship between feared consequences of falling and avoidance of activity in community-living older people. Gerontologist 42:17–23

Yardley L, Donovan-Hall M, Francis K, Todd C 2006 Older people's views of advice about falls prevention: a qualitative study. Health Education Research 21(4):508–517

Yerg J E 2nd, Seals D R, Hagberg J M, Holloszy J O 1985 Effect of endurance exercise training on ventilatory function in older individuals. Journal of Applied Physiology 58:791–794

Young A 1986 Exercise physiology in geriatric practice. Acta Medica Scandinavica 711 (Suppl):227–232

Young A 1997 Ageing and physiological functions. Philosophical Transactions of the Royal Society of London B: 352(1363):1837–1843

Young A 2001 For a healthier old age. In: Young A, Harries M (eds) Physical activity for patients. An exercise prescription. Royal College of Physicians, London

Young A, Dinan S 2005 Active in later life. In: McLatchie G, Harries M, Williams C, King J (eds) ABC of sports medicine, 2nd edn. London: British Medical Journal Books, London

Zhu W, Chodzko-Zajko W J 2006 Measurement issues in aging and physical activity. Human Kinetics, Champaign, IL

Further reading

Jones C J, Rose D J (eds) 2005 Physical activity instruction of older adults. Human Kinetics, Champaign, IL

Lord S R, Sherrington C, Menz H B 2001 Falls in older people: risk factors and strategies for prevention. Cambridge University Press, Cambridge

Spirduso W (ed) 2005 Physical dimensions of aging. Human Kinetics, Champaign, IL

Young A, Harries M (eds) 2001 Physical activity for patients. an exercise prescription. Royal College of Physicians, London

Chapter 7

Bone health

Jacky J Forsyth and Rachel C Davey

CHAPTER CONTENTS

Learning objectives 225
Background information on bone tissue
    and bone remodelling 226
Background to diseases of poor bone
    health – osteoporosis and
    osteopenia 228
    Assessment of osteoporosis 231
Physical activity and bone health 231
Dose response 234
Dose response – exercise mode 235
    Jumping 235
    Walking 235
    Resistance training 236
Dose response – frequency, intensity and
    duration 236
Application of training principles to a
    bone health programme 237
    Specificity 237

Progressive overload 237
Reversibility 237
Principle of initial values and the
    principle of diminishing
    returns 238
Practical issues for prescribing
    exercise for bone health and gaps
    in the research 238
Children, adolescents and young
    adults 240
Dietary advice associated with bone
    health 240
Conclusion 241
Review and task 241
Key points 242
References 242
Further reading 247

LEARNING OBJECTIVES

After studying this chapter, you should be able to:

1. Describe the structure of bone, and gain a basic understanding of the physiological processes involved in the bone remodelling process.
2. Define osteoporosis and osteopenia, and describe how these diseases are assessed.
3. Identify possible risk factors for osteoporosis and osteopenia, and critically analyse how exercise and physical activity can prevent or ameliorate these conditions.
4. Critically appraise the evidence base for recommendations on physical activity for bone health in terms of exercise mode, frequency, intensity and duration.
5. Identify gaps in the evidence base and highlight key areas for future research.

BACKGROUND INFORMATION ON BONE TISSUE AND BONE REMODELLING

The functions of bone are to support and protect tissues of the body, to provide a framework for movement, to give the body shape, to produce blood cells, and to provide a metabolic reservoir of ions (in particular calcium and phosphate). There are two types of bone tissue – cortical bone (also known as compact bone) and trabecular bone (also called cancellous bone or spongy bone). Approximately 80% of the skeleton consists of cortical bone, and 20% of trabecular bone. Cortical bone is found on the outer surfaces of most bones and in the shafts of long bones (Fig. 7.1). Trabecular bone is found mainly at the ends of long bones (Fig. 7.1), and in the internal portions of other bones, such as the spine, pelvis, skull and ribs. Composition of a particular bone depends on its function. Cortical bone provides strength, structure and support to the skeleton, deriving its strength from dense mineralization. The structural unit of cortical bone is the Haversian system or osteon, which usually runs parallel to the

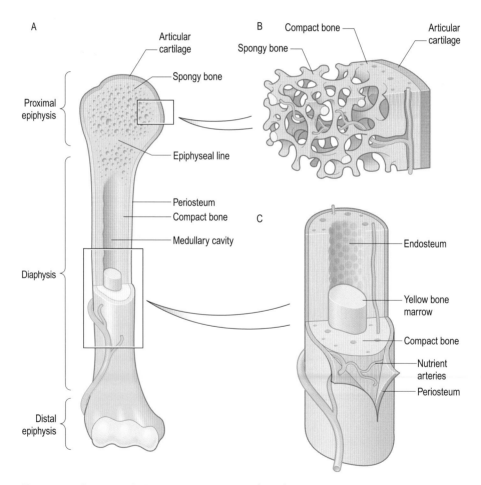

Figure 7.1   Structure of a long bone. From Marieb (2004), with permission of Pearson Benjamin Cummings, Pearson Education.

long axis of the bone (Fig. 7.1). Trabecular bone consists of a criss-cross matrix, the elements of which are called trabeculae, which give this bone its honeycomb appearance. The trabeculae are positioned in such a way as to maximize strength and minimize weight. Bone marrow fills the spaces (lacunae) between the trabeculae, with only about 15–25% of the bone being calcified. This bone marrow is red where haemopoiesis is active, yellow where it is not. Trabecular bone has a higher turnover rate, and a higher age-associated loss than cortical bone.

Bone remodelling involves the systematic renewal and repair of bone that occurs throughout adult life, and takes place predominantly within trabecular bone. Bone contains osteoblasts ('bone germinators'), which are bone-forming cells, and osteoclasts ('bone breakers') or bone-absorbing cells. Osteoblasts are derived from mesenchymal stem cells, and osteoclasts from mononuclear or phagocytic cells. Remodelling is triggered by microtrauma, possibly in response to chemical or mechanical stimuli. Osteoclasts are attracted to the site where the remodelling is required, and remove bone (bone resorption). Osteoblasts are then recruited to these sites (resorption pits) and bone formation begins. Osteoblasts secrete collagen and various proteins, creating osteoid, which is uncalcified bone tissue. Osteoblasts assist with calcification of the osteoid, a process that is not fully understood, but involves secretion of alkaline phosphatase, osteocalcin and osteonectin. Some of the osteoblasts become embedded in the matrix of the bone tissue to become osteocytes, which are mature bone cells. A schematic representation of bone remodelling is shown in Figure 7.2.

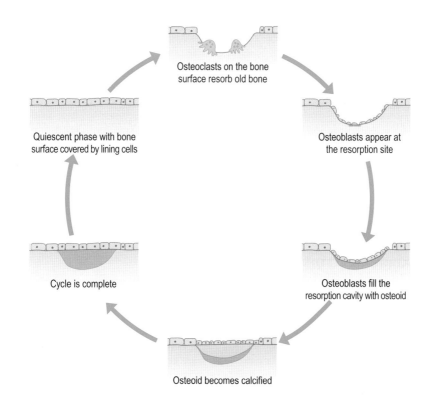

Figure 7.2   Schematic representation of the bone remodelling process.

Parathyroid hormone (PTH), produced by the parathyroid gland, and calcitonin, from specialized cells within the thyroid gland, are together responsible for the homeostatic maintenance of ionized calcium in the blood, and so play an important role in the bone remodelling process. A fall in calcium ions stimulates a release of PTH from the parathyroid; this stimulates osteoclasts to reabsorb bone mineral, resulting in an increase in calcium in the bloodstream. A fall in calcium ions or an increase in PTH, therefore, results in loss of bone tissue. When blood calcium levels rise, the thyroid secretes calcitonin, which inhibits bone resorption, leading to more calcium being deposited and so retained in the bone.

Ossification (the process of bone formation) can be classified according to where the bone develops. Endochondral (or intra-cartilaginous) ossification occurs within cartilage, with this process most commonly occurring in long bones, and initiating in the fetus. Intramembranous ossification occurs within a fibrous membrane and results in the formation of most bones of the skull and clavicle. Bone growth occurs at the epiphyseal plates (epiphyseal line as depicted in Fig. 7.1) in childhood and early adulthood, serving to increase the length of the bone. Width of the bone increases via intramembranous or subperiosteal bone formation, the periosteum being the membrane of connective tissue that covers the outside of the bone. Bone growth is greatest during infancy and around puberty. Peak bone mass is usually reached by 30 years of age, after which time bone mass decreases by 1% per year (Riggs et al 1986), with an accelerated phase of bone loss occurring among women in the perimenopausal and menopausal periods, associated with the decline in oestrogen. Bone mass in men decreases at a steadier rate with increasing age. The exact time at which peak bone mass is reached differs according to the region of the body. For instance, peak bone mass is reached by age 16 in the femoral neck, but does not occur until the third decade in the lumbar spine. In general, peak bone mass is reached in girls earlier than in boys, coinciding with the onset of menstruation (Bailey 1997). Trabecular bone degenerates first, starting in the third decade, whilst cortical bone continues to increase into the fifth decade (Marcus et al 1983, Riggs et al 1986). The difference in the occurrence of peaks in bone mass has implications for exercise and training, and may modify bone response to the stimulus of exercise. Essentially, though, there are two main mechanisms that determine adult bone health:

1. the maximum attainment of peak bone mass achieved during growth and early adulthood, where there is as much as a 40–70% increase in bone density during the pubertal years, thus an important period for skeletal development, and
2. the rate of bone loss with advancing age, especially pronounced during the menopause for women.

BACKGROUND TO DISEASES OF POOR BONE HEALTH – OSTEOPOROSIS AND OSTEOPENIA

The diseases most commonly associated with poor bone health are osteoporosis and osteopenia. Other diseases, such as Paget's disease (which involves excessive osteoblast activity resulting in bone deformity), osteomalacia and rickets (in which calcification of the osteoid is inhibited as a result of a deficiency in vitamin D) will not be included in this chapter, since they are fairly rare conditions.

Osteoporosis is characterized by low bone mass, low bone mineral content (BMC), and architectural deterioration of bone tissue (Drinkwater 1994), affecting both trabecular and cortical bone. Simply, it occurs when osteocyte activity exceeds osteoblast

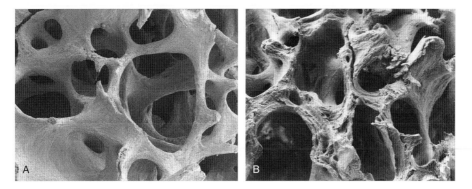

Figure 7.3   The effect of osteoporosis on trabecular bone. (A) Healthy bone tissue (Picture Number P105/212 Dee Breger/Science Photo Library). (B) Bone tissue from a patient suffering from osteoporosis (Picture Number M230/344 Dee Breger/Science Photo Library).

activity. The effects of osteoporosis on trabecular (spongy) bone are depicted in Figure 7.3. Osteoporosis is diagnosed and defined using T-scores derived from dual energy X-ray absorptiometry (DEXA). Bone mineral density (BMD), which is measured using DEXA, is the amount of mineral per unit area or volume of bone tissue (Kahn et al 2001). The T-score is the difference between an individual's BMD and that of a young, normal adult of the same sex and ethnicity at peak bone mass. The T-scores are expressed as a standard deviation (SD), with a BMD of more than 2.5 SD below the mean for a young, normal, adult population representing osteoporosis (World Health Organization 1994). It has, however, been suggested (Kahn et al 2002, Kohrt et al 2004) that this definition for osteoporosis may be too stringent, and may not be applicable to everyone. The onset of this disease, therefore, may be overlooked in individuals who might otherwise benefit from early intervention through exercise. Osteopenia is defined as a BMD of between 1.0 and 2.5 SD below the mean for a young, normal, adult population. Since individuals diagnosed with osteopenia at an early age are at increased risk of osteoporosis later in life, osteopenia is a key variable to determine.

Osteoporosis and osteopenia are major public health issues (Woolf & Pfleger 2003) because low BMD is usually associated with increased fracture risk (Nguyen et al 2005). Osteoporotic fractures occur in over 200 000 people annually in the UK (approximately 9 million worldwide), with the cost to the National Health Service for treatment being over £940 million per annum (Department of Health 1998, Johnell & Kanis 2006). An osteoporotic fracture is estimated to occur once every 3 minutes (Rutherford 1999), with the prevalence of osteoporosis being higher in women (1 in 3 women) than men (1 in 12 men) (Rutherford 1999). Osteoporotic fractures are common at the lumbar spine, femoral neck, distal radius, and vertebrae, where there is a high proportion of trabecular bone, and such fractures can mean a loss of independence and a reduction in quality of life. In extremis, mortality results, with chances of death increasing to 15–20% in the first year after a hip fracture (Woolf & Pfleger 2003). There are growing numbers of people living into mature age, so this trend is set to continue. Since fractures are common with increasing age, the demographical changes in the UK will mean an abundance of osteoporotic fractures in the future (van Staa et al 2001), which will have a huge impact on healthcare costs. In essence, increasing BMD at an early age through exercise may reduce the risk of a fracture later in life. For an overview of recommendations on preventing osteoporotic fractures, see Gass & Dawson-Hughes (2006). Further consideration of fracture risk in an older population may also be found in Chapter 6 of this book.

Current pharmacological treatments for osteoporosis include: hormone replacement therapy (HRT); bisphosphonates (anti-resorptive treatment, which prevents or slows the normal osteoclastic activity); calcitonin (an inhibitor of osteoclastic activity); selective oestrogen receptor modulators or SERMs (which act in a similar way to oestrogen, but without the reported side effects of HRT); vitamin D and calcium supplementation; recombinant DNA parathyroid hormone; and fluoride. For a review of the efficacy of these particular treatments, refer to Delaney (2006). In the UK, pharmacological treatments are usually only given to postmenopausal women, with no treatments being widespread for women prior to this age who may be at risk of developing osteoporosis later in life, or for men. Even if treatments were available for everyone, physical activity is more advantageous than pharmacological intervention, as it can be used as a preventative strategy, whereas treatments are usually only given once individuals have symptoms or suffer an osteoporotic fracture. Furthermore, physical activity concomitantly can increase fitness, beneficial for general health, and can improve balance, coordination and muscular strength, which together may decrease the risk of falls, and hence fractures, in an older population.

Risk factors (other than physical inactivity) for osteoporosis and osteopenia, are listed in Table 7.1 (Elgán et al 2003, Kahn et al 2001, Kanis 2002). In the aetiology of osteoporosis, genetic factors account for approximately 70–85% of cases (Ralston 1997). Various genes have been identified, including polymorphisms of the gene for the vitamin D receptor, interleukin genes, and genes for collagen type I. Genes

Table 7.1 Possible risk factors for osteoporosis and osteopenia

Non-modifiable risk factors
Sex (being female)
Age (more prevalent in older population)
Race (Caucasian/Asian)
Genetics
Modifiable risk factors
Low body mass, in particular fat-free mass (those of slight build or underweight, or a body mass index of ≤ 19 kg/m^2)
Premature menopause (prior to 45 years of age)
Early hysterectomy
Prolonged absence of menstruation (amenorrhoea)
Delayed menarche
Early menopause
Women who have borne no children
Chronic smoking (which reduces oestrogen levels)
Excessive alcohol consumption
Low dietary intake
Poor or calcium-deficient diet
Insufficient absorption of calcium and vitamin D, due to gastrointestinal disturbances, liver or bowel disease
Time spent outdoors
Depression
Corticosteroid use

may modify bone turnover, and may predispose individuals with a certain allele defect to greater bone loss and lower bone gain as a result of physical activity and exercise (Rabon-Stith et al 2005). Although there has been much development in our knowledge of genetics, it is not known precisely how genes interact with one another, and how genetics and the environment interact, meaning that modifiable lifestyle factors are still important determinants of bone health.

Assessment of osteoporosis

Dual energy X-ray absorptiometry (DEXA) is the primary tool for assessing BMD within a healthcare context and within research on bone health, although there are limitations inherent in the use of this technology, in particular, that BMD provides only an estimate of actual bone strength. In DEXA scans, the orientation of the bone needs to be replicated on repeat scans to ensure the same area projection. The scans also do not distinguish between BMD in trabecular bone and that in cortical bone, and provide no measure of bone geometry. Conversely, computed tomography (CT) allows for measurement of volumetric BMD, usually of the spine, with trabecular bone and cortical bone being distinguishable. This technique is, however, expensive and not widely available. A preferable alternative is broadband ultrasound attenuation of the calcaneus (and also radius and finger), which provides an indication of bone stiffness. This technique is easy to use, portable and allows for a bone scan without any exposure to ionizing radiation. Increasingly, biochemical markers of bone formation (such as bone-specific alkaline phosphatase and osteocalcin) and bone resorption (such as deoxypyridinoline and parathyroid hormone) are being utilized. Bone markers can identify acute changes in bone turnover in response to exercise, but are influenced by biological rhythms, such as time of day and menstrual cycle phase, and are not site specific.

The focus of this chapter will be on prevention of osteoporosis and osteopenia, rather than on treatment, because once osteoporosis is detected, it is often too late to do anything about it. Osteoporosis is, in this respect, a 'silent disease', since it is not usually diagnosed until a fracture has occurred. The two key factors to consider in prevention are maximizing peak bone mass in childhood and early adulthood, and minimizing the rate of bone loss with age. If physical activity is low among the young, the number of osteoporotic fractures is likely to rise in the future. Prioritizing prevention, by enhancing bone health in the young and delaying the age-associated loss are, therefore, the key issues that will be discussed.

PHYSICAL ACTIVITY AND BONE HEALTH

The idea of enhancing bone strength through exercise is based on Wolff's law, which states that stress or mechanical loading on the bone via muscles and tendons has a direct influence on bone turnover (Chamay & Tschantz 1972). The relevance of stress in determining bone strength can be seen in Figure 7.4. From early studies on bed rest (e.g. Saltin et al 1968) and those carried out in space (e.g. Whedon et al 1975), it was concluded that weight-bearing physical activity was necessary for maintaining bone health. Removing gravity virtually eliminates strain on bone, with astronauts losing up to 19% of their weight-bearing bone (Hughes-Fulford & Lewis 1996). Since these early studies, an abundance of research, both cross-sectional and longitudinal, has been conducted into bone health and exercise. Essentially, findings from studies among children, adolescents and adults have demonstrated the bone-enhancing

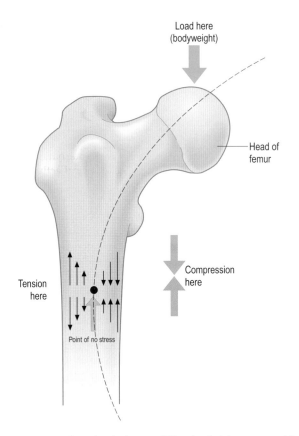

Figure 7.4   Bone anatomy and mechanical stress. When loaded, bones are subjected to bending stress. In this example using the femur of the thigh, bodyweight transmitted to the head of the femur threatens to bend the bone along the indicated arc. This bending compresses the bone on one side (converging arrows) and stretches it on the other side (diverging arrows). Because these two forces cancel each other internally, much less bone material is needed internally than superficially. From Marieb (2004), with permission of Pearson Benjamin Cummings, Pearson Education.

benefit of physical activity, particularly that of a high-impact, weight-bearing nature. Dynamic mechanical loading creates hydrostatic pressure gradients within bone's fluid-filled lacunar–canalicular framework. As the pressure gradients are equilibrated, shear stresses are generated on the plasma membranes of the osteocytes and osteoblasts, which respond by initiating a number of cellular events that increase intracellular calcium, expression of growth factors and ultimately bone matrix production. Before considering the mode, frequency, intensity and duration of exercise that should be recommended, some of the issues with the studies that have been conducted to date will be addressed.

In cross-sectional studies, as well as the limitation of comparing discrete groups of individuals, there is also the issue of cause and effect. In other words, individuals with an already well-developed musculoskeletal system, enhanced strength and fitness, or a genetic predisposition for such, might choose or be chosen to engage in vigorous, high-impact activity. When comparing these individuals with non-active controls, the total body BMD may be exaggerated, leading to a difference in BMD between the athletes and controls of more than 10%. In a study by Nordström et al (2006), there was no significant difference in BMD between the parents of the athletes that were studied and the parents of the controls, but BMD was significantly higher among the athletes (ice hockey and badminton players) compared to controls. In this instance, genetic factors did not seem to predispose the athletes into electing to participate in these sports.

In cross-sectional studies, questionnaires are often used to determine physical activity status. General questionnaires which estimate metabolic rate, such as the Paffenbarger Physical Activity Questionnaire or the International Physical Activity Questionnaire (IPAQ), do not distinguish between physical activity that induces bone growth and that which does not. A more specific Bone Loading History Questionnaire has been developed and validated by Dolan et al (2006), the results of which have been found to be positively associated with femoral neck BMD. Ginty et al (2005) used the European Prospective Investigation into Cancer Questionnaire, which examines impact. These types of questionnaire may be more useful for conducting cross-sectional studies on the history and current status of physical activity which leads to bone accrual, and are also useful for assessing risk of osteoporosis among a general population in a healthcare context.

Results of the effect of exercise on BMD from longitudinal studies are often less impressive than those derived from cross-sectional data. Factors that may account for these results include short duration of the study, an already high bone mass at outset, and problems with compliance (Drinkwater 1994, Rutherford 1999). Genetics may also play a role, and may predispose an individual to greater or lesser gains in BMD in response to an exercise regimen. Intervention studies that have been conducted of less than 6 months in duration might be too short to demonstrate an adaptive response, since bone remodelling takes approximately 3 to 6 months to complete depending on bone site (Humphries et al 2000). Since there is a decline in BMD of 1% per year with age after 30 years, a precision of 2–3% of analysis of BMD may not be accurate enough to detect changes observed as a result of an exercise programme of less than a year in duration (Bergstralh et al 1990). Seasonal variations in BMD also need to be taken into account, since BMD values are higher at the end of the summer compared to the winter both because of sunlight exposure, and because of increased physical activity levels in the summer months (Bergstralh et al 1990). Researchers reporting improvements in BMD in studies where training started in the early spring and finished in the late summer may have overestimated the amount of BMD accrued, if adequate controls were not in place. Although change in BMD is often small in longitudinal studies, bone mass loss is occurring with age, which also needs to be taken into account.

It is important to note that it may not be the physical activity per se that augments BMD, but the associated increase in musculature. Increases observed in BMD as a result of resistance training may, therefore, be a result of the increase in fat-free mass (Layne & Nelson 1999). Although increasing fat-free mass is obviously beneficial for general health purposes, any increase in body mass (whether by fat mass or fat-free mass) is beneficial to bone health. An increase in fat increases circulating levels of oestrogen, which are associated with bone formation. Both fat mass and fat-free mass have, therefore, been found to be related to BMD (Sowers et al 1992). This is of some concern when advising individuals to lose weight, either through exercise or through diet. Salamone et al (1999) found that a modest amount of weight loss (3.2 kg) among premenopausal women, who ranged from being of desirable weight to slightly overweight, led to a loss in BMD at the hip which was twice as great as that observed in the control group who did not lose weight. The loss in BMD was thought to be due to the weight loss directly, or due to the associated decrease in oestrogen and calcium. Physical activity appeared, in this instance, to attenuate the loss in BMD. When the aim is to enhance bone health, advising individuals to lose weight who are only moderately overweight or are of an ideal weight for their height is a decision that must be made on an individual basis. The benefits to general health and well-being as a result of the weight loss may not outweigh the detrimental effects on bone health and vice versa.

DOSE RESPONSE

It is difficult to relate exercise for bone health to any of the seven components of fitness outlined in Chapter 1. Increasing bone strength is not about being able to reach a maximum or being able to exercise at a particular intensity or threshold relative to maximum; rather it is about compressing or deforming the bone, with any force applied to the bone, such as ground-reaction forces, joint-muscle force, or muscle contraction force, being of the essence. Exercise and physical activity can add new bone, and even a relatively small amount of new bone can result in dramatic changes in bone strength if, for example, the new bone is localized to the medial and lateral periosteal surfaces where mechanical strains are greatest. From animal studies (e.g. Lanyon 1984, Rubin et al 2001), dynamic rather than static loads, high strain magnitudes (or intensity), high strain rates (the rate at which strain develops and is released), and unusual frequency distribution, all seem to have osteogenic (bone-forming) effects (Ehrlich & Lanyon 2002, Mosley 2000). The strain imposed also needs to be different from habitual strain, or the strain that the bone is used to in everyday living. Furthermore, trabecular bone appears to be more sensitive to strain than cortical bone (Rubin et al 2001). The results from animal studies have informed the research on dose response for humans. Within the position stand of the American College of Sports Medicine on physical activity and bone health, Kohrt et al (2004) provide recommendations for children and adolescents and for adults, as summarized in Table 7.2.

Table 7.2 Summary of recommendations from the American College of Sports Medicine Position Stand for augmenting bone mineral accrual (Kohrt et al 2004)

Children and adolescents	
Mode	Impact activities, e.g. gymnastics, plyometrics and jumping, and moderate-intensity resistance training; sports that involve running and jumping (e.g. soccer, basketball)
Intensity	High bone-loading forces; for safety reasons, resistance training should be $\leq$60% of 1-repetition maximum (1-RM)
Frequency	$\geq$3 days per week
Duration	10–20 minutes ($\geq$2 times per day may be better)
Adults	
Mode	Weight-bearing endurance activities (tennis, stair climbing, jogging); jumping activities (volleyball, basketball); resistance training
Intensity	Moderate to high bone-loading forces
Frequency	Weight-bearing endurance activities 3–5 times per week; resistance training 2–3 times per week
Duration	30–60 minutes a day of combined activities

DOSE RESPONSE – EXERCISE MODE

In general, studies that have examined high-impact activity have shown the most favourable results. Activities that are weight-supported, such as swimming, cycling and rowing, involve less mechanical strain on the bone, and are generally not advisable for bone health. Stewart & Hannan (2000), for instance, found that athletes who cycled exclusively had a significantly lower spine BMD than runners, athletes who both ran and cycled, and non-exercising controls. Stewart and Hannan suggested that cycling does not induce strains on the bone that are above a 'threshold' for remodelling, since there is no impact on the legs and the upper body is supported substantially by the handlebars.

Jumping

Jumping is often recommended as an activity that enhances bone health (Bassey & Ramsdale 1994, Fuchs et al 2001, Heinonen et al 1996, McKay et al 2005, Shibata et al 2003). Bassey & Ramsdale (1994), for instance, reported significant gains in BMD at the trochanter for a group of premenopausal women who engaged in a programme of jumping for only 60 seconds a day. Heinonen et al (1996) carried out a prospective, randomized controlled trial lasting 18 months, which involved jumping and stepping activities three times per week among premenopausal women (aged 35 to 45 years). The activities elicited peak forces between 2.1 and 5.6 times bodyweight. They observed a significant increase in BMD at the femoral neck compared to a control group. In a school-based programme (McKay et al 2005), BMC increased in young children who undertook 10 jumps at three discrete times a day on at least 2 days of the week, compared with age-matched controls. As with animal studies, the rapid strain reversal, low repetitions and high magnitude through the great ground-reaction forces elicited by jumping explain the significant increases observed in these studies. A very simple, low-cost and time-efficient jumping programme could, therefore, be recommended to both young children and adults (provided that jumping is not contraindicated for the particular individual) to augment bone health. The programme should involve a small number of jumps (between 10 and 20 jumps) repeated two to three times per day, daily or on at least 2 days of the week. To increase the impact, once the programme has been followed for 6 months or more, jumping may be performed from a box or with weighted vests (Fuchs et al 2001, Winters-Stone & Snow 2006). Any sport that involves jumping is also recommended for enhancing bone health. Suitable activities include tennis, high-impact aerobics, basketball, dance, gymnastics, netball, plyometrics, skipping, soccer and volleyball. Obviously, there are problems with recommending high-impact sport to the unaccustomed exerciser, in that individuals may not adhere to the training programme prescribed, or may become injured. It is, therefore, important to ensure that any programme introduced is gradual.

Walking

Walking is often recommended for cardiovascular health, but has not been advocated for enhancing bone health (Bassey 2001, Drinkwater 1994, Rutherford 1999). From a meta-analysis of ten studies, Palombaro (2005) concluded that there was no meaningful increase in BMD (measured using effect sizes) as a result of walking, and that walking-only interventions should not be recommended for maintaining BMD in men and women over the age of 50. Some of the studies on walking have, however, been carried out on active individuals, rather than sedentary non-walkers, which may explain the lack of significant increase in BMD. Brisk, as opposed to normal-paced walking, may be more suitable for attenuating the age-related loss in BMD (Brooke-Wavell et al 1997, Coupland et al 1999), with significant differences being evident between postmenopausal controls and walkers at the calcaneus, a site that is more specific than, for instance, the lumbar spine (Brooke-Wavell et al 1997). The advantage of walking, though, is that it is inexpensive and accessible. Shibata et al (2003) investigated the effect of a programme to encourage premenopausal women to walk 10 000 steps per day. An increase from a mean of 6422 steps to a mean of 7723 steps per day was sufficient to increase BMD at certain sites, and to increase markers of bone formation. Increases were more pronounced, however, for the group of 17 women who also undertook jumping activity (one two-footed jump, 10 times per day). In conclusion, walking may not be sufficient enough to induce an adaptive response, possibly due to the bone becoming desensitized to the repetitive nature of this activity, and because most people already include some amount of walking in their everyday lives. The same may be said for running, although the impact here is much greater. Walking may, however, be recommended for the very inactive or for those who have been bedridden through illness or injury.

Resistance training

Weight training may not be the most effective exercise for increasing mechanical stress, and hence increasing BMD (Gleeson et al 1990, Pruitt et al 1992, Rutherford 1999), since the strain caused by muscle contraction forces is generally less than that produced by ground-reaction forces (Rubin et al 2001). The most significant findings have been with lower repetitions, greater resistance, faster speeds, or with novel training methods, in parallel with the findings from animal studies. In a study by Gleeson et al (1990), BMD only increased by 0.81%, which was non-significant, when premenopausal women undertook a low-intensity, resistance training programme (60% of 1-RM). It was concluded that the small gain in BMD observed might not warrant the time, effort and motivation that is required to undertake this type of resistance training programme. In contrast, Stengel et al (2005) reported that BMD of the lumbar spine and proximal hip was significantly greater among a group of 21 postmenopausal women who undertook 'power training' compared to a group who undertook 'resistance training', despite equivalent increases in strength. The power training consisted of a concentric fast/explosive, 4-second eccentric sequence, whereas the resistance training consisted of a 4-second concentric, 4-second eccentric sequence. The high-velocity nature of the power training resulted in high strain rates and frequencies, and high loading magnitudes and amplitudes. These findings reflect the importance of carrying out resistance training at high velocities, to maximize the osteogenic process. For a further review of the effect of resistance training on BMD, refer to Layne & Nelson (1999).

DOSE RESPONSE – FREQUENCY, INTENSITY AND DURATION

The components duration, frequency and intensity may interact. For instance, with increasing frequencies, the magnitude of the force that is required may be less (Rubin et al 2001). Although the magnitude of loading is low in jogging, the volume or duration is often long enough to produce an osteogenic effect, although since the number of strain cycles need only be small, there is little point, from a bone health perspective, in increasing the duration of a particular activity excessively. Kohrt et al (2004) recommend a duration of 10–20 minutes, twice a day, for adults although, as reported previously, increases in BMD have been found with durations of much less than 10 minutes (e.g. Bassey & Ramsdale 1994), with the added benefit that stress fractures and injury can be avoided. As a rule on intensity, the exercise should be prescribed based on estimated strain that is placed on the bone, rather than by a particular percentage of maximum or an exercise intensity such as heart rate or ratings of perceived exertion. In conclusion, it appears that single bouts of dynamic activity, such as fast jumping, repeated throughout the day, and on at least 3 days of the week seem to be most beneficial for enhancing bone health (Kohrt et al 2004, Rubin et al 2001).

APPLICATION OF TRAINING PRINCIPLES TO A BONE HEALTH PROGRAMME

Specificity

The effect of bone loading is site specific (Kannus et al 1995, Winters-Stone & Snow 2006). Specificity has been demonstrated by comparing the dominant arm with the non-dominant arm of athletes who play racket sports. Among 61 male veteran tennis players who had been playing tennis for an average of 40 years, Montoye et al (1980) found that bone width and mineral content of the players' forearms were greater in their dominant arms. Likewise in runners, there is usually an increase in BMD of the lower limbs, with no concomitant increase in BMD of the lumbar spine (MacKelvie et al 2000). Premenopausal women who undertook an exercise programme of the lower body had increases in BMD of the hip only, but not the spine, whereas those who undertook both an upper and lower body programme (consisting of a variety of jumps and upper and lower body resistance exercises) also gained in BMD at the spine (Winters-Stone & Snow 2006). Even if strain is considered, therefore, the loading effect will still be site-specific, and may even vary according to bone type – cortical or trabecular bone.

Progressive overload

This principle applies to bone accrual, with the need to begin a programme of exercise at a sufficient impact or intensity to induce an osteogenic response. The programme should then be modified in stages, to ensure continued increases in bone mass, or for older individuals, to prevent bone loss. As an example, for someone who has been confined to bed a walking programme may be of sufficient intensity initially, but after several months of this type of activity the bone will be inadequately loaded if progression is not made. The load must, therefore, be greater than the individual is used to at any particular stage.

Reversibility

The principle of reversibility suggests that BMD gained with physical activity will revert back to pre-exercise levels if exercise is stopped (Dalsky et al 1988). From a 27-year analysis of participation levels in physical activity during youth and adulthood, van Langendonck et al (2003) concluded that continued participation in high-impact sports was necessary to ensure positive bone health during adult-hood. The reduction in BMD with cessation of exercise may also be greater in weight-bearing bones, compared to non-weight-bearing bones (Gustavsson et al 2003). It has been suggested by Nordström et al (2006), however, that BMD gained in youth as a result of intensive training may be retained. They monitored BMD of athletes (badminton and ice hockey players) 5 years after the cessation of their training and found that the 'retired athletes' did not lose BMD at the proximal femur and humerus in comparison with both controls and active athletes. A high BMD achieved when younger through engagement in high-impact activity may, therefore, reduce the risk of osteoporosis in the future. In this respect, it appears that although the principle of reversibility may be applicable in the long term, in the short to medium term, cessation of an exercise programme may not be detri-mental to bone health, although obviously the goal should be for continued participation.

Principle of initial values and the principle of diminishing returns

The greatest benefits of a bone-enhancing exercise programme are for those who have the lowest BMD to begin with, although the caveat is that if BMD is too low, it is not possible to elicit a sufficient mechanical response to initiate bone accretion – this is why prevention is key. There is also a point beyond which minimal improvement will occur. For instance, for runners reporting over 95 km of running per week, mean values for BMD at the proximal femur were no different from those observed in active (but not trained) controls (MacKelvie et al 2000), and were actually lower than those observed in the runners who averaged between 64 and 80 km per week. This finding reinforces the idea that intensity of the strain is more important than frequency of repetition.

PRACTICAL ISSUES FOR PRESCRIBING EXERCISE FOR BONE HEALTH AND GAPS IN THE RESEARCH

If, having been prescribed an exercise programme of a high-impact nature to aug-ment bone health, a female subject becomes amenorrhoeic (no menstrual period for more than 3 months), paradoxically, she may actually lose bone. Amenorrhoeic athletes have significantly lower levels of BMD compared to eumenorrhoeic athletes and even compared to sedentary controls (Drinkwater et al 1990). Rencken et al (1996) found that 7 out of 49 amenorrhoeic athletes met the diagnostic criteria of being osteoporotic and 14 had osteopenia. The long duration of the amenorrhoea and late age at menarche (onset of menstruation) were important predictors of low BMD. Punpilai et al (2005) found that menstrual dysfunction, including irregular periods, among female athletes engaged in high-impact, weight-bearing activity (basketball and volleyball) was related to low BMD at the lumbar spine. Even high-impact, weight-bearing exercise, therefore, does not appear to compensate for the BMD lost through menstrual dysfunction.

Subdermal implant systems, such as Implanon, and injectable contraception, namely depot medroxyprogesterone acetate (DMPA), provide a sustained release of low levels of progestins, and are prescribed frequently for contraceptive pur-poses (Dorflinger 2002). Depot medroxyprogesterone acetate acts by inhibiting the secretion of oestrogen causing anovulation and alteration of the endometrium. There is an increasing body of knowledge derived from large-scale prospective and cross-sectional studies on premenopausal women and adolescent girls that use of progesterone-only contraception, in particular DMPA, has an adverse effect on bone health (Cromer et al 2004, Lara-Torre et al 2004, Rome et al 2004), particularly with sustained use and advancing age (Shaarawy et al 2006). From a review of 39 studies, Curtis & Martins (2006) reported that, in general, DMPA users had a lower mean BMD and greater reductions in BMD over time. A similar decrement in BMD has been found among adolescents taking a low-dose (20 µg ethinyl oestradiol) oral contraceptive (Cromer et al 2004).

A few studies have examined the combined effects of using progesterone-only or low-dose oral contraception and physical activity on BMD. Weaver et al (2001) found that women (aged 18 to 31 years) who exercised using oral contraception (OC) had reduced spine BMD and BMC compared to OC users who did not exercise. Hartard et al (1997) found that among a group of individuals who had been using OC for ≥ 3 years, combined with long-term exercise for ≥ 2 hours per week, BMD was comparable to non-OC users who did less exercise. Egan et al (2006) reported a significantly lower BMD at trochanter and total hip regions in athletes who used OC, compared to those who did not. For women who use contraception that is low in oestradiol or that is progesterone only, exercise, therefore, may not be sufficient to counter the contraceptive-related loss in BMD. The lack of oestrogen may counteract the effect of exercise by inhibiting bone formation in response to mechanical stress (Zaman et al 2000). Further research into this area is warranted.

Low levels of oestrogen, associated with progesterone-only contraception, are considered to be equivalent to the loss in oestrogen associated with the menopause (Clark et al 2001). In studies on menopausal women, even intense levels of exercise have been shown to be insufficient to prevent the menopause-related loss in BMD (Bassey et al 1998, Dalsky et al 1988, Humphries et al 2000, Tomkinson et al 2003). Bassey et al (1998), for instance, found no significant increases in BMD among postmenopausal women, despite there being increases in premenopausal women who undertook the same exercise programme. In contrast, an exercise intervention conducted in Erlangen, Germany (Erlangen Fitness Osteoporosis Prevention Study or EFOPS) has been in operation since 2002, with Kemmler et al (2005) reporting favourable consequences in terms of BMD in response to exercise among post-menopausal women. The exercise programme is multifaceted, including group and home-based exercise sessions consisting of resistance training, skipping and jumping. Forty-eight women have continued with the programme (3 years), and have exercised on average at least twice a week. This particular frequency and type of activity appear to offset the loss in BMD that is associated with postmenopausal ageing. It may be that the intervention studies carried out to date among contraceptive users and individuals who have menstrual dysfunction have not identified the specific mode, frequency, intensity and duration of activity that is required for these particular individuals.

The decrease in BMD associated with menopause, contraceptive use and amenorrhoea occurs primarily due to the decrease in endogenous oestrogen. Osteoclastic activity accelerates, and activity of the osteoblasts reduces. The precise mechanism is described elsewhere (Ehrlich & Lanyon 2002, Riggs 2000) and in Chapter 8. The loss of BMD, however, may also be because of a low body mass index (BMI), associated with reduced energy availability (Zanker & Swaine 1998), particularly common in amenorrhoeic athletes. Other factors, such as a reduction in insulin-like growth factor (IGF-1) and leptin levels, may contribute to reduced bone accretion among athletes (Warren & Pelroth 2001).

CHILDREN, ADOLESCENTS AND YOUNG ADULTS

Physical activity that stresses the bone is particularly important during puberty and adolescence. Since consideration is being given to prevention rather than treatment, and since relatively less BMD accrues in later adulthood, recommendations for physical activity to enhance bone health that are specific for children, adolescents and young adults will be given special consideration. Consistent with research findings on other population groups, active children and adolescents have a higher BMD than their inactive counterparts, and this is higher still if children participate in high-impact sports such as gymnastics, ballet dancing, jumping, skipping, plyometrics, running and weightlifting compared to non-impact sports such as swimming (Bassey et al 1998, Cassell et al 1996, MacKelvie et al 2000, Petit et al 2002). The starting age for enhancing bone health is crucial. The benefit to bone is at least doubled if physical activity is started before or at puberty rather than after it (Kannus et al 1995, Sabatier et al 1999). Results from a school curriculum-based exercise programme (Malmö Pediatric Osteoporosis Prevention Study), where pre-menarcheal school girls aged 7 to 9 years just took part in more lessons of physical education (PE) rather than increasing the intensity of the activity performed, showed promising significant increases in BMC, areal BMD and bone width at the 2-year follow-up (Linden et al 2006). These findings suggest that the usual government-prescribed PE of one or two sessions of 30 minutes a week is not enough to benefit bone health. In the Malmö study, the intervention group did 40 minutes of PE every day. In contrast, McKay et al (2005) suggest that a simple intervention of 10 jumps undertaken three times a day within the school time ('Bounce at the Bell' initiative) was sufficient to induce an increase in bone health. This type of programme does not require any specialist equipment, and only takes approximately 3 minutes to complete, which is far less time-consuming than increasing the duration of the PE lesson.

DIETARY ADVICE ASSOCIATED WITH BONE HEALTH

Dietary recommendations are worth mentioning, since often when prescribing exercise it is common to also consider dietary intake, as physical activity and diet are both linked with energy balance. Calcium intake has been found to correlate with BMD (Kyriazopoulos et al 2006), although calcium cannot replace or prevent loss of bone matrix. Recommended calcium intake in the UK is 700 mg a day for adults over 19 years (Committee on the Medical Aspects of Food and Nutrition Policy 1998), with a recommended intake for breastfeeding women of 1250 mg per day. Recommended intake for boys up to 18 years of age is 1000 mg per day, and for girls of the same age is 800 mg per day. Good food sources include dairy products, green vegetables, dried figs, canned sardines, white and brown flour, and bread (the latter two food types being fortified with calcium). Conversely, excessive meat, salt, caffeine and alcohol consumption may inhibit absorption. There are no recent data about calcium intake in primary school children (Department of Health 1998), but values among secondary school children appear to be lower than recommended. Matkovic et al (2005) found a positive effect of calcium supplementation (670 mg per day above that usually ingested) on BMD among children during their pubertal growth spurt, although after this age, the benefit of calcium supplementation diminished. In a review by Winzenberg et al (2006), which included studies on children aged from 3 to 18 years, it was concluded that calcium supplementation had little effect on BMD, with a small increase in BMD in the upper limb not being of any clinical significance in terms of current and future fracture risk. The combined effect of physical activity and calcium supplementation on bone health, however, needs to be investigated further.

Vitamin D aids calcium absorption, and therefore bone health, yet there are no recommendations for dietary intake of vitamin D for individuals aged between 4 and 64 years of age, as it is assumed that enough sunlight exposure will ensure adequate synthesis. Sunlight causes the photoconversion of 7-dehydrocholesterol, an inactive form of vitamin D, which is then stored in the liver and kidneys for later use. During the winter, stores built up in the summer are utilized. Melin et al (2001) suggested that individuals at risk of vitamin D deficiency, because of inadequate cutaneous generation of vitamin D, include those who spend less than 3 hours per day out of doors, especially in the winter months, and those living in northerly latitudes, such as Scandinavia. Individuals who wear clothing that prevents penetration of sunshine, such as those following a strict Islamic dress code, or those using a high factor sunscreen, are also at risk (Hatun et al 2005). Other individuals vulnerable to vitamin D deficiency include children under the age of 3 years, lactating women and people over 65 years, all of whom have been found to have lower intakes than recommended (Department of Health 1998), as well as those with diets poor in vitamin D, such as those excluding meat and oily fish.

Other nutrients, including vitamins A, C and K, sodium, protein and phytooestrogens, may also enhance bone health. In particular, protein intake has been found to be an important determinant of bone health, being linked to fracture incidence in an older population (Hannan et al 2000, Munger et al 1999). Vegans may have an increased risk of osteoporosis, owing to lower amounts of calcium and vitamin D, particularly from animal products, in the diet (Smith 2006). For more extensive reviews in this area, refer to Nieves (2005) and Winzenberg et al (2006).

CONCLUSION

Whilst 30 minutes of moderate-intensity exercise per day is recommended for improving general health, and for reducing the risk of mortality from various diseases, this type of cardiovascular exercise is of little use for bone health. Yet, doing some very simple, bone-loading activities in childhood and into adulthood may be all that is required to prevent osteoporosis. Exercises, such as performing some small, two-footed jumps, or squeezing a tennis ball for only a minute a day, may be all that is required. If going to the gym is already a part of the daily routine, then incorporating some dynamic wrist curls, or spending a minute or two at the punch bag, could be beneficial for BMD improvements in the upper body. It is quite unusual, however, for such bone-enhancing activities to be prescribed to the average gym-goer, or the average sedentary individual who wishes to start an exercise programme. To avoid premature death as a result of an osteoporotic fracture, and to bring down the cost of osteoporosis to the National Health Service generally, more specific, bone-enhancing exercise needs to be prescribed. Consideration should also be given to individual factors that may affect bone accrual, such as disruptions to the menstrual cycle, restricted dietary intake, and the effects of limited sunlight exposure.

REVIEW AND TASK

A 35-year-old woman wishes to improve her bone health, as she has a family history of osteoporosis. She is already fairly active, walking the dog every day for 30 minutes. Based on your reading on bone health and exercise, select and justify a programme of activities that she might partake in to improve her bone health on a weekly basis. Critically consider the confounding factors that may influence the extent to which she will improve her chances of avoiding osteoporosis in the future.

KEY POINTS

1. Bone remodelling involves the systematic renewal and repair of bone that occurs throughout adult life, involving activity of osteoblasts, osteoclasts, parathyroid hormone and calcitonin.
2. Peak bone mass is usually reached by 30 years of age, depending on sex, type of bone tissue and region of the body, with a loss of approximately 1% of bone mass occurring per year thereafter.
3. Osteoporosis is defined as a BMD (assessed via, for instance, DEXA) of >2.5 SD below the mean for a young, normal, adult population, and is associated with increased fracture risk, potentially resulting in loss of independence, and premature death.
4. Two key factors in the preventing osteoporosis are to maximize peak bone mass in childhood and early adulthood, and minimize the rate of bone loss with advancing age.
5. High-impact, weight-bearing, dynamic and non-habitual exercise seem to be effective in maximizing peak bone mass and minimizing bone loss, specific to the site being exercised.
6. Factors such as low oestrogen for women, a low body mass, chronic smoking, a genetic predisposition for osteoporosis, and a calcium-poor diet may limit the amount of bone mass that can be attained, and/or may accelerate bone loss.
7. These key points should be considered when prescribing exercise for the prevention of osteoporosis.

References

Bailey D A 1997 The Saskatchewan bone mineral accrual study: bone mineral acquisition during the growing years. International Journal of Sports Medicine 18(Suppl 3):S191–S194

Bassey E J 2001 Exercise for prevention of osteoporotic fracture. Age and Ageing 30-S4:29–31

Bassey E J, Ramsdale S J 1994 Increase in femoral bone density in young women following high-impact exercise. Osteoporosis International 4(2):72–75

Bassey E J, Rothwell M C, Littlewood J J, Pye D W 1998 Pre-and postmenopausal women have different bone mineral density responses to the same high-impact exercise. Journal of Bone and Mineral Research 13(112):1805–1813

Bergstralh E, Sinaki M, Offord K P et al 1990 Effect of season on physical activity score, back extensor muscle strength, and lumbar bone mineral density. Journal of Bone and Mineral Research 5(4):371–377

Brooke-Wavell K, Jones P R M, Hardman A E 1997 Brisk walking reduces calcaneal bone loss in post-menopausal women. Clinical Science 92:75–80

Cassell C, Benedict M, Specker B 1996 Bone mineral density in elite 7- to 9-yr-old female gymnasts and swimmers. Medicine and Science in Sports and Exercise 28(10):1243–1246

Chamay A, Tschantz P 1972 Mechanical influences in bone remodelling. Experimental research on Wolff's law. Journal of Biomechanics 5(2):173–180

Clark M K, Sower M, Levy B T, Tenhundfeld P 2001 Magnitude and variability of sequential estradiol and progesterone concentration in women using depot medroxyprogesterone acetate for contraception. Fertility and Sterility 75:871–877

Committee on Medical Aspects of Food and Nutrition Policy 1998 Nutrition and bone health with particular reference to calcium and vitamin D. HMSO, London

Coupland C A C, Cliffe S J, Bassey E J et al 1999 Habitual physical activity and bone mineral density in postmenopausal women in England. International Journal of Epidemiology 28:241–246

Cromer B A, Stager M, Bonny A et al 2004 Depot medroxyprogesterone acetate, oral contraceptives and bone mineral density in a cohort of adolescent girls. Journal of Adolescent Health 35:434–441

Curtis K M, Martins S L 2006 Progesterone-only contraception and bone mineral density: a systematic review. Contraception 73:470–487

Dalsky G P, Stocke K S, Ehsani A A et al 1988 Weight-bearing exercise training and lumbar bone mineral content in postmenopausal women. Annals of Internal Medicine 108(6):824–828

Delaney M F 2006 Strategies for the prevention and treatment of osteoporosis during early postmenopause. American Journal of Obstetrics and Gynecology 194(2 Suppl):S12–S23

Department of Health 1998 Report on Health and Social Studies. 49 Nutrition and bone health: with particular reference to calcium and vitamin D. The Stationery Office, London

Dolan S H, Williams D P, Ainsworth B E, Shaw J M 2006 Development and reproducibility of the Bone Loading History Questionnaire. Medicine and Science in Sports and Exercise 38(6):1121–1131

Dorflinger L J 2002 Metabolic effects of implantable steroid contraceptives for women. Contraception 65(3):47–62

Drinkwater B L 1994 Does physical activity play a role in preventing osteoporosis? Research Quarterly for Exercise and Sports 65(3):197–206

Drinkwater B L, Bruemner B, Chestnut C H 1990 Menstrual history as a determinant of current bone density in young athletes. Journal of the American Medical Association 263:545–548

Egan E, Reilly T, Giacomoni M et al 2006 Bone mineral density among female sports participants. Bone 38:227–233

Ehrlich P J, Lanyon L E 2002 Mechanical strain and bone cell function: a review. Osteoporosis International 13:688–700

Elgán C, Samsioe G, Dykes A-K 2003 Influence of smoking and oral contraceptives on bone mineral density and bone remodelling in young women: a 2-year study. Contraception 67:439–447

Fuchs R K, Bauer J J, Snow C M 2001 Jumping improves hip and lumbar spine bone mass in prepubescent children: a randomized controlled trial. Journal of Bone and Mineral Research 16(1):148–156

Gass M, Dawson-Hughes B 2006 Preventing osteoporosis-related fractures: an overview. American Journal of Medicine 119(4A):3S–11S

Ginty F, Rennie K L, Mills L et al 2005 Positive, site-specific associations between bone mineral status, fitness, and time spent at high-impact activities in 16- to 18-year-old boys. Bone 36(1):101–110

Gleeson P B, Protas E J, LeBlanc A D et al 1990 Effects of weight lifting on bone mineral density in premenopausal women. Journal of Bone and Mineral Research 5(2):153–158

Gustavsson A, Olsson T, Nordström P 2003 Rapid loss of bone mineral density of the femoral neck after cessation of ice hockey training: a 6-year longitudinal study in males. Journal of Bone and Mineral Research 18:1964–1969

Hannan M T, Tucker K L, Dawson-Hughes B et al 2000 Effect of dietary protein on bone loss in elderly men and women: the Framingham Osteoporosis Study. Journal of Bone and Mineral Research 15(2):2504–2512

Hartard M, Bottermann P, Bartenstein P et al 1997 Effects on bone mineral density of low-dosed oral contraceptives compared to and combined with physical activity. Contraception 55:87–90

Hatun S, Islam Ö, Cizmecioglu F, Kara B et al 2005 Subclinical vitamin D deficiency is increased in adolescent girls who wear concealing clothing. Journal of Nutrition 135:218–222

Heinonen A, Kannus P, Sievänen H et al 1996 Randomised controlled trial of effect of high-impact exercise on selected risk factors for osteoporotic fractures. Lancet 348:1343–1347

Hughes-Fulford M, Lewis M L 1996 Effects of microgravity on osteoblast growth activation. Experimental Cell Research 224(1):103–109

Humphries B, Newton R U, Bronks R et al 2000 Effect of exercise intensity on bone density, strength, and calcium turnover in older women. Medicine and Science in Sports and Exercise 32(6):1043–1050

Johnell O, Kanis J A 2006 An estimate of the worldwide prevalence and disability associated with osteoporotic fractures. Osteoporosis International 17(12):1726–1733

Kahn K, McKay H, Kannus P et al 2001 Physical activity and bone health. Human Kinetics, Champaign, IL

Kahn K M, Liu-Ambrose T, Sran M M et al 2002 New criteria for female athlete triad syndrome? British Journal of Sports Medicine 36(1):10–13

Kanis J A 2002 Diagnosis of osteoporosis and assessment of fracture risk. Lancet 359:1929–1936

Kannus P, Haapasalo H, Sankelo M et al 1995 Effect of starting age of physical activity on bone mass in the dominant arm of tennis and squash players. Annals of Internal Medicine 123(1):27–31

Kemmler W, von Stengel S, Weineck J et al 2005 Exercise effects on menopausal risk factors of early postmenopausal women: 3-yr Erlangen Fitness Osteoporosis Prevention Study results. Medicine and Science in Sports and Exercise 37(20):194–203

Kohrt W M, Bloomfield S A, Little K D et al 2004 American College of Sports Medicine Position Stand: Physical activity and bone health. Medicine and Science in Sports and Exercise 36(11):1985–1996

Kyriazopoulos P, Trovas G, Charopoulos J et al 2006 Lifestyle factors and forearm bone density in young Greek men. Clinical Endocrinology 65(2):234–238

Lanyon L E 1984 Functional strain as a determinant for bone remodelling. Calcified Tissue International 36:S56–S61

Lara-Torre E, Edwards C P, Perlman S, Hertweck S P 2004 Bone mineral density in adolescent females using depot medroxyprogesterone acetate. Journal of Pediatric Adolescent Gynecology 17:17–21

Layne J E, Nelson M E 1999 The effects of progressive resistance training on bone density: a review. Medicine and Science in Sports and Exercise 31(1):25–30

Linden C, Ahlborg H G, Besjakov J et al 2006 A school curriculum-based exercise program increases bone mineral accrual and bone size in prepubertal girls: two-year data from the pediatric osteoporosis prevention (POP) study. Journal of Bone and Mineral Research 21(6):826–835

McKay H A, MacLean L, Petit M et al 2005 'Bounce at the Bell': A novel programme of short bouts of exercise improves proximal femur bone mass in early pubertal children. British Journal of Sports Medicine 39:521–526

MacKelvie K J, Tanunton J E, McKay H A, Khan K M 2000 Bone mineral density and serum testosterone in chronically trained, high mileage 40–55 year old male runners. British Journal of Sports Medicine 34:273–278

Marcus R, Kosek J, Pfefferbaum A, Horning S 1983 Age-related loss of trabecular bone in premenopausal women: a biopsy study. Calcified Tissue International 35(4–5):406–409

Marieb E N 2004 Human anatomy and physiology, international edn – 6th edn. Pearson Benjamin Cummings, Pearson Education, San Francisco, CA

Matkovic V, Goel P K, Badnhop-Stevens N E et al 2005 Calcium supplementation and bone mineral density in females from childhood to young adulthood: a randomized controlled trial. American Journal of Clinical Nutrition 81(1):175–188

Melin A, Wilske J, Ringertz H, Sääf M 2001 Seasonal variations in serum levels of 25-hydroxyvitamin D and parathyroid hormone but no detectable change in femoral neck bone density in an older population with regular outdoor exposure. Journal of the American Geriatrics Society 49:1190–1196

Montoye H J, Smith E L, Fardon D F, Howley E T 1980 Bone mineral in senior tennis players. Scandinavian Journal of Sports Sciences 2(1):26

Mosley J R 2000 Osteoporosis and bone functional adaptation: mechanobiological regulation of bone architecture in growing and adult bone, a review. Journal of Rehabilitation Research and Development 37(2):189–199

Munger R G, Cerhan J R, Chiu B C 1999 Prospective study of dietary protein intake and risk of hip fracture in postmenopausal women. American Journal of Clinical Nutrition 69(1):147–152

Nguyen N D, Pongchaiyakul C, Center J R et al 2005 Identification of high-risk individuals for hip fracture: a 14-year prospective study. Journal of Bone Mineral Density Research 29(11):1921–1928

Nieves J W 2005 Osteoporosis: the role of micronutrients. American Journal of Clinical Nutrition 81(5):1232S–1239S

Nordström A, Olsson T, Nordström P 2006 Sustained benefits from previous physical activity on bone mineral density in males. Journal of Clinical Endocrinology and Metabolism 91(7):2600–2604

Palombaro K M 2005 Effects of walking-only interventions on bone mineral density at various skeletal sites: a meta-analysis. Journal of Geriatric Physical Therapy 28(3):102–107

Petit M A, McKay H A, MacKelvie K J et al 2002 A randomized school-based jumping intervention confers site and maturity-specific benefits on bone structural properties in girls: a hip structural analysis study. Journal of Bone and Mineral Research 17(3):363–372

Pruitt L A, Jackson R D, Bartels R L, Lehnhard H J 1992 Weight-training effects on bone mineral density in early postmenopausal women. Journal of Bone and Mineral Research 7(4):179–185

Punpilai S, Sujitra T, Ouyporn T et al 2005 Menstrual status and bone mineral density among female athletes. Nursing and Health Sciences 7:259–265

Rabon-Stith K M, Hagberg J M, Phares D A et al 2005 Vitamin D receptor FokI genotype influences bone mineral density response to strength training, but not aerobic training. Experimental Physiology 90(4):653–661

Ralston S H 1997 Science, medicine, and the future: osteoporosis. British Medical Journal 315:469–472

Rencken M L, Chesnut C D, Drinkwater B L 1996 Bone density at multiple skeletal sites in amenorrheic athletes. Journal of the American Medical Association 276(3):238–240

Riggs B L 2000 The mechanisms of estrogen regulation of bone resorption. Journal of Clinical Investigation 106:2203–2204

Riggs B L, Wahner H W, Melton L J et al 1986 Rates of bone loss in the appendicular and axial skeletons of women. Evidence of substantial vertebral bone loss before menopause. Journal of Clinical Investigation 77(5):1487–1491

Rome E, Ziegler J, Secic M et al 2004 Bone biochemical markers in adolescent girls using either depot medroxyprogesterone acetate or an oral contraceptive. Journal of Pediatric and Adolescent Gynecology 17:373–377

Rubin C T, Sommerfeldt D W, Judex S, Qin Y-X 2001 Inhibition of osteopenia by low magnitude, high-frequency mechanical stimuli. Drug Discovery Today 6(16):848–858

Rutherford O M 1999 Is there a role for exercise in the prevention of osteoporotic fractures? British Journal of Sports Medicine 33(6):378–386

Sabatier J P, Guaydier-Souquieres G, Benmalek A, Marcelli C 1999 Evolution of lumbar bone mineral content during adolescence and adulthood: a longitudinal study in 395 healthy females 10–24 years of age and 206 premenopausal women. Osteoporosis International 9(6):476–482

Salamone L M, Cauley J A, Black D M et al 1999 Effect of a lifestyle intervention on bone mineral density in premenopausal women: a randomized trial. American Journal of Clinical Nutrition 70:97–103

Saltin B, Blomqvist G, Mitchell J H et al 1968 Response to exercise after bed rest and after training. Circulation 38(Suppl 7):1–78

Shaarawy M, El-Mallah S Y, Seoudi S et al 2006 Effects of long-term use of depot medroxyprogesterone acetate as hormonal contraceptive on bone mineral density and biochemical markers of bone remodelling. Contraception 74:297–302

Shibata Y, Ohsawa I, Watanabe T et al 2003 Effects of physical training on bone mineral density and bone metabolism. Journal of Physiological Anthropology and Applied Human Science 22(4):203–208

Smith A M 2006 Veganism and osteoporosis: a review of the current literature. International Journal of Nursing Practice 12:302–306

Sowers M R, Kshirsagar A, Crutchfield M M, Updike S 1992 Joint influence of fat and lean body composition compartments on femoral bone mineral density in premenopausal women. American Journal of Epidemiology 136:257–265

Stengel S V, Kemmler W, Pintag R et al 2005 Power training is more effective than strength training for maintaining bone mineral density in postmenopausal women. Journal of Applied Physiology 99(10):181–188

Stewart A D, Hannan J 2000 Total and regional bone density in male runners, cyclists, and controls. Medicine and Science in Sports and Exercise 32(8):1373–1377

Tomkinson A, Gibson J H, Lunt M et al 2003 Changes in bone mineral density in the hip and spine before, during and after the menopause in elite runners. Osteoporosis International 14(6):462–468

Van Langendonck L, Lefevre J, Claessens A L et al 2003 Influence of participation in high-impact sports in adolescence and adulthood on bone mineral density in middle-aged men: a 27-year follow-up study. American Journal of Epidemiology 158(6):525–533

Van Staa T P, Dennison E M, Leufkens G M, Cooper C 2001 Epidemiology of fractures in England and Wales. Bone 29(6):517–522

Warren M P, Perlroth N E 2001 The effects of intense exercise on the female reproductive system. Journal of Endocrinology 170:3–11

Weaver C M, Teegarden D, Lyle R M et al 2001 Impact of exercise on bone health and contraindication of oral contraceptive use in young women. Medicine and Science in Sports and Exercise 33(6):873–880

Whedon G D, Lutwak L, Reid J et al 1975 Mineral and nitrogen balance study: results of metabolic observations on Skylab II 28-day orbital mission. Acta Astronaut 2(3–4):297–309

Winters-Stone K M, Snow C M 2006 Site-specific response of bone to exercise in premenopausal women. Bone 39(6):1203–1209

Winzenberg T M, Shaw K, Fryer J, Jones G 2006 Calcium supplementation for improving bone mineral density in children. Cochrane Database of Systematic Reviews 2, Art No. CD005119

Woolf A D, Pfleger B 2003 Burden of major musculoskeletal conditions. Bulletin of the. World Health Organization 81(9):646–656

World Health Organization Study Group 1994 Assessment of fracture risk and its application to screening for postmenopausal osteoporosis. WHO Technical Report Series 843, 1–129. WHO, Geneva

Zaman G, Cheng M Z, Jessop H L et al 2000 Mechanical strain activates estrogen response elements in bone cells. Bone 27(2):233–239

Zanker C L, Swaine I L 1998 Relation between bone turnover, oestradiol, and energy balance in women distance runners. British Journal of Sports Medicine 32(2):167–171

Further reading

Bonaiuti D, Shea B, Iovine R et al 2002 Exercise for preventing and treating osteoporosis in postmenopausal women. Cochrane Database of Systematic Reviews, 2, Art. No. CD000333

Borer K T 2005 Physical activity in the prevention and amelioration of osteoporosis in women: interaction of mechanical, hormonal and dietary factors. Sports Medicine 35:779–830

Kohrt W M, Bloomfield S A, Little K D et al 2004 American College of Sports Medicine Position Stand: Physical activity and bone health. Medicine and Science in Sports and Exercise 36(11):1985–1996

Rutherford O M 1999 Is there a role for exercise in the prevention of osteoporotic fractures? British Journal of Sports Medicine 33(6):378–386

Chapter **8**

The exercising female

Karen M Birch and Joseph I Esformes

CHAPTER CONTENTS

Learning objectives   249
Introduction   250
Physiology of the exercising
   female   250
   The menstrual cycle   250
   The menopause   252
   Pregnancy   253
Special considerations for the exercising
   female   253
   The female athlete triad   253
   Physical activity guidelines for the
      female athlete triad   258

The premenstrual syndrome and
   dysmenorrhoea   259
Pregnancy   259
   Physical activity guidelines for the
      pregnant female   261
The postmenopausal female   262
   Physical activity guidelines for the
      postmenopausal female   263
Key points   265
References   265

LEARNING OBJECTIVES

After studying this chapter, you should be able to:

1. Understand the basic physiological fluctuations associated with the menstrual cycle, menopause and pregnancy.
2. Evaluate how these fluctuations might influence physical performance and the physiological responses to performance.
3. Understand and critique the female athlete triad.
4. Understand how disordered eating and/or aberrations in menstrual cycle functioning influence the long-term risk of osteoporosis.
5. Analyse the increased risk of cardiovascular disease associated with being sedentary in postmenopausal women.
6. Reflect upon how the physiological alterations during pregnancy impact upon the potential to exercise.
7. Describe the considerations that need to be given to exercise prescription for premenopausal, postmenopausal and pregnant women.

INTRODUCTION

At first sight, the immediate physiological responses of female exercisers normally differ from those of their male counterparts only in a manner dictated by body size and organ differences. However, the cyclical nature of the menstrual cycle on a monthly and lifespan basis provides some special considerations for the exercising female. The rhythmic nature of reproductive hormonal fluctuation has been seen to influence both performance (e.g. muscle strength, time to fatigue) and physiological responses to exercise (e.g. blood lactate production, carbohydrate metabolism, minute ventilation, heart rate); however, these aspects will not be covered in this chapter (for review see Constantini et al 2005). Of more importance in relation to the exercising female and exercise prescription are the considerations that need to be given to low and high fit pre- and postmenopausal women in order to avoid the 'female athlete triad' of disordered eating, osteoporosis and amenorrhoea. In addition, of course, of great relevance to the exercising female are the special considerations pertinent to exercise training during and following pregnancy. This chapter will review the reproductive physiology of the female menstrual cycle and pregnancy and the interrelationship between reproductive hormone fluctuations, physical activity and health.

PHYSIOLOGY OF THE EXERCISING FEMALE

The menstrual cycle

The female menstrual cycle is characterized by cyclical fluctuations in the anterior pituitary hormones (the gonadotrophins), follicle-stimulating hormone (FSH) and luteinizing hormone (LH), and the ovarian steroid hormones oestrogen and progesterone (Fig. 8.1). Each menstrual cycle lasts approximately 26 to 35 days and is simplistically divided into two phases by the mid-cycle occurrence of ovulation. The first half of the cycle is characterized by the growth of a primordial follicle within the ovary and higher concentrations of FSH and LH. Towards the end of the phase oestrogen reaches its peak concentrations. This phase, referred to as the *follicular phase*, begins on the first day of menstrual bleeding (day one) and continues until ovulation. Ovulation, or the release of the ovum into the fallopian tubes, occurs at approximately day 14 and continues until the next menstrual blood loss. The second half of the cycle is characterized by the presence of both oestrogen and progesterone and is referred to as the *luteal phase*. In addition, the 4 to 5 days of menstrual blood loss are referred to as *menses*, whilst the 72 hours prior to menses are known as *premenses*.

The rhythmic nature of the menstrual cycle is controlled by a series of feedback loops between the hypothalamic–pituitary axis and the ovaries (Fig. 8.2). The hypothalamus and anterior pituitary glands (the hypothalamic–pituitary axis) communicate principally through the portal blood vessels that run between them. At the onset of puberty, or *menarche*, the existing pulsatile release of gonadotrophin-releasing hormone (GnRH) from the median eminence of the hypothalamus increases in magnitude and rhythm. This maturation in GnRH cycling enhances the sensitivity of the anterior pituitary to the gonadotrophins, produces the first period in female adolescents (menarche) and then controls the cycle on a monthly basis. The average age of menarche in the UK is approximately 12 years. Each month the pulsatile release of GnRH causes the synthesis and release of FSH and LH from the anterior pituitary gland. FSH released into the circulation targets receptor cells in the ovaries that respond by releasing 17-β-oestradiol

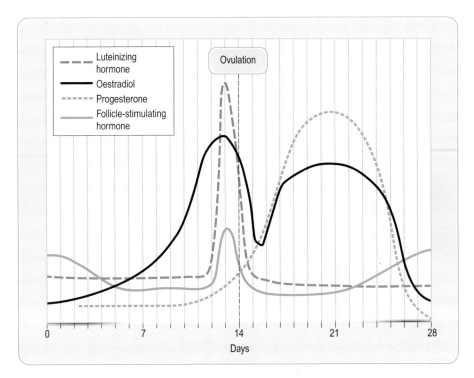

Figure 8.1 The menstrual cycle.

into the circulation. Circulating oestradiol concentrations are monitored via the hypothalamic–pituitary axis via a positive feedback loop leading to a mid-cycle surge in
LH that is responsible for the release of the ovum from the ovary. At this stage the
remaining cells within the ovary, the *corpus luteum*, begin to secrete 17-β-oestradiol
and progesterone.

The circulating concentrations of oestradiol and progesterone at this stage of
the cycle act via a negative feedback loop to the hypothalamic–pituitary axis
to inhibit the release of FSH and LH from the anterior pituitary. However, the
corpus luteum is dependent upon LH for its survival, so once LH is suppressed
the corpus luteum begins to involute and die. As oestradiol and progesterone concentrations thus begin to decrease, the feedback loop inhibiting FSH and LH release
from the anterior pituitary is removed, the lining of the womb (the endometrium) is
shed in menses, and the cycle begins again. It is noteworthy that these feedback loops
work in exactly the same way when concentrations of oestrogen and progesterone
are elevated through consumption of the oral contraceptive pill, or by contraceptive
implants.

The menstrual cycle normally continues from menarche (approximately age 11–14
years) to the climacteric or menopause (approximately age 53–56 years), during
which time females have exposure to high levels of oestrogen for approximately
14–16 days each month. Females experiencing regular and healthy menstrual cycles
are referred to as being *eumenorrhoeic*, whilst those experiencing irregular menstrual
cycles are referred to as being *oligomenorrhoeic*. A loss of menstrual cycles for a period
of 6 months or more following successful menarche is referred to as *secondary*

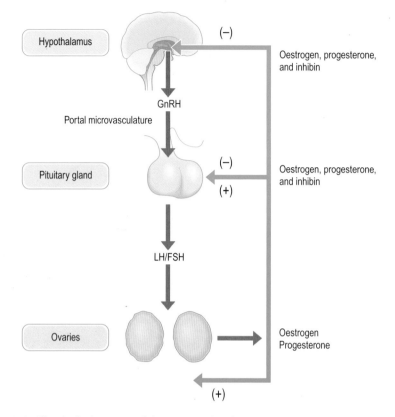

Figure 8.2   The rhythmic nature of the menstrual cycle.

amenorrhoea. If this loss is non-pathological and deemed to be associated with participation in high-intensity or high-volume physical exercise, it has been referred to as *athletic amenorrhoea.* Some women experience painful menses usually due to cramps initiated by high concentrations of prostaglandins. This disorder is known as *dysmenorrhoea* and differs from the little understood syndrome of premenstrual tension, or *premenstrual syndrome* (PMS), that occurs in the few days prior to menses. The physiology of the menstrual cycle can be reviewed in Guyton & Hall (2006).

The menopause

The cessation of menstruation occurs primarily because of a decline in the number of primordial follicles within the ovary. Initially this results in increasing failure to ovulate and a compensatory increase in gonadotrophin secretion. Despite this effort to maintain hormonal concentrations there is a gradual decline in hormone production and the falling oestrogen levels commonly result in hot flushes and night sweats (vasomotor symptoms), sleep disturbance and vaginal dryness. Levels of the steroid hormones begin to fall approximately 5–10 years prior to the menopause. During this time the luteal phase of the cycle may shorten, menses may become irregular and menstrual blood flow may be lighter. Eventually the cycle will become anovulatory (lack of ovulation), as follicular maturation becomes inadequate to trigger ovulation.

The physiology of the menopause can be reviewed in Guyton & Hall (2006) and may have some impact upon cardiovascular and bone health in sedentary women.

Pregnancy

If the ovum released into the fallopian tubes following ovulation is fertilized by ejaculated sperm and then is successfully implanted into the endometrial lining, the menstrual cycle will cease throughout pregnancy. The corpus luteum is maintained for the first 3 to 4 months of pregnancy and continues to secrete oestrogen and progesterone, an action that will inhibit further secretion of the gonadotrophins. Following this time the high levels of these hormones required throughout pregnancy are produced by the placenta. The chorion of the placenta also secretes human chorionic gonadotrophin (hCG). This hormone provides a stimulus for the continued production of progesterone from the corpus luteum, which is necessary for the continued connection of the embryo and fetus to the endometrium. The placenta produces oestrogen from about 4 weeks into pregnancy, and takes over from the corpus luteum in the production of both oestrogen and progesterone from approximately 4 months. At this stage the production of hCG is greatly reduced.

Both the placenta and the ovaries also secrete relaxin. This hormone relaxes the symphysis pubis and the ligaments of the sacroiliac and sacrococcygeal joints in order to aid delivery. The physiology of pregnancy can be reviewed in Guyton & Hall (2006).

SPECIAL CONSIDERATIONS FOR THE EXERCISING FEMALE
The female athlete triad

The 'female athlete triad' describes a model (Fig. 8.3) utilized to identify exercising females presenting with one or more of three disorders – amenorrhoea, disordered eating and osteoporosis. These disorders are interlinked and can seriously impact upon exercise performance and long-term health. A female may enter the triad most likely displaying amenorrhoea or disordered eating, as osteoporosis is more likely to be a consequence of the former disorders. Importantly, identifying an exercise performer as having entered the triad implies that the cause of the identified disorder is related to participation in high-volume or high-intensity physical activity, and not to another departure from normality (a different pathology, or pregnancy).

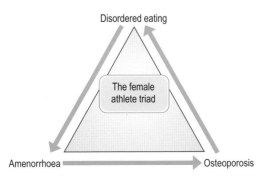

Figure 8.3   The female athlete triad.

In the general population the incidence of secondary amenorrhoea is approximately 5%. However, in a population of female exercise participants the incidence has been reported to be anywhere between 10% and 80%. It is important to note that the female athlete triad is not only found in elite female athletes. On the contrary, disorders which are part of the triad have been identified in club level athletes and in exercising females who utilize exercise training as a means to control body mass (Torstveit & Sundgot-Borgen 2005). The loss of oestrogen production in athletic or secondary amenorrhoea has been associated with infertility, an increased risk of osteopenia and/or osteoporosis plus related stress fractures, and an increased risk of cardiovascular disease. Whereas infertility is reversible on reattainment of menstruation, the participant must understand that bone loss and disease risk may be controllable, but are not fully retrievable.

Athletic amenorrhoea

The aetiology of athletic amenorrhoea appears to be multifactorial in nature. Primarily, amenorrhoea is caused by down-regulation of the hypothalamic–pituitary axis. The pulse frequency of GnRH is decreased whilst its amplitude is increased (Warren & Shantha 2000) such that the pulsatile release of LH from the anterior pituitary is inhibited. Altered LH pulsatility may impact upon the cycle by inducing luteal phase suppression. In effect, the lowered production of LH means that the corpus luteum involutes earlier, oestrogen and progesterone production decrease and menses occurs at an earlier point in the cycle (shortened luteal phase). A healthy luteal phase should have duration of greater than 10 days. The complete down-regulation of LH secretion from the anterior pituitary results in failure to develop a dominant follicle within the ovary, and thus anovulation (lack of ovulation). The pathophysiology of athletic amenorrhoea can be reviewed in Redman & Loucks (2005).

A popular theory explaining the aetiology of amenorrhoea has been that females who lose weight through exercise, and/or participate in sports where aesthetics require a low body mass (e.g. ballet, gymnastics), display an exceedingly low percentage body fat, which in turn leads to amenorrhoea. Historically, it was felt that 17% body fat was required to initiate menarche, whilst 22% body fat was required to maintain menstruation (Frisch & McArthur 1974). However, this theory has been thoroughly refuted, although the identification of a low percentage body fat does serve to signpost that athletic amenorrhoea may be present. In other words low body fat may be correlated with the prevalence of amenorrhoea; however, it is not the cause of amenorrhoea. Other theories have reported down-regulation of the hypothalamic–pituitary axis as a result of elevated β-endorphins following high duration exercise, and indeed administration of a β-endorphin antagonist (naloxone) has been seen to reverse amenorrhoea (Szabo et al 1987). The GnRH pulse generator may also be suppressed by the hypothalamic–adrenal axis as increased levels of corticotrophin-releasing factor (CRF) and adrenocorticotrophic hormone (ACTH) have both been seen to decrease GnRH pulse frequency. Certainly ACTH and cortisol are elevated during exercise and ACTH and cortisol rhythms have been seen to be dysfunctional in amenorrhoeic athletes, probably as a result of sustained (not rhythmic) activation of CRF (De Souza et al 1994). Thus one cause of down-regulation of the hypothalamic–pituitary axis may be stress-induced by competitive action.

Bullen et al (1984) attempted to initiate down-regulation of the hypothalamic–pituitary axis in a prospective study that involved women endurance training for 4.5 hours per week at 85% maximal heart rate (approximately 70% $\dot{V}O_2$max) over

2 to 3 months. Although diminished urinary oestradiol concentrations were found in half of the group participants, no change in cycle length or ovulatory capacity occurred. This and similar studies of the day concluded that moderate-intensity exercise was not a great enough stimulus to induce down-regulation of the axis. Bullen et al (1985) randomly assigned 28 college women to either a weight-loss training group, or a weight maintaining group for a study that covered two consecutive menstrual cycles. Weight loss was limited to 0.45 kg/week and training consisted of running 6.4 km/day during the first week, increasing to 16 km/day by the fifth to eighth week at heart rates corresponding to 70–80% $\dot{V}O_2$max. In addition, all participants engaged in 3.5 hours of moderate-intensity sports activity daily. Forty-four per cent of the participants proceeded from abnormal luteal function in cycle 1 to amenorrhoea in cycle 2, with a significantly greater number presenting as amenorrhoeic in the weight-loss group. It thus appeared that more vigorous intensity and/or higher volume physical activity was more likely to induce amenorrhoea.

Interestingly, Bullen et al (1985) did not match energy balance (energy consumption less energy utilization) between the two groups of participants. In fact the weight-loss group necessarily consumed many fewer calories than their energy expenditure. Historically, researchers in this area began to ponder the impact of a negative energy balance upon the hypothalamic–pituitary axis. It was contended that a 'metabolic arrest' was induced by a negative energy balance aimed at conserving energy (Donen 1994). Indeed, maintenance of the luteal phase of the cycle requires a basal metabolic rate of between 0.7 and 1.0 kcal/min more than that of the follicular phase (Solomon et al 1982). Certainly some hibernating animals are seen to conserve energy during hibernation by temporarily 'switching off' the reproductive cycle. Given the prevalence of amenorrhoea in females with anorexia nervosa, it was contended that the down-regulation of the hypothalamic–pituitary axis may thus be related to energy balance.

Loucks et al (1998, 2003) have conducted well-controlled prospective studies to evaluate the impact of energy availability and exercise stress upon LH pulsatility. Eumenorrhoeic women participating in these studies were admitted to a hospital environment where exercise and energy intake were closely controlled. Energy availability was standardized per kilogram of lean body mass (kgLBM) by controlling nutritional intake and energy expenditure through exercise at an energy cost of 30 kcal·kgLBM^{-1}. Thus energy availability was either balanced at 45 kcal·kgLBM^{-1} or deprived at 10 kcal·kgLBM^{-1}. LH pulsatility, measured via repetitive 10-minute blood sampling, was suppressed whether energy availability was reduced by dietary restriction alone, or by energy expenditure alone. Supplementing the diet to replace the energy cost of exercise prevented the disruption of LH pulsatility. Loucks & Thuma (2003) expanded these data by investigating the dose–response effect of restricted energy availability on LH pulsatility in exercising women. Within 5 days of the start of exercising, LH pulsatility was disrupted below a threshold of energy availability between 20 and 30 kcal·kgLBM^{-1}·d^{-1}, a response that was most extreme in women who already displayed shortened luteal phases.

It would thus appear that maintenance of a healthy menstrual cycle in exercising women is entirely possible as long as energy availability is maintained. However, in the women studied by Loucks & Thuma (2003), normal LH pulsatility was demonstrated in women whose energy availability was restricted by 33% to 30 kcal·kgLBM^{-1}·d^{-1}. Loucks & Thuma thus contend that 30 kcal·kgLBM^{-1}·d^{-1} appears to be sufficient energy availability to preserve normal reproductive function, and that screening for athletes/participants with decreased luteal phase lengths will identify females who are at greatest risk of developing amenorrhoea if energy intake is further restricted.

Disordered eating

Of course, restricted energy availability is brought about by participating in high training intensities or volumes whilst restricting dietary intake. It should be noted that although some female athletes may partake in unhealthy dietary practices such as using laxatives etc., the second corner of the 'female athlete triad' is termed 'disordered eating' and not 'eating disorders'. Disordered eating ranges from abnormal eating behaviours to clinical eating disorders such as anorexia nervosa and bulimia nervosa. Clinical eating disorders are identified using the Diagnostic and Statistical Manual of Mental Disorders (DSM-IV: APA 1994) criteria, whilst disordered eating can be identified with the Eating Disorder Inventory Drive for Thinness and Body Dissatisfaction subscales (Espelage et al 2003). Exercising females may be driven to achieve unrealistic and unhealthy body mass through energy restriction, restriction of high fat or high carbohydrate foods, purging, use of diet pills, laxatives or diuretics and over-exercising, and may achieve high scores on the Drive for Thinness and Body Dissatisfaction scales. To be classified as having an eating disorder the participant must show a disturbance of eating habits or weight control behaviour that could result in impairment of physical health or psychosocial functioning (Fairburn & Harrison 2003).

The causes of disordered eating are complicated but, in the population at large, might include social, psychological and physiological factors. In female exercise participants additional factors include expectations of athletic perfection and a belief that low body mass induces better performance. The prevalence of disordered eating in athletic female populations ranges from 10% to 32%, although establishing a correct figure is hampered by the secretive nature of disordered eating and the differing diagnostic criteria used throughout the literature (Sudi et al 2004). The prevalence of pathological eating disorders in exercising females is quite low (approximately 1–3%). However, the markers of nutritional deficiency found in amenorrhoeic female exercise participants, such as increased insulin-like growth factor binding protein-1, cortisol and growth hormone (GH) and low tri-iodothyronine (T_3) and insulin-like growth factor-1, are very similar to the levels found in anorexic patients (Laughlin et al 1998). Additionally, the low levels of leptin found in these women are due to low energy availability, and not the stress of exercise itself.

Osteoporosis

For the exercising female who becomes amenorrhoeic the risk of stress fractures and future osteoporosis significantly increases. The risk of osteoporosis has been found to be related to the life-long exposure to oestrogen, and so given the monthly production of oestrogen that should occur between the years of menarche and the menopause, long periods of amenorrhoea will significantly decrease life-long exposure.

In both sexes oestrogen acts largely at endosteal sites (the inner surface of bone), whereas testosterone in the male also acts upon periosteal sites (the fibrous membranes covering the bone) leading to a larger cortical apposition. After the third decade, bone mass tends to be stable for some 15 years, following which (after approximately 45 years of age) an age-related bone loss ensues. The rate of bone loss for the female will increase during the menopausal years and thus, in order to ensure an adequate bone mass in older years, females are best served by reaching a good peak in bone mass, maintaining a eumenorrhoeic menstrual cycle and having a later menopause. See Borer (2005) for more detailed review.

The hormone oestrogen acts to inhibit bone resorption and thus decreases the rate of bone turnover. Any loss of oestrogen, such as that occurring with down-regulation of the hypothalamic–pituitary axis or with the menopause, leads to resorption being favoured and a subsequent loss of bone mineral. The mechanism by which oestrogen exerts its action is an inhibition of production of the cytokines, interleukin-1 (IL-1) and -6 (IL-6), and tumour necrosis factor alpha (TNF-α) in the marrow. These cytokines induce osteoclastogenesis when unchecked, and thus elevate the rate of bone resorption. Oestrogen also acts to stimulate production of the resorption inhibitor tumour growth factor beta (TGF-β) (for review see Riggs 2000). For amenorrhoeic female exercise participants who are displaying a low energy availability, suppression of the bone trophic hormones IGF-1 and T_3 can also lead to inadequate bone formation.

For the premenopausal female exercise participant who becomes amenorrhoeic, the loss of oestrogen has been seen to increase the prevalence of stress-induced fractures and scoliosis, and these conditions are highly associated with low bone mass. Indeed, amenorrhoeic female athletes have been seen to have 10–20% lower bone mineral densities than their eumenorrhoeic counterparts, with rates of loss as high as 3–5% per year in the first year of amenorrhoea. Importantly, the mechanical effect of physical activity upon bone mineral density still exists in amenorrhoeic exercising females and amenorrhoeic athletes have been seen to have a greater bone mineral density than non-exercising amenorrhoeic women (see also Chapter 7). Resumption of menses has been seen to increase bone mineral density by an initial 6–9.7% per annum, but this rate of increase slowed and then ceased following the first year of resumption (see Warren & Perlroth 2001 for review). In the long term, even after regaining menses and increasing bone mineral density, amenorrhoeic participants remain significantly below normal controls when bone mineral density is examined.

Osteoporosis has existed as the third point of the triangle since the triangle's inception in 1993. Osteoporosis is defined as a bone mineral density that is more than 2.5 SD below the mean of young adults, whilst a bone mineral density between 1 and 2.5 SD below this mean defines osteopenia. Khan et al (2002) re-evaluated a number of journal articles in the literature that had reported the prevalence of osteoporosis in premenopausal exercising females and females diagnosed with anorexia nervosa using dual X-ray absorptiometry in the lumbar spine. The prevalence of osteoporosis reported within the literature was no higher than 13% in the exercising females and 21% in the anorexic females. However, when reanalysed using the above strict SD criteria for osteoporosis and osteopenia, all of the females originally classified as having osteoporosis were reclassified as having osteopenia, mild osteopenia or as having normal bone mineral density.

It would thus appear that osteopenia would be better placed within the female athlete triad and indeed Khan et al (2002) call for osteoporosis to be replaced by osteopenia/osteoporosis as the third corner of the triad. This would perhaps mean that a greater prevalence of bone mass irregularities would be seen in exercising females, and thus the triad would potentially have better clinical utility. What is clear is that female exercise participants who present with osteopenia are at a greater risk of developing osteoporosis later in life than a participant with normal bone mass. Physical activity and optimal nutrition are the key factors to managing osteopenia, and as both of these factors are related to amenorrhoea and disordered eating, defining the triad as a continuum of amenorrhoea, disordered eating and osteopenia/osteoporosis might well be more appropriate.

Physical activity guidelines for the female athlete triad

It is imperative that the existence of any corner of the female athlete triad is identified using valid tools. As previously discussed, evaluation must utilize correct diagnostic criteria and these must be undertaken by medical personnel. The diagnosis of athletic amenorrhoea must rule out other pathology and pregnancy, and should be based upon a detailed medical history, a physical examination, a pelvic examination and laboratory tests. Disordered eating and/or eating disorders should be diagnosed with a full medical history, use of valid diagnostic criteria from the DSM (APA 1994) and other questionnaires and by interview with a psychologist. Bone mineral density should be measured using valid tools, whilst other endocrinological disorders should be identified via laboratory tests. It should not be the role of the coach, trainer or selector to clinically identify an aspect of the triad. However, it is extremely important that coaches, trainers, selectors and parents/spouses are aware of (a) the risk factors associated with entering the female athlete triad, and (b) the signs and symptoms of disordered eating/eating disorders (pathological eating behaviours, mood changes, fatigue, constipation, light-headedness, etc.), amenorrhoea (loss of menstruation, shortened luteal phase) and low bone mass (recurrent stress fractures). For a detailed review of early identification see Waldrop (2005).

Treatment of the exercising female again depends upon the extent to which she has progressed down the continuum of the triad. Assuming low bone mass is present the reader is referred to Bassey & Dinan (2001) and Chapter 6 of the present volume for guidelines on treatment and exercise modification. Management of the female in the triad as a whole centres on changing both eating and exercise behaviour. Changing eating behaviour must be managed with psychological intervention, perhaps using cognitive behaviour change or a 'stages of change' approach. The exercise intervention requires a complete analysis of training history, training intensity, duration and frequency. It is recommended that training volume is decreased initially by 10%, and that this decrease might be either in intensity or in duration. The optimal requirement is a gain of 2–3 kg in body mass. The recommended approach to this management is that a stabilization period of 3 months might involve reduction of exercise volume, whilst following this time an evaluation and counselling period can explore exercise behaviour and knowledge (Prior et al 1992). Certainly many exercising females believe that low body mass will enhance performance, even in the light of low nutritional status and power-to-weight ratio; the endeavour must be to help the triad sufferer adjust her perspective on these factors.

During the evaluation and counselling stage of treatment it may be advisable to increase calcium intake, utilizing 1500 mg/day calcium + 400–800 IU/day vitamin D. If stress fractures are present then the exercise regimen will need to be changed to one using non-weight-bearing activities. Overall, energy availability will also need to be assessed, remembering that athletes can be in a negative energy balance and yet successfully maintain menstruation (and thus oestrogen levels) as long as they do not drop below a threshold of $30 \text{ kcal} \cdot \text{kgLBM}^{-1} \cdot \text{d}^{-1}$ (Loucks & Thuma 2003). It is recommended that the participant should be reassessed every 3–6 months, whilst bone density examinations should be repeated at intervals of 1–2 years.

For the extra complications in team management of the female athlete triad, the reader is referred to the detailed analysis by Joy et al (1997a, 1997b).

THE PREMENSTRUAL SYNDROME AND DYSMENORRHOEA

The prevalence of the premenstrual syndrome (PMS) ranges from 30% to 63% of populations across the age span, whilst premenstrual mood changes have been reported in up to 97% of women. The validity of these numbers is difficult to ascertain given the wide-ranging diagnostic criteria used throughout the literature. Clinical diagnosis of PMS requires a prospective self-report of at least one of six affective complaints (including depression, anxiety and irritability) and one of four somatic complaints (breast tenderness, abdominal bloating, headache and swelling of extremities) in at least two cycles (Warren & Shanghold 1997). The aetiology of these so-called 'moliminal' symptoms is unclear, but it is thought to relate to imbalances in oestrogen and progesterone concentrations late in the cycle, potentially causing a disturbance in calcium regulation (Bertone-Johnson et al 2005). Certainly calcium supplementation has been found to relieve symptoms, whilst serotonin reuptake inhibitors have also been observed to aid treatment.

The evidence suggesting that exercise might alleviate PMS is contentious. Timonen & Procope (1971) reported that active university students had fewer premenstrual emotional symptoms than their less active counterparts, but that self-reports of moliminal symptoms did not differ between the two groups. However, in a comparison of sedentary women who took up regular running, runners training for a marathon and sedentary women, Prior et al (1986) reported decreased breast tenderness, fluid retention and stress in the new runners, decreased breast tenderness, fluid retention, depression and anxiety in the marathon runners and no changes in the non-exercise controls. Lustyk et al (2004) suggested that women with the worst PMS symptoms may reduce these by exercising, while women who exercise often or never do not associate exercise with their symptoms.

The prevalence of dysmenorrhoea (pain accompanying menstruation) in the general population ranges from 47% to 80%, and 58% of these sufferers also complain of PMS. Symptoms include lower abdominal pain that may radiate to the lower back or legs, headache, nausea and vomiting. The aetiology of dysmenorrhoea is again unclear; however, there is a firm belief that raised prostaglandin concentrations lead to uterine contractions and ischaemia (Tzafettas 2006). Certainly prostaglandin inhibitors and oral contraceptives providing progesterone to inhibit prostaglandin synthesis in endometrial cells have been found to alleviate symptoms.

Attempting to identify whether exercise participation might decrease the incidence of dysmenorrhoea is difficult given that an exercise-induced change in mood state might very well influence the experience of and reporting of painful sensations. The effect of physical activity upon the severity of dysmenorrhoea certainly requires more investigation.

PREGNANCY

The physiological alterations experienced throughout pregnancy are driven by the need to support both maternal and fetal well-being and functioning. Maternal system alterations are controlled by the changes in gestational hormones previously reviewed. In the first two trimesters of pregnancy, increased concentrations of oestrogen and progesterone promote β-cell hyperplasia and thus greater insulin sensitivity and secretion. This in turn promotes an increased maternal adiposity until late in gestation when the fetal energy requirements tend towards an adipose tissue decrease (Boden 1996). Weight gain in pregnancy is approximately 12 kg (uterus: 1.0 kg, breasts: 1.5 kg, placenta: 0.7 kg, amniotic fluid 0.8 kg, maternal fluid gain:

2.0 kg, maternal fat: 2.5 kg: fetus: 3.5 kg; Clark 1992), which throughout the period of pregnancy has an impact upon balance, posture and locomotion. Certainly the abdominal protrusion, upward displacement of the diaphragm, flattening of the lower back and forward displacement of the centre of gravity are thought to provide some explanation for why approximately 50% of pregnant women suffer with low back pain. Additionally, the increased secretion of the reproductive steroid hormones and relaxin are associated with ligamentous and connective tissue laxity, which may predispose the pregnant female to ligament strain and further pain.

The endocrine responses to pregnancy lead to significant changes in the cardiovascular system. Increased aldosterone secretion leads to sodium and water retention that cause a 40–50% increase in blood volume (a major contribution to the 2 kg maternal fluid gain), whilst red cell mass increases by 17–25% (Longo 1983). Both systolic and diastolic blood pressures fall during the first trimester but rise again towards term. Cardiac output rises by approximately 40% during the first trimester due to an increased heart rate and stroke volume (enhanced left ventricular end-diastolic volume and contractility). Much of this increased cardiac output is directed towards the uteroplacental circulation, whilst blood flow to the skin and breasts is also increased. Renal blood flow increases by up to 80% in the first trimester but again falls towards term. The third trimester is associated with a reduced venous return because of the mechanical depression of the inferior vena cava by the gravid uterus. This is particularly a problem in the supine position and pregnant women are advised not to lie, and certainly not to exercise, in this position.

The above-mentioned physiological alterations are associated with an increase in resting $\dot{V}O_2$ of 20–30%, whilst the increased insulin secretion leads to reduced lipolysis and a greater reliance upon carbohydrate metabolism. Certainly metabolic homeostasis requires an additional 300 kcal per day. Late in pregnancy insulin resistance develops and there is a reduced carbohydrate use, increased lipolysis and greater use of maternal fat stores. The increased insulin resistance may well develop into gestational diabetes; however, this disorder does not always continue postpartum. The increase in resting $\dot{V}O_2$ is mostly due to fetal oxygen consumption and is aided by the increased red cell mass and a 40% increase in minute ventilation. Minute ventilation is increased solely via an increase in tidal volume as a result of a progesterone-mediated increase in CO_2 sensitivity. The increase in pulmonary ventilation leads to an increase in arterial PO_2 to approximately 100 mmHg, whilst arterial PCO_2 drops to 30–32 mmHg (Templeton & Kelman 1976), a respiratory alkalosis not entirely compensated for.

Participation in steady-state exercise during pregnancy has been seen to induce physiological responses similar to those observed at rest. Maternal heart rate, stroke volume, cardiac output, tidal volume and minute ventilation are all greater, whilst PCO_2 and pH are lower than would be expected in the non-pregnant state. Blood pressure responses are unchanged at a given absolute work rate. Net $\dot{V}O_2$ of non-weight-bearing activities is also unchanged, whilst weight-dependent activities elicit an increased oxygen cost. In late pregnancy stroke volume and cardiac output may well be reduced during exercise due to the compression of the vena cava by the gravid uterus. For more detailed review see Davies et al (2003).

Absolute $\dot{V}O_2$max is unchanged throughout pregnancy, unless physical activity levels are particularly reduced. Expression of $\dot{V}O_2$max relative to body mass, however, indicates a declining maximal aerobic capacity throughout pregnancy. Maximal heart rate has been seen to be reduced during late pregnancy probably due to blunted sympathoadrenal responses to exercise, and as resting heart rate is increased there is a reduced heart rate reserve. It would appear that the $\dot{V}O_2$ at the ventilatory threshold is not affected by being pregnant; however, peak exercise respiratory exchange ratio, blood lactate concentration and excess post-exercise oxygen consumption following maximal exercise are all reduced in pregnancy. This is thought to be due to a decreased ability to exercise anaerobically because of reduced availability of carbohydrates as a result of decreased maternal liver glycogen stores or glycogenolysis and blunted sympathoadrenal responses to exercise. In prolonged strenuous exercise these maternal factors may well decrease availability to the fetus leading to decreased birthweight. The reader is referred to a further review by Morris & Johnson (2005).

The two major concerns for the fetus during maternal exercise are fetal hypoxia and fetal hyperthermia. Fetal oxygen delivery is aided by compensatory mechanisms that favour the fetus against the mother; these include haemoconcentration of maternal blood during exercise, redistribution of uteroplacental blood flow and an increased uteroplacental arteriovenous oxygen difference (Wolfe et al 1994). The fetus is protected from heat gain by further maternal compensations such as enhanced peripheral vasodilatation, reduced sweating threshold and increased ventilatory heat loss. The fetal temperature is usually approximately 0.5°C higher than the maternal core temperature, and thus prevention of an increase in maternal core temperature acts to protect the fetus during exercise.

The fetal heart rate increases during maternal aerobic exercise and takes approximately 20 minutes to return to resting values post exercise. The magnitude of increase is dependent upon exercise intensity and duration. The effect of heavy-intensity exercise upon fetal heart rate has been evaluated in a small number of studies indicating minimal responses. Exercise in the supine or semi-supine position results in fetal bradycardia and should, as previously noted, be avoided in late pregnancy.

Physical activity guidelines for the pregnant female

Exercise prescription for the pregnant female is dependent upon pre-pregnancy fitness level and/or physical activity status. Whether previously sedentary or active, all pregnant women should be examined by medical personnel prior to beginning their exercise programme and may be screened using the Physical Activity Readiness Medical Examination (PARmed-X) for Pregnancy questionnaire (Canadian Society for Exercise Physiology 2002). Contraindications to exercising during pregnancy have been published by the American College of Obstetricians and Gynecologists (2002). General advice for exercise during pregnancy is that participation in a wide range of recreational activities is safe as long as the participant avoids abdominal trauma, exercising in the heat or in the supine position, exercise above an altitude of 6000 feet and breath-holding activities such as scuba diving. Vigorous activity should be avoided in the third trimester. On the whole it is the mother that will benefit from long-term exercise but the fetus that will pay the price for her over-exercising.

The use of heart rate training zones to set levels of exercise intensity requires adjustment during pregnancy because of the reduced HR reserve (HRR). Wolfe (Canadian Society for Exercise Physiology 2002) recommends that the upper end of the age-related non-pregnant (60–75% maximal HRR) training zone be lowered for the pregnant state. Given that the non-pregnant training zone represents a width of approximately 20 beats/minute, the width of the pregnant zone should be decreased to 15 beats/minute by decreasing the top end by 5 beats/minute. Those women who were sedentary prior to pregnancy are recommended by the American College of Sports Medicine (ACSM 2006) to begin aerobic training at 20–39% HRR, with low-impact activities such as walking or swimming. RPE is a valid tool to utilize during pregnancy as an adjunct to heart rate monitoring. The ACSM recommend 'light' to 'somewhat hard' (11–13) on the Borg 6–20 scale. In the absence of medical or obstetric complications, 30–40 minutes or more of moderate-intensity activity is recommended on most, if not all days per week, whilst a minimum of 15 minutes per session is required for a conditioning stimulus. Previously sedentary women can then increase duration by 1–2 minutes per week during the second trimester, to a maximum of 30 minutes.

Exercise for muscle strength and endurance and flexibility during pregnancy is complicated by the potential ligament laxity associated with the release of relaxin and the need to avoid raising blood pressure by a large magnitude. Flexibility exercises need to be controlled and non-ballistic, whilst strength training should consist of high repetition but low resistance exercises conducted in the upright position and with avoidance of the Valsalva manoeuvre (breath holding). Supine exercises should be avoided and abdominal exercises should be avoided so as not to aggravate any tearing of the linea alba. Balance training in pregnancy should be avoided due to the obvious risks of falls and related complications.

The rate of return to physical activity following delivery is dependent upon postpartum health and mode of delivery (particularly a caesarean). Following an uncomplicated normal delivery the participant may return to aerobic exercise once vaginal bleeding has stopped and her postpartum check-up is normal. She should attempt to start training at a similar HRR as when pregnant. Following caesarean section, the participant is advised not to return to aerobic exercise for at least 10 weeks, or until all complications have healed. Resistance exercises can be started after vaginal bleeding has ceased and Kegel exercises for the pelvic floor are recommended. These exercises involve contractions of the vaginal muscles for repeated 10 second periods. Abdominal exercises can be conducted in the supine position but only if diastasis recti (division of the abdominal muscles felt with the fingertips) has healed. Exercise has no detrimental effects upon milk composition, milk volume or maternal health.

THE POSTMENOPAUSAL FEMALE

The physiological changes that occur with ageing have been reviewed in Chapter 6, and indeed the postmenopausal female exercise participant will (on the whole) be over 50 years of age. Consequently, physical performance and physiological responses to exercise will vary according to age and physical activity/fitness status. However, the postmenopausal female brings with her a number of factors related specifically to the loss of oestrogen following the menopausal transition.

A recent UK birth cohort study indicated that at 53 years of age body mass index (BMI), waist circumference, total cholesterol (TC), low-density lipoprotein (LDL) and HbA_{1c} concentration (blood marker of glucose control) varied between pre- and postmenopausal women (all being greater post menopause), and that TC and HbA_{1c} increased across the menopausal transition before and after adjustment for BMI, smoking, lifestyle and socioeconomic circumstances (Kuh et al 2005). In addition, Zaydun et al (2006), in a study of 3149 women, added that being postmenopausal significantly increased the risk of arterial stiffness independently of age, hypertension, hypercholesterolaemia, diabetes mellitus, obesity and smoking, whilst Taddei et al (1996) associated the menopause with endothelial dysfunction. Each of these reported variations is associated with an increased risk of cardiovascular disease following the menopausal transition, whilst studies by Rossi et al (2005a, 2005b) have also indicated that the menopausal transition might well increase the risk of both hypertension and type 2 diabetes.

Participation in physical activity in postmenopausal women has been shown to have positive effects upon risk factors associated with cardiovascular disease. In cross-sectional analyses of physical activity status, LDL and high-density lipoprotein (HDL) cholesterol levels have been more favourable in active than non-active women, irrespective of HRT utilization (Green et al 2004). Physical activity interventions have resulted in decreases in BMI and waist circumference, decreases in LDL, fasting blood glucose, HbA$_{1c}$, C-reactive protein (CRP: marker of inflammation) and TC concentrations, and increases in insulin sensitivity and arterial compliance in women, whether utilizing or not utilizing HRT. These results have been seen in studies as short as 2 and 12 weeks in duration and in those which have utilized walking as the exercise stimulus. Changes in fat mass, especially visceral adiposity, lipoprotein subfractions and markers of glucose control (HbA$_{1c}$) and inflammation (CRP), are all indicative of a decrease in the risk of cardiovascular disease and this decrease appears to be independent of HRT utilization (Green et al 2004). HRT use may have an additive effect upon the favourable alterations in these risk factors; however, this evidence needs to be weighed against the known risks of HRT.

The loss of oestrogen following the menopause also places the exercising female at risk of osteopenia and osteoporosis. The mechanisms for this increase in risk have been covered above. In brief, oestrogen deficiency accelerates bone resorption, and thus women who have low bone mass prior to the menopause have a significantly greater risk of developing osteoporosis in later years. Comparisons of pre- and postmenopausal athletes suggest that even participation in vigorous physical activity does not prevent the loss in bone mineral density that occurs at the menopause. Indeed, data from the Nurses' Health Study (Feskanich et al 2002) suggested that the risk of hip fracture was reduced by 60–70% in women using hormone replacement therapy (HRT), regardless of physical activity level, compared to sedentary women not using HRT. Among those women not using HRT, those in the highest quintile of physical activity (>24 METs, hours per week) also had a 67% reduction in hip fracture risk, suggesting an additional benefit of physical activity above the effect upon bone mass.

The effect of physical activity upon bone mass and bone mineral density in postmenopausal women has received considerable attention over the last three decades. The influence of physical activity upon bone turnover in hypo-oestrogenic conditions has become of even greater importance in the last decade due to the newly observed detrimental health effects of HRT. The recent attention to HRT-induced coronary events and incidence of breast cancer has induced contentious results and reports (for review see Tormey et al 2006). What is clear, however, is that HRT is no longer recommended for the attenuation of bone loss in postmenopausal women. Recently recommended courses of action are bisphosphonates, selective oestrogen receptor modulators, raloxifene and, of course, physical activity (Delaney 2006).

Physical activity guidelines for the postmenopausal female

Exercise prescription for the postmenopausal woman and the seven components of fitness discussed in Chapter 1 does not differ from the details discussed in other chapters within this book. The factors indicating an increased risk of cardio-vascular disease at the menopausal transition (e.g. markers of glucose control, inflammation, insulin sensitivity, visceral adiposity, LDL, TG and TC, endothelial dysfunction and arterial stiffness) will respond more to physical activity aimed at enhancing cardiorespiratory endurance (see Asikainen et al 2004 for further review). This means, for these special considerations, the postmenopausal and indeed perimenopausal female should be partaking in high-volume, low–moderate-intensity, longer duration aerobic activities. The reader is referred to Chapters 1, 2, 3, 6 and 7 for further guidelines that relate to females of differing ages or relevant health conditions.

The special considerations for the postmenopausal woman do not only include the menopause-related increase in the risk of cardiovascular disease. Indeed, the postmenopausal woman, if already sedentary, may well also be at an increased risk of osteopenia, osteoporosis and related stress fractures and falls. The reader is referred to Chapter 6 for further information regarding guidelines for increasing muscle strength and balance in an older population. Bassey & Dinan (2001) provide guidelines on the recommendations for safely increasing bone mineral density using exercise or physical activity.

The literature evaluating the influence of physical activity upon bone mass in postmenopausal women has utilized a range of different exercise modes, intensities and durations. Walking interventions have been seen to provide only modest effects at best. Daily walking at an intensity equivalent to 50% $\dot{V}O_2$max, for a duration of 1 hour per day with at least 8000 steps, 4 days per week over 12 months induced an increased bone mineral density of the lumbar spine in women with osteopenia (Yamazaki et al 2004). An evaluation of elite female runners not using HRT before, during and after the menopause revealed an expected age-related decrease in bone mineral density from the femoral neck and spine, but a reduced rate of bone loss in the femoral trochanter and almost no bone loss in the calcaneus (Tomkinson et al 2003). It would thus appear that oestrogen loss has a greater effect upon the femoral neck and spine than the trochanter, even when mechanical stress is constant.

Given that bone responds positively to stresses of multiple amplitudes and directions, physical activity interventions in postmenopausal women have attempted to use multiple exercise modes to increase bone mass. The Erlangen Fitness Osteoporosis Prevention study (Engelke et al 2006), cited in Chapter 7, examined the impact of a vigorous combined high-impact, strength and endurance programme over 2 years upon bone mineral density in postmenopausal women with osteopenia. Bone mineral density increased by 1.3% at the lumbar spine, whilst no change occurred in the hip and femoral neck. At 3 years bone mineral density was increased in the spine, hip and calcaneus but not in the forearm. Similar studies using high-impact but low-volume training have reported identical results. Stengel et al (2005) compared power training to strength training in postmenopausal women over a period of 12 months. As noted in Chapter 7, the power-trained women maintained bone mineral density at the spine and total hip, whereas the strength-trained women lost density at both sites. Hip bone mineral density has also been seen to be maintained in postmenopausal women parti-cipating in jumping whilst wearing a weighted vest and it thus appears that for women in a hypo-oestrogenic condition bone responds best to higher-volume and high-speed mechanical stresses. Of course if osteoporosis is already present, the use of exercise to increase bone mineral density should be tailored to protect the low starting point.

KEY POINTS

1. The menstrual cycle, pregnancy and menopause are associated with major physiological and endocrinological fluctuations that indicate key considerations for exercise prescription.
2. The 'female athlete triad' describes a unique set of disorders that place the exercising female at risk of decreased health and performance.
3. Disordered eating that induces a negative energy balance can lead to loss of the secretion of oestrogen (often indicated by amenorrhoea) and thus increase the risk of stress fractures and osteopenia/osteoporosis.
4. Negative energy balance can be avoided in exercising females, typically by a modest reduction in training volume coupled with an altered eating pattern.
5. Pregnancy requires attention to the type and intensity of exercise undertaken and can influence fetal safety or birthweight if guidelines are not followed.
6. The menopausal transition may well be associated with a detrimental cardiovascular disease profile, and with progressive decline in bone strength, in sedentary females.
7. Consideration given to each of the key points above will ensure that the female can exercise or train effectively and safely.

References

ACOG 2002 Exercise during pregnancy and the postpartum period. American College of Obstetricians and Gynecologists Committee Opinion No 267. Obstetrics and Gynecology 99:171–173

ACSM 2006 American College of Sports Medicine's guidelines for exercise testing and prescription, 7th edn. Lippincott Williams & Wilkins, Philadelphia

APA 1994 Diagnostic and statistical manual of mental disorders, 4th edn. American Psychiatric Association, Washington DC

Asikainen T M, Kukkonen-Harjula K, Miilunpalo S 2004 Exercise for health for early postmenopausal women: a systematic review of randomised controlled trials. Sports Medicine 34:753–778

Bassey J, Dinan S 2001 Exercise for strong bones: a step-by-step program to prevent osteoporosis and stay fit and active for life. Carroll & Brown Publishers, London

Bertone-Johnson E R, Hankinson S E, Bendich A et al 2005 Calcium and vitamin D intake and risk of incident premenstrual syndrome. Archives of Internal Medicine 165:1246–1252

Boden G 1996 Fuel metabolism in pregnancy and in gestational diabetes mellitus. Obstetrics and Gynecology Clinics of North America 23:1–10

Bonen A 1994 Exercise-induced menstrual cycle changes. A functional, temporary adaptation to metabolic stress. Sports Medicine 17:373–392

Borer K T 2005 Physical activity in the prevention and amelioration of osteoporosis in women: interaction of mechanical, hormonal and dietary factors. Sports Medicine 35:779–830

Bullen B A, Skrinar G S, Beitins I Z et al 1984 Endurance training effects on plasma hormonal responsiveness and sex hormone excretion. Journal of Applied Physiology 56:1453–1463

Bullen B A, Skrinar G S, Beitins I Z et al 1985 Induction of menstrual disorders by strenuous exercise in untrained women. New England Journal of Medicine 312:1349–1353

CSEP 2002 Physical activity readiness medical examination for pregnancy (PARmed-X for pregnancy). Available from Canadian Society for Exercise Physiology, Ontario, Canada

Clark N 1992 Shower your baby with good nutrition. Physician and Sports Medicine 20:39–45

Constantini N W, Dubnov G, Lebrun C M 2005 The menstrual cycle and sport performance. Clinical Sports Medicine 24(2):e51–e82, xiii–xiv

Davies G A, Wolfe L A, Mottola M F et al 2003 SOGC Clinical Practice Obstetrics Committee, Canadian Society for Exercise Physiology Board of Directors. Exercise in pregnancy and the postpartum period. Journal of Obstetrics and Gynaecology Canada 25:516–529

Delaney M F 2006 Strategies for the prevention and treatment of osteoporosis during early postmenopause. American Journal of Obstetrics and Gynecology 194:S12–S23

De Souza M J, Luciano A A, Arce J C et al 1994 Clinical tests explain blunted cortisol responsiveness but not mild hypercortisolism in amenorrheic runners. Journal of Applied Physiology 76:1302–1309

Engelke K, Kemmler W, Lauber D et al 2006 Exercise maintains bone density at spine and hip EFOPS: a 3-year longitudinal study in early postmenopausal women. Osteoporosis International 17:133–142

Espelage D L, Mazzeo S E, Aggen S H et al 2003 Examining the construct validity of the Eating Disorder Inventory. Psychological Assessment 15:71–80

Fairburn C G, Harrison P J 2003 Eating disorders. Lancet 361:407–416

Feskanich D, Willett W, Colditz G 2002 Walking and leisure-time activity and risk of hip fracture in postmenopausal women. Journal of the American Medical Association 288:2300–2306

Frisch R E, McArthur J W 1974 Menstrual cycles: fatness as a determinant of minimum weight for height necessary for their maintenance or onset. Science 185:949–951

Green J S, Stanforth P R, Rankinen T et al 2004 The effects of exercise training on abdominal visceral fat, body composition, and indicators of the metabolic syndrome in postmenopausal women with and without estrogen replacement therapy: the HERITAGE family study. Metabolism 53:1192–1196

Guyton A C, Hall J E 2006 Textbook of medical physiology, 11th edn. Elsevier/Saunders, Philadelphia

Joy E, Clark N, Ireland M et al 1997a Team management of the female athlete triad: part 1: what to look for, what to ask. Physician and Sports Medicine 25:94–111

Joy E, Clark N, Ireland M et al 1997b Team management of the female athlete triad: part 2: optimal treatment and prevention tactics. Physician and Sports Medicine 25:65–69

Khan K M, Liu-Ambrose T, Sran M M et al 2002 New criteria for female athlete triad syndrome? As osteoporosis is rare, should osteopenia be among the criteria for defining the female athlete triad syndrome? British Journal of Sports Medicine 36:10–13

Kuh D, Langenberg C, Hardy R et al 2005 Cardiovascular risk at age 53 years in relation to the menopause transition and use of hormone replacement therapy: a prospective British birth cohort study. British Journal of Obstetrics and Gynaecology 112:476–485

Laughlin G A, Dominguez C E, Yen S S 1998 Nutritional and endocrine-metabolic aberrations in women with functional hypothalamic amenorrhea. Journal of Clinical Endocrinology and Metabolism 83:25–32

Longo L D 1983 Maternal blood volume and cardiac output during pregnancy: a hypothesis of endocrinologic control. American Journal of Physiology 245:R720–R729

Loucks A B, Thuma J R 2003 Luteinizing hormone pulsatility is disrupted at a threshold of energy availability in regularly menstruating women. Journal of Clinical Endocrinology and Metabolism 88:297–311

Loucks A B, Verdun M, Heath E M 1998 Low energy availability, not stress of exercise, alters LH pulsatility in exercising women. Journal of Applied Physiology 84:37–46

Lustyk M K, Widman L, Paschane A et al 2004 Stress, quality of life and physical activity in women with varying degrees of premenstrual symptomatology. Women and Health 39:35–44

Morris S N, Johnson N R 2005 Exercise during pregnancy: a critical appraisal of the literature. Journal of Reproductive Medicine 50:181–188

Prior J C, Vigna Y, Alojada N 1986 Conditioning exercise decreases premenstrual symptoms. A prospective controlled three month trial. European Journal of Applied Physiology 55:349–355

Prior J C, Vigna Y M, McKay D W 1992 Reproduction for the athletic woman. New understandings of physiology and management. Sports Medicine 14:190–199

Redman L M, Loucks AB 2005 Menstrual disorders in athletes. Sports Medicine 35:747–755

Riggs B L 2000 The mechanisms of estrogen regulation of bone resorption. Journal of Clinical Investigation 106:1203–1204

Rossi R, Cioni, E, Nuzzo A et al 2005a Endothelial-dependent vasodilation and incidence of type 2 diabetes in a population of healthy postmenopausal women. Diabetes Care 28:702–707

Rossi R, Chiurlia E, Nuzzo A et al 2005b Flow-mediated vasodilation and the risk of developing hypertension in healthy postmenopausal women. Journal of the American College of Cardiology 44:1636–1640

Solomon S J, Kurzer M S, Calloway D H 1982 Menstrual cycle and basal metabolic rate in women. American Journal of Clinical Nutrition 36:611–616

Stengel S V, Kemmler W, Pintag R et al 2005 Power training is more effective than strength training for maintaining bone mineral density in postmenopausal women. Journal of Applied Physiology 99:181–188

Sudi K, Ottl K, Payerl D et al 2004 Anorexia athletica. Nutrition 20:657–661

Szabo E, Annus J, Zalanyi S Jr et al 1987 Disparate effects of naloxone in hypothalamic amenorrhoea of athletes. Functional Neurology 2:315–321

Taddei S, Virdis A, Ghiadoni L et al 1996 Menopause is associated with endothelial dysfunction in women. Hypertension 28:576–582

Templeton A, Kelman G R 1976 Maternal blood-gases, PAO$_2$–PaO$_2$, physiological shunt and VD/VT in normal pregnancy. British Journal of Anaesthesia 48:1001–1004

Timonen S, Procope B J 1971 Premenstrual syndrome and physical exercise. Acta Obstetrica et Gynecologica Scandinavica 50:331–337

Tomkinson A, Gibson J H, Lunt M et al 2003 Changes in bone mineral density in the hip and spine before, during, and after the menopause in elite runners. Osteoporosis International 14:462–468

Tormey S M, Malone C M, McDermott E W et al 2006 Current status of combined hormone replacement therapy in clinical practice. Clinical Breast Cancer 6(Suppl 2):S51–S57

Torstveit M K, Sundgot-Borgen J 2005 Participation in leanness sports but not training volume is associated with menstrual dysfunction: a national survey of 1276 elite athletes and controls. British Journal of Sports Medicine 39:141–147

Tzafettas J 2006 Painful menstruation. Pediatric Endocrinology Reviews 3:160–163

Waldrop J 2005 Early identification and interventions for female athlete triad. Journal of Pediatric Health Care 19:213–220

Warren M P, Perlroth N E 2001 The effects of intense exercise on the female reproductive system. Journal of Endocrinology 170:3–11

Warren M P, Shanghold M M 1997 Sports gynecology. Problems and care of the athletic female. Blackwell Science, Cambridge, MA

Warren M P, Shantha S 2000 The female athlete. Baillière's Best Practice Research. Clinical Endocrinology and Metabolism 14:37–53

Wolfe L A, Brenner I K, Mottola M F 1994 Maternal exercise, fetal well-being and pregnancy outcome. Exercise and Sport Science Reviews 22:145–194

Yamazaki S, Ichimura S, Iwamoto J et al 2004 Effect of walking exercise on bone metabolism in postmenopausal women with osteopenia/osteoporosis. Journal of Bone Mineral Metabolism 22:500–508

Zaydun G, Tomiyama H, Hashimoto H et al 2006 Menopause is an independent factor augmenting the age-related increase in arterial stiffness in the early postmenopausal phase. Atherosclerosis 184:137–142

Chapter **9**

Neurological and neuromuscular disorders, a guide to pathological processes and primary symptoms

Helen Dawes

CHAPTER CONTENTS

Learning objectives   270
Introduction   270
Stroke and traumatic brain injury   271
  Pathophysiology   271
  Cardiorespiratory fitness   273
  Muscle endurance   273
  Strength/power/speed   274
  Flexibility   274
  Balance/skill/coordination   274
  Exercise in primary prevention   274
  General health and secondary
    prevention   275
  Strength of evidence summary   277
Parkinson's disease (PD)   278
  Pathophysiology   278
  General fitness   278
  Cardiorespiratory fitness   278
  Muscle endurance   279
  Muscle strength/speed/power   279
  Flexibility   279
  Skill and coordination   279
  Exercise in primary prevention   279
  General health and secondary
    prevention   279
  Strength of evidence summary   281
Multiple sclerosis (MS)   282
  Pathophysiology   282
  General fitness   282
  Cardiorespiratory fitness   282
  Muscle endurance   283
  Muscle strength/power/speed   283
  Flexibility   283
  Skill and coordination   283

General health and secondary
  prevention   283
Strength of evidence
  summary   285
Neuromuscular disorders and allied
  conditions   286
Pathophysiology   286
General fitness   286
Cardiorespiratory fitness   286
Muscle endurance   287
Muscle speed/strength/power   287
Flexibility   287
Balance/skill/coordination   287
General health and secondary
  prevention   287
Strength of evidence
  summary   289
Selecting the mode and dose   289
Mode   289
Dose   289
Frequency   290
Duration   290
Intensity   290
Overload   291
Specificity   291
Summary of the gaps in the
  evidence; components, mode
  and dose of exercise   291
Typical co-morbidities   292
Key points   296
References   296
Further reading   306

LEARNING OBJECTIVES

After studying this chapter, you should be aware of:

1. The epidemiology and pathology affecting people with neurological and neuromuscular disorders in general and more specifically, stroke, traumatic brain injury, Parkinson's disease, multiple sclerosis and neuromuscular disorders.
2. The primary symptoms and possible co-morbidities of neurological and neuromuscular disorders.
3. The suitable mode, components and dose for effective exercise prescription in the above conditions.
4. The evidence regarding safe, effective exercise prescription and gaps in the evidence with regard to effectively designing training interventions in these clinical groups.

INTRODUCTION

Working with individuals with neurological and neuromuscular conditions is both challenging and rewarding. These conditions often present with functional effects that lead to immobility and secondary deconditioning. The level of severity and progression may vary. Some diseases are slowly progressive (muscular dystrophies), some have a sudden onset (stroke), some may relapse and remit (multiple sclerosis), and therefore the disease presentation and progression needs careful consideration when profiling an individual and delivering effective exercise prescription. This chapter aims to cover the more commonly found conditions including multiple sclerosis (MS), traumatic brain injury (TBI), stroke, Parkinson's disease (PD) and neuromuscular disorders (NMD). In these conditions the underlying pathological process, possible co-morbidities and likely functional effects that require consideration when prescribing exercise will be outlined. Whilst outside the remit of this text, awareness of the basic anatomical structure and function of the neuromuscular system will enable a better understanding of the possible difficulties facing people with neurological and neuromuscular conditions and facilitate more effective exercise prescription.

Texts providing good guides to basic structure are Fuller & Manford (1999) for neurological problems and Enoka (2002) for the neuromuscular system. Pathologies affecting neurological and neuromuscular function may be divided (Fuller & Manford 1999) into:

1. systemic (metabolic, toxic, nutritional, immunological or endocrine disorders), e.g. diabetic neuropathy
2. intrinsic (metabolic, infectious, neoplastic, degenerative, paroxysmal, immunological and genetic), e.g. multiple sclerosis, Parkinson's disease, motor neuron disease, neuromuscular disorders
3. vascular, e.g. stroke; and
4. extrinsic (trauma to the nervous system), e.g. traumatic brain injury (TBI).

People with neurological and neuromuscular disorders may present confusing pictures, with changes in components of fitness either due to the primary disease process or as secondary consequences of the enforced physical inactivity (Fig. 9.1).

Fitness will be considered in this chapter under sections on cardiorespiratory fitness, muscle strength/power/speed, muscle endurance, flexibility, and skill and

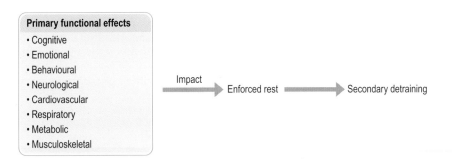

Primary functional effects

- Cognitive
- Emotional
- Behavioural
- Neurological
- Cardiovascular
- Respiratory
- Metabolic
- Musculoskeletal

Impact ➡ Enforced rest ➡ Secondary detraining

Figure 9.1   Overview of the functional effects of neurophysiological/neuromuscular disorders on physical activity.

coordination. Health and social benefits have been observed as a result of exercise in these conditions and exercise prescription in neurological/neuromuscular disorders is an exciting and rapidly developing specialty. Exercises such as treadmill walking, muscle strengthening and circuit training have been shown to improve mobility and can be delivered effectively in the home or the community (Ada et al 2003). To date, people with neurological conditions have had limited access to leisure-time physical activities. Some people may receive short periods of hospital-based rehabilitation but afterwards there is minimal initiation of community activity or focus on preventing secondary complications (Saunders et al 2004). Not surprisingly, factors affecting exercise participation in people with disabilities have been shown to mirror findings from the general population (Trost 2002). Specific barriers have been highlighted as: lack of provision of appropriate fitness facilities, lack of disability awareness among facility staff, lack of knowledge amongst disabled people of the benefits of exercise, decreased self-efficacy and negative attitudes to exercise, barriers of the health condition itself, lack of energy and perceived lack of available expertise (Kinne et al 1999, Rimmer et al 2004, 2005). For effective prescription, barriers highlighted by individuals should be addressed (Rimmer et al 2004).

The incidence and prevalence of neurological conditions in the UK is shown in Table 9.1.

STROKE AND TRAUMATIC BRAIN INJURY

Pathophysiology

A stroke is caused by a disruption in the flow of blood to the brain or spinal cord (Winer & Goetz 1999). A stroke most commonly affects the cerebral hemispheres and subcortical structures. Stroke is grouped into two major categories that reflect the mechanism of the insult: primary ischaemia (a blood clot occludes an artery interrupting the brain's blood supply) and primary haemorrhage (a blood vessel ruptures causing bleeding, the resulting pressure directly damaging cells or preventing blood flow). Primary ischaemic stroke accounts for approximately 80% and haemorrhagic stroke for 20% of cases (Winer & Goetz 1999). The terms 'transient ischaemic attack (TIA)' and 'minor stroke' are often used synonymously, but with TIA there should be no residual impairments 24 hours after an episode, whereas the effects of minor stroke will be substantially longer lasting, if they ever resolve.

The resulting effect on function depends on the size and location of the area of the brain affected, but commonly one side of the body is affected with function generally

Table 9.1 Incidence and prevalence of some neurological conditions (Office of Health Economics, 1989, http://www.ohe.org/page/index.cfm; Health Survey for England, 1991, Office for National Statistics (ONS), http://www.statistics.gov.uk/ssd/surveys/health_survey_england.asp)

Condition[a]	Incidence (new cases per year per 100 000 of population)	Prevalence (cases per 100 000 of population)	Approximate total numbers
Cerebral palsy	N/k	186	110 000
Charcot–Marie–Tooth disease	N/k	40	23 600
Dystonia[b]	N/k	65	38 000
Early onset dementia[c]	N/k	N/k	18 000
Epilepsy[d]	24–58	430–1 000	182 750–425 000
Essential tremor	N/k	850	500 000
Huntington's disease	N/k	13.5	6000–10 000
Migraine[e] (England)	400	15 000	8 000 000
Motor neuron disease	2	7	4000
Multiple sclerosis[f]	3–7	100–120	52 000–62 000
Muscular dystrophy	N/k	50	30 000
Parkinson's disease	17	200	120 000
Post-polio syndrome	N/k	N/k	120 000
Spinal cord injury[g]	2[h]	50	36 000
Spina bifida and congenital hydrocephalus	N/k	24	14 000
Young onset stroke[i]	55	N/k	N/k
Traumatic brain injury	175	1200	420 000

[a]Unless indicated otherwise, this table is based on figures in 'Neuro numbers: a brief review of the numbers of people in the UK with a neurological condition', published 2002 (see www.neural.org.uk/docs/annual_reports/NA2003AN.PDF). This table includes a selected number of neurological conditions. See publication for details on other conditions such as ataxia, brain tumour, Guillain–Barré syndrome and narcolepsy. Where additional and comparable information has become available, it is added with a footnote.

[b]Primary idiopathic, i.e. not associated with another condition.

[c]For Alzheimer's disease/dementia, the incidence is 25 000 per 100 000 in over 65s, prevalence 1000 per 100 000 in the general population and approximate total numbers 700 000. Alzheimer's disease and other dementias are covered in the National Service Framework (NSF) for Older People (see http://www.doh.gov.uk/nsf/olderpeople.htm).

[d]Figures for England and Wales from National Institute for Health and Clinical Excellence (NICE) guidelines (see http://www.nice.org.uk/search/guidancesearchresults.jsp?keywords=epilepsy&searchType=guidance).

[e]Steiner T J et al 1999 Epidemiology of migraine in England. Cephalalgia 19:305–306.

[f]Figures from NICE guidelines for England and Wales (see http://www.nice.org.uk/search/guidancesearchresults.jsp?keywords=multiple+sclerosis&searchType=guidance).

[g]Kurtzke J F 1978 Epidemiology of spinal cord injury. Neurología, Neurocirugía, Psiquiatría 18:157–191.

[h]The Spinal Injury Association gives 666 new patient admissions to spinal cord injury centres in the UK and Ireland in 2000 (equivalent to about 2 in 100 000).

[i]For stroke in all ages the incidence is 204, prevalence 800, and approximate total numbers 300 000. Stroke is covered in the NSF for Older People.

reduced most in the arm (Schiemanck et al 2005). For a detailed understanding of the degree of damage, time course of recovery and underlying mechanism, see Kwakkel et al (2004a). Longitudinal studies show that almost all stroke patients experience some functional recovery in the first 6 months although the recovery process in relation to time is often non-linear (Kwakkel et al 2004a). Several mechanisms are presumed to be involved in recovery, such as healing of penumbral tissues, neural plasticity (where the brain changes in order to adapt to the stroke) resolution of diaschisis (inhibition of function as a result of stroke in areas of the brain that lie at a distance from the original injury, but are anatomically connected with it through fibre tracts) and finally behavioural compensation strategies (Kwakkel et al 2004a). Recovery within the first 12 weeks will indicate the degree of damage and likely outcome, with further improvements after 6 months being probably due mainly to behavioural compensation strategies (Kwakkel et al 2004a).

TBI commonly affects younger individuals (~15–25 years), often as a result of motor vehicle accidents. In older individuals (75+ years) it is often a consequence of falling (http://www.headway.org.uk). The initial injury to the brain and haemorrhage from the resulting trauma may lead on to secondary damage from oedema, ischaemia and metabolic changes. TBI usually results in more diffuse brain injury than observed with stroke and is often associated with widespread traumatic injuries to the body. Brain injury may be classified into 'mild', 'moderate', 'severe' and 'persistent vegetative state' (Fuller & Manford 1999). The functional effect and general outcome will depend on the size and location of the damage.

Cardiorespiratory fitness

Reduced aerobic fitness, ~50–60% of predicted peak $\dot{V}O_2$, has been reported after both stroke (Kelly et al 2003) and brain injury (Bateman et al 2001), with substantial limitations in exercise capacity persisting even in individuals who receive standard physiotherapy (MacKay-Lyons & Makrides 2004). When considering factors limiting cardiovascular exercise, both stroke and TBI populations are generally unable to exercise to the physiological and psychological intensities expected in healthy populations (Dawes et al 2003c, 2006b, Macko et al 1997). However, within the range attainable, heart rate, oxygen consumption, blood lactate and rating of perceived exertion (RPE) increase linearly during submaximal exercise and behave similarly to measures observed in sedentary healthy populations (Dawes et al 2003c, 2006b, Macko et al 1997, Saltin & Landin 1975, Yates et al 2004). Exercise intensity measures are higher and succinate dehydrogenase (SDH) activity (indicating aerobic capacity) lower during exercise involving hemiparetic limbs (Saltin & Landin 1975). However, the efficiency of work production by paretic and spastic lower limb muscles has been suggested to be normal (Stoquart et al 2005). Exercise limitations in this group of individuals are multifactorial and complex, but higher fatigue levels have been shown to relate to the attainment of lower heart rates at test termination. In addition, lower quadriceps strength has been shown to relate to lower peak power output (Dawes 2005).

Muscle endurance

The evidence is limited but individuals with brain injury; TBI and stroke may have increased muscle fatiguability, as measured by cutaneous electrical stimulation, similar to changes observed in disuse (Bateman et al 1999).

Strength/power/speed

Following a stroke, approximately 90% of patients experience persistent motor deficits (Hesse & Werner 2003, Lin 2005). Indeed, loss of isometric and isotonic strength has been proposed to contribute, more than loss of dexterity, to physical activity limitation (Canning et al 2004, Hsu et al 2003). Muscle strength deficits in both limbs have been shown to impact on function (Bohannon 1991). Specifically, ankle plantar and hip flexor strength have been related to walking speed (Nadeau et al 1999a, 1999b), isometric quadriceps strength to peak bicycle power output (Dawes 2006b) and shoulder flexor and handgrip strength to upper limb function (Mercier & Bourbonnais 2004). The speed at which contractions can be generated may be important for function (Kim et al 2003), with explosive leg power correlating strongly with walking performance, particularly when there is asymmetry between limbs (Dawes et al 2005).

Flexibility

Spasticity (continuous contraction of muscles, resulting in limb stiffness) is often a consequence of stroke and TBI (Noth 1997). In the upper limb, stiffness caused by spasticity correlates with a reduction in hand dexterity (Lin & Sabbahi 1999) and treatments to reduce spasticity assist function (Francis et al 2004), but in the lower limb the impact of spasticity is less clear (Bressel & McNair 2002).

Balance/skill/coordination

Following stroke and TBI, skill, dexterity and coordination are often affected, with increased incidence of falls and impaired coordination between limb segments (Swinnen et al 2002). Both upper and lower limb actions may require more physical and cognitive effort (Eastridge & Mozzoni 2005, Jorgensen et al 2002, Kawahira et al 2005a, 2005b, Yamanaka et al 2005). Indeed people may experience difficulty in talking and interacting at the same time as performing physical tasks (Dawes et al 2003b, Haggard et al 2000).

Table 9.2 summarizes the common symptoms that may be present in people with stroke and TBI.

Exercise in primary prevention

Ischaemic strokes (cerebral infarction and transient ischaemic attack (TIA)) account for ≈88% of all strokes. Risk factors for ischaemic stroke may be classified (Shinton & Sagar 1993) into four major groups:

1. non-modifiable risk factors (including age, race, gender and family history)
2. well-documented modifiable risk factors (including previous transient ischaemic attack, carotid artery disease, atrial fibrillation, coronary artery disease (CAD))
3. other types of cardiac disease, hypertension, cigarette smoking, hyperlipidaemia, diabetes mellitus and sickle cell disease); and
4. less well-documented, potentially modifiable risk factors (including physical inactivity, obesity, alcohol abuse, hyperhomocysteinaemia, drug abuse, hypercoagulability, hormone replacement therapy, oral contraceptive use and inflammatory processes).

Table 9.2   Summary of common symptoms that may be present in people with stroke and TBI

Motor	Weakness, primarily on the side of the body contralateral to the brain lesion in stroke, bilateral in TBI
	Spasticity (continuously contracted muscles) of the affected limbs. Moving the limbs may be hard, especially fast movements
	Apraxia (difficulty in sequencing movement)
	Ataxia (unsteady and clumsy motion) in people with TBI
Somatic/autonomic	Incontinence (difficulty controlling the bladder and bowels) is relatively uncommon after the initial recovery period
Perception	Difficulty recognizing familiar objects or knowing how to use them (e.g. telling the time)
Vision	Diplopia (double vision) or hemianopia (loss of half of the field of vision)
Skill	Poor skill with a high incidence of falls
Swallowing	Dysphagia (about 50% of people have difficulty with swallowing after a stroke)
General health	Fatigue (extreme tiredness) in the first few weeks, which may persist
Communication	Reduction/loss of the ability to communicate; receptive and expressive aphasia/dysphasia (difficulty understanding speech or text or speaking)
Neuropsychological	Altered attention span, concentration, memory and information processing
	Altered personality, loss of insight and self-restraint, particularly in TBI
Mood	Depression, sadness, anger, anxiety, low self-esteem, loss of confidence and difficulty in controlling emotion
Sensation	Over-sensitive to colour, sound and light. Reduced sensation to heat or sharp objects

Sources: http://www.stroke.org.uk/index.html (accessed December 2007); http://www.headway.org.uk (accessed December 2007).

There is evidence that intensive exercise in the 20s protects against stroke, and exercising into the 50s gives further protection (Ohkubo et al 2004, Rodgers et al 1998). When considering haemorrhagic stroke (intracerebral and subarachnoid haemorrhage), although there is no direct evidence of the preventative effect of exercise, a link between high blood pressure and pathology has been established, suggesting that exercise may play a preventative role (Rodgers et al 1998).

General health and secondary prevention

After a transient ischaemic attack or stroke, people are at increased risk of recurrent cerebrovascular events. Approaches to the prevention of recurrent strokes and acute cardiac events is through lifestyle modification, appropriate pharmacological therapy and, if indicated, carotid endarterectomy (Saunders et al 2004). To date, with insufficient studies, there is no strong evidence for the effectiveness of secondary prevention on either death or dependency (Flemming & Brown 2004) or of exercise on the prevention of reoccurrence or secondary conditions (Karmisholt & Gotzcshe 2005) although preliminary evidence suggests aerobic exercise may reduce insulin resistance and prevent diabetes (Ivey et al 2007). A review by the American Heart Association provides helpful guidelines and recommendations for physical activity after stroke (Gordon et al 2004). What is clear is that exercise can be safely performed in community settings and can improve performance during everyday activities.

Cardiorespiratory exercise training

Typical physiotherapy after stroke or TBI is not at an intensity to induce an aerobic training effect and the patient may have reduced aerobic capacity after this stage of rehabilitation (MacKay-Lyons & Makrides 2004). Reasonably strong evidence demonstrates increased aerobic capacity and cardiovascular fitness following aerobic training both early and late (up to 6 months) (Pang et al 2006). Cardiorespiratory training has been shown to be more effective in improving fitness and functional mobility than regular physiotherapy (Macko et al 2005). A range of modes that include hydrotherapy, cycling and treadmills can be used and certainly techniques that enable individuals to train, such as strapping feet during cycling and bodyweight support during walking, should be employed. Selecting the mode of exercise is important, as training has been shown to improve performance of the activity trained (Gordon et al 2004). Treadmill training is a popular mode of exercise, with or without bodyweight support, as it enables intense walking practice, which can achieve both cardiovascular and repetitive motor skill training (Brown et al 2005, Macko et al 2005). As yet it is not clear if age or time since injury more substantially affect the degree of change observed, but the later or longer. The use of submaximal exercise tests is appropriate for individuals with moderate motor deficits (Yates et al 2004) but in more impaired individuals altered movement economy and inability to attain/maintain work rates may invalidate their use. At this point there is not enough evidence for reliable conclusions to be drawn as to how effective training is at improving performance of everyday tasks and general activity levels, and no trials report data on death and dependency effects (Karmisholt & Gotzcshe 2005, Saunders et al 2004).

Muscle strength/speed/power/endurance

Concern has been expressed in the past by physiotherapists that high-intensity exercise increases spasticity, is detrimental to performance and should not be used. However, recent evidence contradicts this dogma and has shown that high-intensity exercise does not detrimentally affect spasticity or motor performance (Dawes et al 2003a, Sharp & Brouwer 1997, Teixeira-Salmela et al 1999). Rather, a recent review of randomized controlled trials (RCTs) suggests that there is strong evidence in favour of using high-intensity strengthening exercises of the lower paretic limb after stroke (Van Peppen et al 2004). Certainly progressive resistance training increases muscle strength and reduces musculoskeletal impairments after stroke and brain injury (Morris et al 2004). A 12-week endurance training programme in individuals with brain injury elicited performance changes, though no changes were observed in muscle fatigue characteristics (Bateman et al 2000). In particular, programmes that utilize task-orientated strength training, such as sitting to standing (squats), possibly included in circuit training, are effective but the exercise mode needs careful consideration as benefits are mainly restricted to tasks directly trained (Van Peppen et al 2004). An investigation of repetition of an exercise, with added weight compared to no weight, highlighted the importance of the repetitive movement itself in neuropathological populations (Moreland et al 2003).

Flexibility training

Although there are no controlled trials examining the effectiveness of flexibility training, it should be considered as part of programmes as both active and passive stretching have been shown to improve movement (Selles et al 2005) and walking (Bressel & McNair 2002). Active and passive stretches delivered as part of a hydrotherapy programme have also been effectively employed; improving walking speed and oxygen (Zamparo & Pagliaro 1998).

Coordination/skill training skill

A review of different physiotherapy approaches to rehabilitation after stroke, neurophysiological, motor learning and mixed approaches, found no clear evidence of the best approach for improving leg strength, skill, walking speed or the ability to perform everyday tasks (Pollock et al 2003). Training benefits are mainly restricted to the tasks directly trained, i.e. skill and gait and task-related circuit training improves performance of locomotor tasks (Dean et al 2000). A review of the training literature suggests that task-orientated exercise training both induces brain plasticity (Johansen-Berg et al 2002) and is particularly effective when applied intensively and early after stroke (Kwakkel et al 2004b, Van Peppen et al 2004). Although there is no evidence, interventions after the initial recovery period may be better directed to compensation strategies that aim to optimize independence, such as training the least affected muscles.

Strength of evidence summary

(See Table 9.3 for evidence ratings.)

- Cardiovascular components:
  Increased endurance in activity trained   *Strong*
  Decreased likelihood of secondary stroke   *None*
- Muscle strength, to improve performance in trained activities   *Strong*
- Muscle speed/power to improve performance in activities of   *Low*
  daily living (ADLs)
- Skill/balance training of specific daily living tasks   *Moderate*
- Active and passive flexibility exercises   *Low*
- Muscle endurance   *None*

Table 9.3 Rating of strength of scientific evidence to date to support the use of each suggested fitness component

None	No studies showing evidence of effect
Low	Uncontrolled, non-randomized studies favourable
Moderate	One favourable randomized controlled trial (RCT)
Strong	More than one favourable RCT

PARKINSON'S DISEASE (PD)

Pathophysiology

Parkinson's disease, named after Dr James Parkinson (1755–1824), is a progressive neurological condition affecting movements such as walking, talking and writing (Eldar & Marincek 2000). Usually symptoms first appear after the age of 50, although one in 20 of people diagnosed will be aged under 40. It affects 0.3% of the 55–64 age group, 10% of the 65–74 age group, 3.1% of the 75–84 age group, and 4.3% of the 85–94 age group, and is greater in males (Zhang & Roman 1993). Parkinson's disease occurs when neurons in the substantia nigra of the basal ganglia die or become impaired (Fuller & Manford 1999). Normally, these cells produce dopamine, a neurotransmitter that signals to the striatum (Fuller & Manford 1999). The striatum has a prominent role in selecting which motor programme should be called into action to perform a given movement (Grillner et al 2005). When 60–80% of these dopamine-producing cells are lost, symptoms develop (Grillner et al 2005).

At present there is no cure for Parkinson's, but there are a range of treatments available to help control the symptoms and maintain quality of life for people with the condition. The main management is the use of drug treatments. Levodopa is generally given, often in combination with other medications, as nerve cells can use levodopa to make dopamine and replenish the brain's dwindling supply. More detailed information is available in the publication, 'The drug treatment of Parkinson's disease' (http://www.parkinsons.org.uk). Surgery is also sometimes used. Surgical procedures include deep brain stimulation, via a wire electrode, of the thalamus, globus pallidus or subthalamic nucleus, or rarely lesioning of some cells in the thalamus or globus pallidus.

General fitness

Activity limitations fluctuate during and from day to day, often related to blood medication levels. The timing of medication in relation to exercise testing and training needs careful consideration as anti-parkinsonian medication levels may affect muscle strength, walking speed, skill strategies (Nallegowda et al 2004), anaerobic threshold (Lewitt et al 1994) and the ability to learn new physical skills (Soliveri et al 1997). Fatigue and reduced energy are also commonly reported (Pentland et al 1992), which may result from both the disease and medication.

Cardiorespiratory fitness

Cardiovascular fitness has been shown to inversely relate to fatigue levels in people with PD (Garber & Friedman 2003) but not to disease severity (Canning et al 1997) Individuals mildly to moderately affected record normal cycle ergometer tests with expected peak oxygen consumption and work rates, with people who are more sedentary producing lower scores. During submaximal exercise, oxygen uptake may be higher than expected in healthy individuals but physiological indices of energy demand increase linearly and correlate with work output (Saltin & Landin 1975) although blood pressure and blood lactate concentrations may be lower than expected in healthy individuals (Reuter & Engelhardt 2002). Succinate dehydrogenase (SDH) activity may also be lower than expected in healthy individuals during exercise, particularly in more affected muscles, suggesting that detraining may in part contribute to the observed reduced work capacity (Saltin & Landin 1975).

Muscle endurance

Weakness and a propensity to fatigue quickly (lack of endurance) are symptoms commonly reported alongside abnormalities in skeletal muscle utilization and decreased efficiency of energy utilization (Lewitt et al 1994, Ziv et al 1998). Muscle fatigue has been shown to relate to reduced mobility and be improved by anti-parkinsonian medication (Ziv et al 1998).

Muscle strength/speed/power

Muscle strength may be reduced in the back, hip and ankle in people with Parkinson's disease (Nallegowda et al 2004). A person's ability to respond, move fast and powerfully will generally be reduced (Paasuke et al 2002). Strength reductions in leg muscles relate to functional activities such as the ability to rise from a chair (Inkster et al 2003). Initially one side may be more affected (Kakinuma et al 1998, Nogaki et al 1999). As the disease progresses, the difference between sides may become less obvious in slow movements but remain at faster speeds (Kakinuma et al 1998, Nogaki et al 1999).

Flexibility

A lack of dynamic trunk flexibility (Schenkman et al 2000), increased spinal stiffness and impaired knee flexibility (Horak et al 2005), typically observed in PD, may reduce functional reach and postural stability. Reduced flexibility and slow movement appear to be related to reduced coordination and more effortful movements (Winogrodzka et al 2005).

Skill and coordination

In people with PD, movements are slower, less skilled and coordinated in both upper and lower limbs (Kurillo et al 2004). There may be a reduced ability to generate forces quickly (Paasuke et al 2002), lower executive function (the ability to manage organization, priority-setting, time management, and decision making), impaired skill responses, and reduced interlimb coordination (Rochester et al 2004, Winogrodzka et al 2005). Altered skill strategies (Inkster & Eng 2004) and reduced postural stability (Horak et al 2005) are also reported. The effect of altered physical and executive skill may be a reduced ability to perform two tasks simultaneously (Canning 2005, Yogev et al 2005a, 2005b, 2005c). The ability to learn new skills may be comparable to healthy controls, but prolonged practice improvement (improvement after 2 weeks) and long-term retention of skills is often reduced (Agostino et al 2004, Mochizuki-Kawai et al 2004, Piemonte et al 2004). Table 9.4 summarizes the common symptoms that may be present in people with Parkinson's disease.

Exercise in primary prevention

It has been tentatively suggested that higher levels of physical activity may lower the risk of PD in men or that men predisposed to PD tend to avoid strenuous physical activity in their early adult years (Chen et al 2005).

General health and secondary prevention

A review of the evidence in 2000 suggested that it was not possible to draw conclusions regarding the efficacy of exercise for people with Parkinson's disease

Table 9.4 Common symptoms that may be present in people with Parkinson's disease

Tremor	Typically, a rhythmic back-and-forth motion of the thumb and forefinger (~8 Hz) that usually disappears during sleep and improves with intentional movement
Rigidity	The muscles remain constantly contracted so that the person aches or feels stiff or weak and there is resistance to movement. Limbs move in ratchet-like or short, jerky movements (cogwheel rigidity), leading to problems turning round, getting out of chair, turning over in bed, or making fine finger movements (fastening a button)
Bradykinesia	There is a slowing down and loss of spontaneous and automatic and routine movements
Impaired skill and coordination	Individuals may get stuck mid-stride (freeze), walk with quick, small shuffling steps, find it difficult to adapt quickly to changes in their environment, stop when walking and easily lose skill. Driving may become problematic
Mood	Individuals may be more irritable or uncharacteristically pessimistic, have memory loss, slow thinking, lose motivation for socializing
Difficulty in swallowing and chewing	Food and saliva may collect in the mouth and back of the throat, which can result in choking or drooling
Speech changes	Individuals may speak too softly, in a monotone, hesitate before speaking, slur, repeat their words or speak too fast. They may have a lack of facial expression, affecting communication
Autonomic dysfunction	Some people may become incontinent while others have trouble urinating. Constipation may occur. Individuals may have sexual dysfunction
General health	There may be difficulty sleeping (restlessness, nightmares, hallucinations and emotional dreams) and drowsiness during the day
Dyskinesias	Involuntary movements (twitching, nodding and jerking) may develop in people taking large doses of levodopa over an extended period. Severity varies in relation to time since medication

Sources: http://www.ninds.nih.gov/index.htm (accessed December 2005); http://www.parkinsons.org.uk/ (accessed December 2005).

(Eldar & Marincek 2000). Certainly there is limited evidence, but in general it appears that exercise may benefit people with mild-to-moderate Parkinson's disease (Ellis et al 2005, Smidt et al 2005) and this exercise prescription can be effectively provided in a community setting (Lun et al 2005).

Cardiorespiratory

There is limited evidence of the effect of aerobic exercise in people with PD. A few small studies are positive and have shown that aerobic exercise training may increase aerobic capacity and improve a subject's ability to initiate and perform movement patterns (Baatile et al 2000, Bergen et al 2002). Exercise modes utilized have included striding using walking poles, treadmill training, cycling and fast treadmill training. Inspiratory muscle performance may be improved by inspiratory muscle training (Inzelberg et al 2005). Treadmill training without (Herman et al 2005) or with bodyweight support has been shown to produce greater improvement in activities of daily living, motor performance and ambulation than physical therapy (Miyai et al 2000, 2002) and is an attractive mode of delivery as it trains a functional activity.

Muscle strength/speed/power/endurance

To date there is no evidence of the effectiveness of strength training if delivered on its own. However, people with mild-to-moderate Parkinson's disease can increase strength and walking performance similarly to healthy adults of the same age (Scandalis et al 2001). Resistance training, when delivered alongside skill exercises, has been shown to increase strength and skill and this combination has a greater impact on walking than skill exercises on their own (Hirsch et al 2003).

Flexibility training

There is evidence that 10 weeks of stretching improves spinal mobility and physical performance in people in the early and midstages of PD (Schenkman et al 1998). Carry-over to functional tasks has not yet been established.

Coordination/skill training

Coordination exercises alongside conventional fitness training and repetitive training may benefit people with PD. Skill training has been shown to improve skill, particularly if skill is trained alongside strength (Hirsch et al 2003). Training task-specific activities is indicated, such as walking training on a treadmill which improves walking performance (Frenkel-Toledo et al 2005). There is strong evidence that it is helpful for auditory cues (e.g. metronome beat) to be used to improve performance in tasks such as walking, but insufficient evidence of the carry-over benefit to other activities, community ambulation, or of sustainment (Lim et al 2005). People with PD who are learning to perform new motor skills may have difficulty transferring them to long-term motor memory (Agostino et al 2004) and so retaining their new skills (Mochizuki-Kawai et al 2004). This may be frustrating for both participant and trainer.

Strength of evidence summary

(See Table 9.3 for evidence ratings.)

- Cardiovascular component with the aim of decreasing secondary complications   *None*
- Increasing mobility   *Strong*
- Muscle strength to improve performance in ADL   *Moderate*
- Muscle endurance   *None*
- Skill/balance training of specific tasks of ADL   *Moderate*
- Active and passive exercises   *Low*

MULTIPLE SCLEROSIS (MS)

Pathophysiology

Multiple sclerosis (MS) is a chronic demyelinating disorder in which axon insulation, myelin, is lost from nerves in the central nervous system (CNS). The disease may affect various parts of the CNS, including the spinal cord, brainstem, cerebellum, cerebrum and optical nerves, but the peripheral nerves are not affected (Thompson 2001). Although the aetiology is unknown, an abnormal immune response against oligodendrocytes and myelin is believed to contribute to the disease. Lesions, scattered throughout the CNS white matter, cause multiple, varied symptoms and signs of neurological dysfunction (Thompson 2001). The essential feature of these lesions is loss of the myelin sheath with perivascular inflammation and relative sparing of the axons (Thompson 2001). The presence of inflammation in MS plaques and of oligoclonal immunoglobulin bands suggests an autoimmune basis of the disease (Thompson 2001). The major cause of negative symptoms during relapses (e.g. paralysis, blindness and numbness) is conduction block, caused mainly by demyelination and inflammation, and possibly also by defects in synaptic transmission (Thompson 2001). Recovery from symptoms during remissions is due mainly to the restoration of axonal function, either by remyelination, resolution of inflammation, or paradoxical restoration of conduction to axons that persist in the demyelinated state (Thompson 2001).

MS is progressive, characterized by exacerbations and remissions. Nerve conduction alters with variations in sclerosis and inflammation. Symptoms and the rate of progression of the disease differ between people. At times there may be a plateau or slight improvement in symptoms due to reduction of inflammation, whereas at other times a sudden deterioration may occur due to rapid demyelination. MS is often classified by its clinical course (Ebers 2001). Benign MS is characterized by mild intermittent relapses with nearly complete resolution. Secondary progressive MS starts with a relapsing–remitting course, with symptoms becoming more severe with less complete recovery of function after each exacerbation (Ebers 2001). Patients may then enter a chronic progressive phase, characterized by a step-like downhill course. MS that begins with a slow progression of signs and symptoms is classified as 'primary progressive MS' (Ebers 2001).

General fitness

MS tends to progress over years to decades, in general affecting quality rather than duration of life. Fatigue is an overriding symptom for many individuals, affecting their ability to perform everyday activities.

Cardiorespiratory fitness

Exercise capacity has been shown to be reduced in people with MS (Petajan et al 1996), possibly due to deficits in cardiorespiratory fitness, the high energy cost of moving, altered cardiovascular control, and/or respiratory muscle weakness (Olgiati et al 1986, Ponichtera-Mulcare 1993, Sutherland & Andersen 2001). Expiratory muscle strength has been shown to be significantly reduced and to relate to general function (Gosselink et al 2000). Walking distance in people with mild activity limitation does not appear to be related to perceived fatigue levels, dyspnoea or cardiorespiratory factors but rather to muscle strength and muscle oxidative capacity and neurological disability (White & Dressendorfer 2005).

Muscle endurance

It has been suggested that aerobic capacity may be limited in people with MS due to peripheral factors such as muscle weakness (Ponichtera et al 1992), reduced muscle oxidative capacity (White & Dressendorfer 2005) and changed muscle fibre type in the direction of disuse (Garner & Widrick 2003). When observing moderately impaired subjects with MS the myosin heavy chain (MHC) and fibre-type characteristics appear similar to those of age-matched sedentary controls (Carroll et al 2005). It would appear that in moderately impaired individuals there is a subtle shift, characteristic of disuse, with observed increases in fast more fatiguable MHC isoform coexpression, but at the same time there may be a modest reduction in cross-bridge number and density with no change in maximal cross-bridge cycling rate or susceptibility to intracellular metabolites (Garner & Widrick 2003) and slower relaxation times and left-shifted force–frequency relationships (Ng et al 2000). To date, the underlying muscle changes are not clear or easily understood but individuals with MS have been shown to generally recover from exercise sessions normally, although altered skeletal muscle performance and greater fatiguability should be considered when prescribing (KentBraun et al 1997).

Muscle strength/power/speed

Weakness is common in people with MS, even allowing for age, body and fat-free mass, spasticity and muscle fatigue differences from the normal (Iriarte 1998). Muscle weakness has been suggested to impair $\dot{V}O_2$ peak and functional activity levels (Sutherland & Andersen 2001). The lower limb tends to be affected before and more than the upper limb (de Ruiter et al 2001). Weakness in certain muscle groups may directly relate to problems with specific activities such as walking (Iriarte 1998). In particular there may be difficulty generating fast powerful movements, caused by impaired central activation (Ng et al 2004).

Flexibility

Spasticity in muscle groups that reduces limb and trunk mobility is a common complaint of people with MS (Noth 1997). However, the effect of reduced limb flexibility on function is less clear, as spasticity may reduce dexterity in the upper limb, and mobility generally, but in the lower limbs may help sustain function in people with muscle weakness (Holt et al 1996).

Skill and coordination

skilled tasks such as walking may be affected by reduced motor control (McCarthy et al 2005) with the effort of walking, measured by oxygen cost, up to three times higher in people with MS than in controls (Olgiati et al 1988). The effect of altered motor control and reduced ability to sustain attention may be particularly noticeable during more skilled activities, with reduced automation and difficulty dividing attention during activities such as walking (Hausdorff et al 2005, McCarthy et al 2005). Table 9.5 summarizes the common symptoms that may be present in people with multiple sclerosis.

General health and secondary prevention

In an effort to help minimize the risk of exacerbations and symptoms of fatigue, individuals have until recently been advised to restrict physical activity (Solari et al 1999).

Table 9.5   Common symptoms that may be present in people with multiple sclerosis

Eye	Optic neuritis (inflammation or demyelination of optic nerve) may cause: diplopia (double vision), visual blurring, decreased acuity and colour perception, discomfort, disorientation, flashes of light, exercise- or heat-induced visual deterioration, or hemianopia (loss of vision in one half of the visual field)
Sensation	Sensory loss, tingling and/or pain
Motor	Muscle weakness, spasticity (continuously contracted muscles), and muscle cramping
Somatic/ autonomic	Autonomic symptoms (e.g. bladder, bowel, sexual dysfunction) experienced early on
Cerebellar	Ataxia (inability to coordinate movements) a tremor (involuntary, oscillating movement) present when moving
General health	A consuming feeling of fatigue may occur in ~70% of individuals Dizziness and heat intolerance
Neuropsychological	Altered attention span, concentration, memory and information processing
Mood	Depression or euphoria, with ~5–10% of people developing clinical depression or dementia
Communication	Receptive and expressive aphasia/dysphasia (difficulty in understanding speech or text, or in speaking) Dysarthria (decreased coordination of the muscles of speech) Dysphagia (weakness of muscle of swallowing)

Source: http://www.nationalmssociety.org/ (accessed December 2007).

However, a Cochrane review of exercise therapy in general, by Reitberg et al (2005), found that exercise therapy improved muscle strength, exercise tolerance and mobility-related activities, with no evidence of deleterious effects. It has also been suggested that exercise therapy may improve mood. In summary, short- and long-term exercise interventions may improve health for people with MS not experiencing an exacerbation, but more evidence is needed over the long term. Unfortunately, fatigue and physical limitations may in themselves hinder exercise participation (Becker & Stuifbergen 2004).

Cardiorespiratory training

Effective cardiovascular (CV) programmes can be delivered using a variety of modes including combined arm and leg ergometry, treadmills, bicycle exercise and water aerobics, and may be combined with circuit training or programmes including aerobic, strength and/or flexibility training. There are limited RCTs of the effect of aerobic programmes when they are delivered in isolation. However, a 15-week aerobic cycling programme improved cycling and benefited health (increasing aerobic capacity and upper and lower extremity strength, and decreasing skinfolds, circulating triglyceride, very-low-density lipoproteins (VLDL), depression, anger and fatigue) (Petajan et al 1996). Shorter programmes have increased performance of the trained task, improved factors related to quality of life and started to reduce fatigue (Mostert & Kesselring 2002, Van den Berg 2005). Other effects included a drop in resting oxygen consumption, reductions in oxygen cost during walking, associated with increased walking speed and distance and improved coordination (Schulz et al 2004, Van den Berg 2005). Severely impaired individuals have also benefited from expiratory muscle training (Gosselink et al 2000).

Muscle strength/speed/power/endurance training

There is strong evidence in favour of general exercise therapy, compared to no exercise, improving muscle power, exercise tolerance and mobility-related activities without increasing fatigue levels (Rietberg et al 2005, White & Dressendorfer 2004). A few studies have shown strength training in isolation to be effective in MS but more evidence is needed (DeBolt & McCubbin 2001, 2004, Gutierrez et al 2005, Jones et al 1999). Combined programmes that include strength training amongst aerobic and/or flexibility exercises are safe and recommended as effective for those with mild-to-moderate activity limitation (Carter & White 2003, Romberg et al 2004, Solari et al 1999, Wiles et al 2001). Programmes can be effectively delivered at home or in community centres. Faster contraction speed, concentric strengthening programmes have been found to be more effective (Ponichtera et al 1992).

Flexibility training

There are no controlled trials examining the effectiveness of flexibility training, but combined programmes that include flexibility training can be safe and effective (Carter & White 2003, Solari et al 1999). Interventions using Iyengar yoga, tai chi, stretching exercises with drug treatments for spasticity, and active and passive movements during hydrotherapy, have all been reported to have beneficial effects.

Coordination/skill training

When skills are trained within aerobic cycling and walking training programmes, coordination and style improve in the tasks directly trained (Cattaneo et al 2005, Schulz et al 2004, Van den Berg et al 2005). A study comparing task-orientated training and training that facilitated movements found that they both led to improvements in skill (Lord et al 1998). Skill can be improved with task-specific training and for optimal functional carry-over programmes should include activities targeted as important by the individual clients.

Strength of evidence summary

(see Table 9.3 for evidence ratings.)

- Cardiorespiratory component with the aim of decreasing secondary complications — *None*
- Increasing endurance in activity trained, health and quality of life — *Strong*
- Muscle strength to improve performance in ADLs — *Strong*
- Skill/balance training of specific ADLs — *Low*
- Muscle endurance — *None*
- Respiratory training improving respiratory function — *Moderate*
- Muscle speed/power to improve performance in ADLs — *Moderate*
- Active and passive flexibility exercises — *Low*

NEUROMUSCULAR DISORDERS AND ALLIED CONDITIONS
Pathophysiology

There are over 60 different types of neuromuscular disorders and allied conditions, which are characterized by progressive muscle wasting and weakness (http://www.muscular-dystrophy.org).

Most of the conditions are genetic although some are autoimmune (http://www.muscular-dystrophy.org).

The major diseases affecting the neuromuscular system can be classified into:

- *Atrophies* – the central nervous system is affected and the upper and lower motor neurons waste away (e.g. adult spinal muscular atrophy).
- *Neuropathies* – the peripheral nervous system is affected (e.g. Charcot–Marie–Tooth disease and Friedreich's ataxia).
- *Dystrophies* – muscular dystrophy and allied conditions caused by mutations in the genes encoding for the production of muscle membrane proteins, which results in muscle damage and weakness. Disruptions in membrane proteins lead to sarcolemma instability and muscle cell necrosis (Barnes et al 2003). Different types of muscular dystrophy are caused by distinct protein deficiencies. The possible presentation varies between conditions and is complex. Conditions can be categorized in accordance with the distribution of muscle weakness, with certain muscular dystrophies having a more proximal or distal pattern. For more information, students should consult the Muscular Dystrophy Campaign (MDC) website: http://www.muscular-dystrophy.org/.

General fitness

The range of possible effects of neuromuscular disorders (NMD) include those on fatigue (Carter et al 1995a), intellectual function and neuropsychological profiles. For most forms of NMD intellect is normal (Carter et al 1995b, Johnson et al 1995, Kilmer et al 1995, McDonald et al 1995a, 1995b) but individuals with myotonic dystrophy may develop limitations (Carter et al 1995a). Individuals may first develop symptoms of neuromuscular disorder in adult life and may be coming to terms with managing the condition alongside their work and social commitments. People with NMD have been shown to be more obese and sedentary than healthy controls (McCrory et al 1998) and to have cardiovascular and metabolic risk factors, with low high-density lipoprotein cholesterol, high body mass index (BMI) and high triglyceride being the most common; indeed 55% of the NMD group satisfied the criteria for metabolic syndrome, versus 0% of a control group (Aitkens et al 2005, Chaudhuri & Behan 2004). Information detailed in the following sections on specific fitness components has been assimilated from Carter et al (1995b), Johnson et al (1995), Kilmer et al (1995, 2000), McDonald et al (1995a, 1995b) and Nogues et al (2002).

Cardiorespiratory fitness

Pulmonary and cardiac abnormalities may be present in individuals with neuromuscular disorders, particularly those presenting with myotonic dystrophy, Becker's muscular dystrophy, hereditary motor and sensory neuropathy types I and II (HMSN), spinal muscular atrophy (SMA) types II and III, limb-girdle syndrome (LGS) and with pulmonary symptoms in facioscapulohumeral muscular dystrophy

(FSHMD). Symptoms can develop as the above diseases progress and exercise professionals should consult with their client's medical consultant in order to determine their status regarding safe exercise. Possible symptoms could include abnormal ECG, reduced expiratory respiratory pressures, restrictive lung disease (RLD), increased work of breathing, cardiomyopathy and abnormal cardiopulmonary responses to exercise, and reduced aerobic capacity.

Muscle endurance

Evidence is limited in adults with NMD, but studies of muscle fatigue from animal models of NMD have revealed that slow oxidative (SO) muscle and fast glycolytic (FG) fibres differ from normal fibres, with SO fibres fatiguing more slowly and FG fibres fatiguing more rapidly but fast, oxidative, glycolytic (FOG) muscle fibres do not differ from healthy muscle fibres (Wineinger et al 2002). A study on children with severe neuromuscular disease found their muscles to be both extremely weak and more fatiguable (Scott et al 1985).

Muscle speed/strength/power

The most obvious symptom in NMD is muscle weakness with the distribution of affected muscle groups, rate of progress and associated limitations in function and activity varying within and between conditions. Strength and power deficits translate into reduced performance (Lindeman et al 1998); however, the relationship between strength and performance during everyday tasks is not linear, with imbalance between muscle groups a factor and the effect of changes in strength impacting more in weaker individuals (Willen et al 2004).

Flexibility

Although not a primary complaint, altered mechanics acting on joints, resulting from weakness and fibrosis in some muscle groups whilst others remain strong, may lead to deformities and joint contractures and so reduce flexibility.

Balance/skill/coordination

An altered walking style, characteristic for each condition, secondary to weakness may be observed as the disease progresses. Altered movement control has also been observed, although it is not clear if this is in adaptation to weakness (Bakhtiary et al 2000). Table 9.6 summarizes the common symptoms that may be present in people with neuromuscular disorders and allied conditions.

General health and secondary prevention

Many people with NMD do not receive regular therapy and may have been advised to be careful or avoid exercising; these factors alongside other physical and environmental barriers reduce exercise participation and individuals may be extremely detrained and unused to exercise (Ansved 2003, Eagle 2002, Philips & Mastaglia 2000). However, the importance of physical activity for social health has recently been emphasized in this group (McDonald 2002).

Table 9.6 Possible symptoms to consider with neuromuscular disorders in adults

Senses	In some conditions vision and hearing may be affected (myotonic dystrophy). It may be hard for patients to hold their eyes open for reading, watching television or driving. Cataracts may form
Muscular	Muscle weakness, wastage, fibrosis, cramps and difficulty in relaxing handgrip (myotonic dystrophy) may be present
Joint deformities	Muscle weakness may cause joint or skeletal deformities and problems
Neurological motor and sensory	Reduced coordination, pain and pins and needles
Cardiorespiratory	Breathing difficulties may present latterly and cardiac symptoms may occur associated with fainting, near fainting dizzy spells, low blood pressure (see section on neuromuscular conditions)
Communication	Difficulties with speech and swallowing secondary to respiratory muscle weakness
Neuropsychological	Intellectual and cognitive function (myotonic dystrophy)
General health	Alterations in the rhythm of sleeping and waking and general tiredness Crampy abdominal pain, constipation and diarrhoea may occur

Source: http://www.nationalmssociety.org/ (accessed December 2007).

Cardiorespiratory training

Studies evaluating the effects of various aerobic training programmes in a range of slowly progressive muscle disorders show benefit in activity performance, aerobic capacity, $\dot{V}O_2$ max and exercise tolerance, and no signs of muscle damage (Ansved 2003, Florence & Hagberg 1983, Olsen et al 2005, Tiavassalo et al 1999, Wright et al 1996). However, small sample sizes, no control groups and inclusion of a range of conditions limit conclusions (Ansved 2003, Philips & Mastaglia 2000), in particular for the long term, in these progressive conditions. Combined exercise programmes such as home exercise programmes containing strengthening (Dawes 2006a) or creatine supplementation (Kilmer et al 2005) alongside aerobic walking exercise may be beneficial. Respiratory muscle training has been shown to be effective in patients with neuromuscular weakness, particularly those less severely affected (Gozal & Thiriet 1999, McCool & Tzelepis 1995, Winkler et al 2000). To date, there is not enough evidence to draw conclusions regarding benefit of aerobic training on either general health or mobility but it appears to do no harm (Van der Kooi et al 2004).

Muscle strength/speed/power/endurance training

Resistance strength training has been controversial in NMD patients (Johnson & Braddom 1971, Kilmer et al 1994), with evidence from animal studies indicating muscle damage after eccentric contractions in dystrophic muscles (Childers et al 2002, Petrof 1998) and also that dystrophic muscles are less able to sustain muscle repair (Carter 1997). However, people with slowly progressive dystrophies, neuropathies and atrophies appear to respond to functional strength training similarly to healthy controls (Aitkens et al 1993, Allen 2001, Ansved 2003, Chetlin et al 2004a, 2004b, Kelm et al 2001, Lindeman et al 1995, Philips & Mastaglia 2000, Spector et al 1997), although the use of intense eccentric exercise should probably be avoided (Allen 2001). In conclusion, in myotonic dystrophy and facioscapulohumeral muscular dystrophy (FSHMD), moderate-intensity strength training will do no harm, but there is insufficient evidence that it is beneficial (Van der Kooi et al 2004). There is insufficient evidence to draw conclusions in other disorders (Van der Kooi et al 2004).

Flexibility training

There is no evidence of benefit from stretching alone (Carter 1997), but flexibility training has been included in effective home programmes (Dawes et al 2006a).

Coordination/skill training

Although there is no strong evidence, a short motor learning experimental intervention led to timing and movement improvements in drinking, in people with FSHMD (Bakhtiary et al 2000). As such, training functional activities within exercise programmes should be considered.

Strength of evidence summary

(See Table 9.3 for evidence ratings.)

- Cardiovascular component with the aim of decreasing secondary complications   *None*
- Increasing mobility   *Low*
- Inspiratory muscle training   *Moderate*
- Muscle strength to improve performance in ADLs   *Low*
- Muscle endurance   *None*
- Active and passive flexibility exercises   *None*
- Skill/balance training of specific tasks of ADL   *Low*

SELECTING THE MODE AND DOSE

Mode

The mode of training should relate to activities in which performance gains are desired but should be adapted to accommodate impairments. For example, a treadmill-training programme can attain a cardiovascular response, and in an individual struggling to use a treadmill a support harness can be used. Circuit training may be particularly effective as a range of functional activities can be incorporated.

Dose

Evidence of the dose response is limited in both neurological and neuromuscular populations, but there is no evidence suggesting that training principles from exercise science for healthy sedentary individuals do not hold true. Trainers should follow accepted exercise science guidelines unless otherwise indicated. Warm-up and cool-down should be incorporated into all programmes and, as in other populations, careful baseline testing should be carried out prior to prescription. Details of exercise testing are outside the remit of this text, but modifications may be required, as standard submaximal predictive testing utilized in healthy individuals may not be practical and may generate errors larger than the expected 15% (ACSM 2002). People may be unaccustomed to exercise and thus familiarization with any testing procedure may be needed; otherwise performance gains may occur due to increased familiarity with the test rather than improvements in fitness.

Frequency

To date there are no studies that have directly compared outcome from different training frequencies in this clinical group. However, most published programmes for all fitness components have, in line with practice in healthy individuals, prescribed training not less than five times/week. Intensive programmes with daily 6-hour interventions covering varied components (strength, skill, flexibility) over 2 weeks have been shown to be effective in stroke cases, but are not practical in the long term. Lifestyle and family commitments, individual preference and the degree of cross training should be considered when tailoring programmes.

Duration

There is evidence after stroke, but not as yet from other conditions, that the more hours spent training, the better. However, direct comparisons of different training durations have not been made. Generally, most evidence for all fitness components is from training sessions lasting 20–60 minutes. In individuals after stroke, longer training sessions appear to generate greater gains in endurance parameters (Dawes, unpublished observation). Programmes using intermittent exercise (alternating intervals of 5 minutes training/rest) have been successfully used in all neurological/neuromuscular conditions, particularly in those with limited capacity. Intermittent training may be useful when aiming for performance gains in certain functional tasks, but to date there is little evidence of effect and in general training has worked towards attaining the capacity to sustain 20 minutes of continuous CV exercise, before increasing exercise intensity. Programmes of 1–6 months' duration are reported, and although longer programmes appear to be more effective in TBI, with a suggestion that at least 6 weeks are needed for CV improvements, often only short periods of treatment are available within the NHS. However, intensive programmes with daily 6-hour interventions including components of strength, skill and flexibility for only 2 weeks have also been effective after stroke.

Intensity

There is a need for caution early on in programmes in neurological conditions, as individuals may be extremely detrained, unused to exercising and have co-morbidities such as cardiovascular conditions. It is advised that individuals should initially train at low/moderate CV intensity and progress cautiously (Gordon et al 2004). In practice it may be hard to achieve even moderate intensity levels. Heart rate should be monitored, but from experience even when individuals are going for fast speeds, both on a bike or treadmill, they have trained within safe CV training zones. No evidence is available concerning the effect of training at different HR intensities, but there is evidence that faster movements are better in CV training after stroke, MS and PD, with a suggestion that strengthening exercises should also be performed at faster speeds. Although the measure of intensity is often unclear, there are indications that more intense exercise is more effective after stroke or TBI.

No evidence is available from direct comparisons of different strengthening programmes, but a range of regimens (repetitions/rest/weights) have been shown to produce a training effect specific to the training, and specifically training towards functional activities using guidelines as for healthy individuals should be considered. Strengthening programmes, particularly those involving eccentric exercise, should only be employed in NMD in functional activities and progressed cautiously – gradually progressing up to moderate resistance levels.

In summary, accepted exercise science guidelines for healthy individuals should be followed for CV training zones, flexibility and resistance/repetition levels for strength training according to the desired training effect.

Overload

Standard progression guidelines should be followed, but in initial phases, particularly in NMD, progressions should be cautious and carefully monitored, with 48 hours allowed between sessions to enable exercise responses to be taken into account in guiding progression.

Specificity

Evidence of training effect in different components of fitness has concerned the mode and dose of exercises employed. However, limitations of the condition may necessitate the use of specific or adapted equipment. As would be expected from the experience of healthy subjects, there has certainly been carry-over between trained components (e.g. strength training improving walking endurance).

Summary of the gaps in the evidence; components, mode and dose of exercise

Exercise prescription in people with neurological and neuromuscular conditions is rapidly evolving. The co-morbidities and heterogeneous nature of neurological and neuromuscular conditions and the questionable ethics of giving isolated interventions mean that interventions are often delivered within a package of rehabilitation and it is difficult to unpick the active components. Another major barrier to obtaining strong evidence is the progressive nature of conditions. With a changing picture of limitations and activity, careful control groups are needed in intervention studies. There is a strong placebo effect of exercise interventions and difficulty in blinding individuals from being aware of the specific nature of each intervention. Selecting a suitable control intervention for studies is difficult, with ethical issues requiring careful consideration and the close social grouping often creating difficulty in preventing contamination across exercise groups examining the effect and impact of exercise interventions; there is also a need to develop theoretical models that underpin exercise interventions with underlying physiology and neurophysiology.

Areas where more research is needed

- Long-term observation of fitness, activity, exercise participation and health in patients with neurological and neuromuscular conditions.
- More general research to explore the efficacy and feasibility of training different components of fitness.
- Specific studies to explore how best to train fitness. Which mode of exercise (walking, cycling, swimming), component of fitness (strength, cardiovascular, flexibility), environment (home, centre, hospital) and dose (frequency, intensity, duration – continual/interval and progression) works best?
- Establishment of optimal timing of interventions in relation to pathological onset or exacerbations.
- Establishment of standardized testing batteries.
- Long-term follow-up of interventions.
- Investigations of the threshold for various components of fitness (e.g. threshold muscle strength in muscle groups to perform various functional tasks).
- There is very little evidence in general regarding flexibility (components of flexibility training, i.e. type of stretching (static/ballistic), length of hold, physiological effect, timing of the intervention, effect).
- Investigations of the effectiveness of different strength training programmes (different speeds, resistances, repetitions, sets, rests).
- Investigation of whether to focus on training weak muscles or train stronger components to compensate.
- Seeking evidence of the effect of factors such as medication, temperature, time of day, or age on the exercise response in this group.
- There is little evidence, in any of the above respects, concerning the more impaired patients.
- There is likewise little evidence of any sort concerned with upper limb exercise modes.
- There is a need to stratify populations in an attempt to determine optimal training for different levels of severity or impairment, over different time courses.

TYPICAL CO-MORBIDITIES

Knowledge of the pathologies themselves is helpful in understanding how symptoms may affect individuals. Some conditions have associated specific problems; for example, people with MS experience fatigue and heat intolerance. Symptoms may have a different onset of presentation in some conditions; for example, people with MS may get early bladder complications whilst still relatively unimpaired physically. Understanding of the disease and typical co-morbidities will enable delivery of an effective and safe exercise programme. A thorough knowledge of the background pathology and likely concurrent medical management and possible complications is indicated. Possible co-morbidities are reported under the sections on each neurological condition, and sensible precautions when dealing with clients suggested (see Tables 9.7, 9.8, 9.9 and 9.10). However, anyone considering exercise prescription in any of these conditions must be encouraged to read further on exercise testing and prescription, particularly concerning the effects of medication. Exercise professionals should seek information regarding conditions and utilize the support of medical and health professionals in ensuring safe prescription.

Table 9.7 Stroke and traumatic brain injury

Co-morbidity	Precaution
Coronary artery disease (present in ~75% of individuals after stroke) and peripheral arterial disease (Gordon et al 2004)	Pre-exercise evaluation of complete medical history, physical examination. The American Heart Association scientific statement from the Council on Clinical Cardiology (Gordon et al 2004) recommends a 12-lead ECG graded exercise test (GET) prior to prescription, but there are no guidelines in the UK. The suggestion for individuals who have not undergone a GET is that they should perform light/moderate-intensity exercise at a greater frequency and duration than that normally prescribed in healthy individuals (ACSM 2002)
Medication including: anticoagulants/ platelet inhibiting agents, vasodilators, antihypertensive medication, and anticonvulsant medication and medication to reduce muscle tone	When exercise testing, consider the effect of medications and that individuals may be deconditioned and need to start at very low intensities
Consideration of medication. For details of typical medications and their interaction with exercise see ACSM (2002)
Reduced motor control/weakness	Exercise/testing will need to be adapted to accommodate for physical limitations, i.e. seated positions, use of bodyweight support during treadmill walking, use of arm/toe straps
Coexisting injuries and conditions	Careful assessment of each individual and adaptation to allow for possible limitations
Psychological, cognitive or emotional effects of brain injury	Consideration of a quiet exercise environment, the use of careful instructions and avoidance of too fast or too great a delivery of information. A great deal of support and encouragement may be needed to motivate some individuals

Table 9.8 Multiple sclerosis

Co-morbidity	Precaution
Heat intolerance and fatigue	Exercise/test in cool environment, utilize fans. Evaluate the exercise programme's impact on individuals' fatigue and test and progress cautiously. Morning may be the best testing/ training time
Exacerbation	Consider possible exacerbations and avoid exercise if there is an exacerbation

(Continued)

Table 9.8   Multiple sclerosis—Cont'd

Co-morbidity	Precaution
Prevalence of psychological, cognitive, emotional effects	This may necessitate the use of careful instructions and avoidance of too fast or too great a delivery of information during exercising and when advising. A great deal of support and encouragement may be needed to motivate some individuals
Prevalence of incontinence	Planning of voiding prior to and during sessions
Medication to reduce muscle tone and the number of exacerbations (e.g. baclofen, amantadine, amitriptyline, prednisolone, interferon beta-1a/1b)	The medications may cause a range of symptoms including muscle weakness, sweating, hypertension, diabetes, osteoporosis, generally feeling unwell, reduced exercise tolerance. For details of typical medication and the exercise response in neurological conditions see ACSM (2002)
Physical/coordination limitations	Modifications may be needed to allow for physical limitations, e.g. recumbent ergometer testing or the use of bodyweight support on the treadmill
	Motor tasks may be difficult to learn or coordinate and simplified tasks/activities should be considered

Table 9.9   Parkinson's disease

Co-morbidity	Precaution
Freezing phenomena/poor skill	Careful consideration of timing and safety of exercise (safety harness)
Fluctuating symptoms often related to medication dose. Typically medication includes: dopaminergics (levodopa), anticholinergics (benztropine) and monoamine oxidase type B inhibitors (deprenyl)	Careful consideration of timing in relation to medication administration. Optimal testing and exercise should be timed ~45–60 minutes after medication. Individuals should be tested at different times from administration of medication to observe full clinical picture. The heart rate response may vary according to medication plasma level. Medication may cause some of the following symptoms: exercise bradycardia or tachycardia transiently at peak dose, dyskinesia, gastrointestinal discomfort and drug-related mood swings. Details of typical medication and the exercise response are given elsewhere (ACSM 2002)

(Continued)

Table 9.9 Parkinson's disease—Cont'd

Co-morbidity	Precaution
High prevalence of dysrhythmias, tachycardia and bradycardia	Careful observation of heart rate response to exercise
Neurological/autonomic dysfunction (reduced sweating, orthostatic hypotension, depression, delusions, raised resting metabolic rate)	Care in ensuring safe exercise – consideration of temperature control and care when changing positions quickly Consideration of mood
Age-related conditions	Individualized approach is required that considers joint stiffness and pain
Painful muscles	Consideration when handling individuals' limbs, particularly during flexibility training
Altered motor learning and memory	Repeated demonstrations may be needed with consideration that long-term skill acquisition may be impaired

Table 9.10 Neuromuscular disorders

Co-morbidity	Precaution
Abnormal response to muscle damage	Avoid or use extreme care if prescribing eccentric exercises. Use functional activities such as sit-to-stand, monitor carefully and progress cautiously Some texts suggest the monitoring of creatine kinase (CK) activity during exercise programmes, but this marker is variable and unlikely to be available for patients (Barbiroli et al 1993, Biral et al 2000, Feasson et al 2002). Consultation with the individual's consultant or specialist physiotherapist prior to embarking on an exercise programme is recommended. Support is available through the Muscular Dystrophy Campaign
Muscle pain and contractures (FSHMD)	Flexibility training should be included and testing/training modified appropriately
Possible cardiac complications in some conditions, e.g. cardiomyopathy (LGMD, BMD) and conduction block (EDMD, myotonic dystrophy)	Prior to exercise prescription consultation with the individuals' consultant or specialist physiotherapist will establish cardiac health. Individuals with LGMD, BMD, EDMD and myotonic dystrophy may require specialized cardiac testing prior to participation

(Continued)

Table 9.10   Neuromuscular disorders—Cont'd

Co-morbidity	Precaution
Respiratory deficits due to muscle weakness	Pulmonary function, FEV_1 and FVC should be monitored
Joint problems secondary to muscle weakness may occur	Modify testing/training positions
Fatigue and illness	Encourage individuals to modify exercise participation in line with their general health
Motivational issues (myotonic dystrophy)	Support
Temperature sensitivity	Care with exercise environment. Avoid too cold an exercise environment for some conditions (myotonic dystrophy)
Medication (corticosteroids)	Consider possible side effects and exercise in weight-bearing positions if possible in order to stimulate bone

LGMD, Limb girdle muscular dystrophy; BMD, Becker muscular dystrophy; EDMD, Emery–Dreifuss muscular dystrophy.

KEY POINTS

1. Exercise prescription must be highly individualized in people with neurological and neuromuscular conditions. Exercise prescription will require a flexible approach in order to allow for possible physical, psychological, cognitive and emotional consequences of the disorders.
2. Knowledge of the pathological process, likely symptoms and medical management is essential for safe and effective exercise prescription.
3. Support from specialist clinicians should be sought when developing programmes.
4. Programmes will be more effective if individuals are closely monitored and programmes modified to allow for day-to-day and circadian variability and to accommodate disease progression.

References

ACSM (eds) 2002 ACSM's guidelines for exercise testing and prescription. Guidelines for graded exercise testing and training. Lippincott Williams & Wilkins, Philadelphia

Ada L, Dean C M, Hall J M et al 2003 A treadmill and overground walking program improves walking in persons residing in the community after stroke: a placebo-controlled randomized trial. Archives of Physical Medicine and Rehabilitation 84(10):1486–1491

Agostino R, Curra A, Soldati G et al 2004 Prolonged practice is of scarce benefit in improving motor performance in Parkinson's disease. Movement Disorders 19(11):1285–1293

Aitkens S G, McCrory M A, Kilmer D D et al 1993 Moderate resistance exercise program – its effect in slowly progressive neuromuscular disease. Archives of Physical Medicine and Rehabilitation 74(7):711–715

Aitkens S, Kilmer D D, Wright N C et al 2005 Metabolic syndrome in neuromuscular disease. Archives of Physical Medicine and Rehabilitation 86(5):1030–1036

Allen D G 2001 Eccentric muscle damage: mechanisms of early reduction of force. Acta Physiologica Scandinavica 171(3):311–319

Ansved T 2003 Muscular dystrophies: influence of physical conditioning on the disease evolution. Current Opinion in Clinical Nutrition and Metabolic Care 6:435–439

Baatile J, Langbein W E, Weaver F et al 2000 Effect of exercise on perceived quality of life of individuals with Parkinson's disease. Journal of Rehabilitation Research and Development 37(5):529–534

Bakhtiary A H, Phoenix J, Edwards R H et al 2000 The effect of motor learning in facioscapulohumeral muscular dystrophy patients. European Journal of Applied Physiology 83(6):551–558

Barbiroli B, McCully K K, Iotti S et al 1993 Further impairment of muscle phosphate kinetics by lengthening exercise in DMD/BMD carriers – an in-vivo P-31-NMR spectroscopy study. Journal of the Neurological Sciences 119(1):65–73

Barnes P R J, Hilton-Jones D, Dalakas M C et al 2003 Myopathies in clinical practice. Martin Dunitz; Taylor and Francis, London

Bateman A, Culpan J, Dawes H et al 1999 Exercise tolerance in patients who have suffered recent brain injury. Journal of Sports Science 17:27–28

Bateman A, Greenwood R J, Scott O M 2000 Exercise tolerance, quadriceps strength and fatiguability and functional ability after recent brain injury. Society for Rehabilitation Research, Summer 2000

Bateman A, Culpan F J, Pickering A D et al 2001 The effect of aerobic training on rehabilitation outcomes after recent severe brain injury: a randomized controlled evaluation. Archives of Physical Medicine and Rehabilitation 82(2):174–182

Becker H, Stuifbergen A 2004 What makes it so hard? Barriers to health promotion experienced by people with multiple sclerosis and polio. Family and Community Health 27(1):75–85

Bergen J L, Toole T, Elliott R G et al 2002 Aerobic exercise intervention improves aerobic capacity and movement initiation in Parkinson's disease patients. Neurorehabilitation 17(2):161–168

Biral D, Jakubiec Puka A, Ciechomoka I et al 2000 Loss of dystrophin and some dystrophin-associated proteins with concomitant signs of apoptosis in rat leg muscle overworked in extension. Acta Neuropathologica 100(6):618–626

Bohannon R W 1991 Strength deficits also predict gait performance in patients with stroke. Perceptual and Motor Skills 73(1):146

Bressel E, McNair P J 2002 The effect of prolonged static and cyclic stretching on ankle joint stiffness, torque relaxation, and gait in people with stroke. Physical Therapy 82(9):880–887

Brown T H, Mount J, Rouland B L et al 2005 Body weight-supported treadmill training versus conventional gait training for people with chronic traumatic brain injury. Journal of Head Trauma Rehabilitation 20(5):402–415

Canning C G 2005 The effect of directing attention during walking under dual-task conditions in Parkinson's disease. Parkinsonism and Related Disorders 11(2):95–99

Canning C G, Alison J A, Allen N E et al 1997 Parkinson's disease: an investigation of exercise capacity, respiratory function, and gait. Archives of Physical Medicine and Rehabilitation 78(2):199–207

Canning C G, Ada L, Adams R et al 2004 Loss of strength contributes more to physical disability after stroke than loss of dexterity. Clinical Rehabilitation 18(3):300–308

Carroll C C, Gallagher P M, Seidle M E et al 2005 Skeletal muscle characteristics of people with multiple sclerosis. Archives of Physical Medicine and Rehabilitation 86(2):224–229

Carter G T 1997 Rehabilitation management in neuromuscular disease. Journal of Neurologic Rehabilitation 11(2):69–80

Carter P, White C M 2003 The effect of a general exercise training on effort of walking in patients with MS. 14th International World Confederation for Physical Therapy, Barcelona

Carter G T, Abresch R T, Fowler W M et al 1995a Profiles of neuromuscular diseases, hereditary motor and sensory neuropathy, type-I and type-Ii. American Journal of Physical Medicine and Rehabilitation 74(5):S140–S149

Carter C T, Abresch R T, Fowler W M et al 1995b Profiles of neuromuscular diseases – spinal muscular-atrophy. American Journal of Physical Medicine and Rehabilitation 74(5):S150–S159

Cattaneo D, Ferrari M, Frasson W, Casiraghi A 2005 Head control: volitional aspects of rehabilitation training in patients with multiple sclerosis compared with healthy subjects. Archives of Physical Medicine and Rehabilitation 86(7):1381–1388

Chaudhuri A, Behan P O 2004 Fatigue in neurological disorders. Lancet 363(9413):978–988

Chen H, Zhang S M, Schwarzschild M A et al 2005 Physical activity and the risk of Parkinson disease. Neurology 64(4):664–669

Chetlin R D, Gutmann L, Tarnopolsky M et al 2004a Resistance training effectiveness in patients with Charcot–Marie–Tooth disease: Recommendations for exercise prescription. Archives of Physical Medicine and Rehabilitation 85(8):1217–1223

Chetlin R D, Gutmann L, Tarnopolsky M A et al 2004a Resistance training exercise and creatine in patients with Charcot–Marie–Tooth disease. Muscle and Nerve 30(1):69–76

Childers M K, Okamura C S, Bogan D J et al 2002 Eccentric contraction injury in dystrophic canine muscle. Archives of Physical Medicine and Rehabilitation 83:1572–1578

Dawes H, Bateman A, Culpan F J et al 2003a The effect of increasing effort on movement economy during incremental cycling exercise in individuals early after acquired brain injury. Clinical Rehabilitation 17:528–534

Dawes H, Cockburn J, Roach N K et al 2003b The effect of a perceptual cognitive task on exercise performance: the dual-task condition after brain injury. Clinical Rehabilitation 17(5):535–539

Dawes H, Bateman A, Culpan J et al 2003c Heart rate as a measure of exercise testing early after acquired brain injury. Physiotherapy 89:10–15

Dawes H, Smith C, Collett J et al 2005 A pilot study to investigate explosive leg extensor power and walking performance after stroke. Journal of Sports Science and Medicine 4(4):556–562

Dawes, H, Korpershoek N, Freebody J et al 2006a A pilot randomised controlled trial of a home based exercise programme aimed at improving endurance and function in adults with neuromuscular disorders (NMD). Journal of Neurology, Neurosurgery and Psychiatry online

Dawes H, Scott O M, Roach N K, Wade D 2006b Exertional symptoms and exercise capacity in individuals with brain injury. Disability and Rehabilitation 28(20):1243–1250

de Ruiter C J, Jongen P J H, van der Woude L H V et al 2001 Contractile speed and fatigue of adductor pollicis muscle in multiple sclerosis. Muscle and Nerve 24(9):1173–1180

Dean C M, Richards C L, Malouin F 2000 Task-related circuit training improves performance of locomotor tasks in chronic stroke: a randomized, controlled pilot trial. Archives of Physical Medicine and Rehabilitation 81(4):409–417

DeBolt L S, McCubbin J A 2001 The effect of resistance exercise on fatigue and depression in women with multiple sclerosis. Research Quarterly for Exercise and Sport 72(1): A99–A100

DeBolt L S, McCubbin J A 2004 The effects of home-based resistance exercise on skill, power, and mobility in adults with multiple sclerosis. Archives of Physical Medicine and Rehabilitation 85(2):290–297

Eagle M 2002 Report on the muscular dystrophy campaign workshop: exercise in neuromuscular diseases Newcastle, January 2002. Neuromuscular Disorders 12:975–983

Eastridge D, Mozzoni M P 2005 Fluency and functional motor skills following brain injury. Behavioral Interventions 20(1):77–89

Ebers G C 2001 Natural history of multiple sclerosis. Journal of Neurology, Neurosurgery and Psychiatry 71:II16–II19

Eldar R, Marincek C 2000 Physical activity for elderly persons with neurological impairment: a review. Scandinavian Journal of Rehabilitation Medicine 32(3):99–103

Ellis T, de Goede C J, Feldman R G et al 2005 Efficacy of a physical therapy program in patients with Parkinson's disease: a randomized controlled trial. Archives of Physical Medicine and Rehabilitation 86(4):626–632

Enoka R M 2002 Neuromechanics of human movement. Human Kinetics, London

Feasson L, Stockholm D, Freyssenet D et al 2002 Molecular adaptations of neuromuscular disease-associated proteins in response to eccentric exercise in human skeletal muscle. Journal of Physiology, London 543(1):297–306

Flemming K D, Brown R D 2004 Secondary prevention strategies in ischemic strike: Identification and optimal management of modifiable risk factors. Mayo Clinic Proceedings 79(10).1330–1340

Florence J M, Hagberg J M 1983 Effect of training on the exercise responses of neuromuscular disease patients. Medicine and Science in Sports and Exercise 16(5):460–465

Francis H P, Wade D T, Turner-Stokes L et al 2004 Does reducing spasticity translate into functional benefit? An exploratory meta-analysis. Journal of Neurology, Neurosurgery and Psychiatry 75(11):1547–1551

Frenkel-Toledo S, Giladi N, Peretz C et al 2005 Treadmill walking as an external pacemaker to improve gait rhythm and stability in Parkinson's disease. Movement Disorders 20(9):1109–1114

Fuller G, Manford M R 1999 Neurology: an illustrated colour text. Elsevier Health Sciences, Oxford

Garber C E, Friedman J H 2003 Effects of fatigue on physical activity and function in patients with Parkinson's disease. Neurology 60(7):1119–1124

Garner D J P, Widrick J J 2003 Cross-bridge mechanisms of muscle weakness in multiple sclerosis. Muscle and Nerve 27(4):456–464

Gordon N F, Gulanick M, Costa F et al 2004 Physical activity and exercise recommendations for stroke survivors – An American Heart Association scientific statement from the Council on Clinical Cardiology, Subcommittee on Exercise, Cardiac Rehabilitation, and Prevention; the Council on Cardiovascular Nursing; the Council on Nutrition, Physical Activity, and Metabolism; and the Stroke Council. Stroke 35(5):1230–1240

Gosselink R, Kovacs L, Ketelaer P et al 2000 Respiratory muscle weakness and respiratory muscle training in severely disabled multiple sclerosis patients. Archives of Physical Medicine and Rehabilitation 81(6):747–751

Gozal D, Thiriet P 1999 Respiratory muscle training in neuromuscular disease: long-term effects on strength and load perception. Medicine and Science in Sports and Exercise 31(11):1522–1527

Grillner S, Helligren J, Menard A et al 2005 Mechanisms for selection of basic motor programs – roles for the striatum and pallidum. Trends in Neurosciences 28(7):364–370

Gutierrez G M, Chow J W, Tillman M D et al 2005 Resistance training improves gait kinematics in persons with multiple sclerosis. Archives of Physical Medicine and Rehabilitation 86(9):1824–1829

Haggard P, Cockburn J, Cock J et al 2000 Interference between gait and cognitive tasks in a rehabilitating neurological population. Journal of Neurology, Neurosurgery and Psychiatry 69(4):479–486

Hausdorff J M, Yogev G, Springer S et al 2005 Walking is more like catching than tapping: gait in the elderly as a complex cognitive task. Experimental Brain Research 164 (4):541–548

Herman T, Giladi N, Erlich S et al 2005 Six weeks intensive treadmill training improves gait and quality of life in patients with Parkinson's disease: a pilot study. Journal of the American Geriatrics Society 53(4):S117–S117

Hesse S, Werner C 2003 Poststroke motor dysfunction and spasticity: novel pharmacological and physical treatment strategies. CNS Drugs 17(15):1093–1107

Hirsch M A, Toole T, Maitland C G et al 2003 The effects of skill training and high-intensity resistance training on persons with idiopathic Parkinson's disease. Archives of Physical Medicine and Rehabilitation 84(8):1109–1117

Holt K G, Obusek J P, Fonseca S T 1996 Constraints on disordered locomotion. A dynamical systems perspective on spastic cerebral palsy. Human Movement Science 15(2):177–202

Horak F B, Dimitrova D, Nutt J G 2005 Direction-specific postural instability in subjects with Parkinson's disease. Experimental Neurology 193(2):504–521

Hsu A L, Tang P F, Jan M H 2003 Analysis of impairments influencing gait velocity and asymmetry of hemiplegic patients after mild to moderate stroke. Archives of Physical Medicine and Rehabilitation 84(8):1185–1193

Inkster L M, Eng J J 2004 Postural control during a sit-to-stand task in individuals with mild Parkinson's disease. Experimental Brain Research 154(1):33–38

Inkster L M, Eng J J, MacIntyre D L et al 2003 Leg muscle strength is reduced in Parkinson's disease and relates to the ability to rise from a chair. Movement Disorders 18(2):157–162

Inzelberg R, Peleg N, Nisipeanu P et al 2005 Inspiratory muscle training and the perception of dyspnea in Parkinson's disease. Canadian Journal of Neurological Sciences 32(2):213–217

Iriarte J 1998 Correlation between symptom fatigue and muscular fatigue in multiple sclerosis. European Journal of Neurology 5(6):579–585

Ivey F M, Ryan A S, Hafer-Macko C E et al 2007 Treadmill aerobic training improves glucose tolerance and indices of insulin sensitivity in disabled stroke survivors: a preliminary report. Stroke 38(10):2752–2758

Johansen-Berg H, Dawes H, Guy C et al 2002 Correlation between motor improvements and altered fMRI activity after rehabilitative therapy. Brain 125:2731–2742

Johnson E R, Abresch R T, Carter G T et al 1995 Profiles of neuromuscular diseases – myotonic-dystrophy. American Journal of Physical Medicine and Rehabilitation 74(5): S104–S116

Johnson E W, Braddom R 1971 Over-work weakness in facioscapulohumeral muscular dystrophy. Archives of Physical Medicine and Rehabilitation 52:333–336

Jones R, Davies-Smith A, Harvey L 1999 The effect of weighted leg raises and quadriceps strength, EMG and functional activities in people with multiple sclerosis. Physiotherapy 85(3):154–161

Jorgensen L, Engstad T, Jacobsen B K 2002 Higher incidence of fall in long-term stroke survivors than in population controls – depressive symptoms predict falls after stroke. Stroke 33(2):542–547

Kakinuma S, Nogaki H, Pramanik B et al 1998 Muscle weakness in Parkinson's disease: isokinetic study of the lower limbs. European Neurology 39(4):218–222

Karmisholt K, Gotzcshe P C 2005 Physical activity for secondary prevention of disease – systematic reviews of randomised clinical trials. Danish Medical Bulletin 52(2):90–94

Kawahira K, Shimodozono M, Matsumoto S et al 2005a Evaluation of skilled leg movements in patients with stroke using a computerized motor-skill analyzer for the lower limb. International Journal of Neuroscience 115(3):379–392

Kawahira K, Shimodozono M, Ogata A et al 2005b Impaired visuo-motor skills in the unaffected lower limb of patients with stroke. International Journal of Neuroscience 115 (9):1315–1332

Kelly J O, Kilbreath S L, Davis G M et al 2003 Cardiorespiratory fitness and walking ability in subacute stroke patients. Archives of Physical Medicine and Rehabilitation 84(12): 1780–1785

Kelm J, Ahlhelm F, Regitz T et al 2001 Controlled dynamic weighttraining in patients with neuromuscular disorders. Fortschritte Der Neurologie Psychiatrie 69(8):359–366

KentBraun J A, Ng A V, Castro M et al 1997 Strength, skeletal muscle composition, and enzyme activity in multiple sclerosis. Journal of Applied Physiology 83(6):1998–2004

Kilmer D D, McCrory M A, Wright N C et al 1994 The effect of a high resistance exercise program in slowly progressive neuromuscular disease. Archives of Physical Medicine and Rehabilitation 75:560–563

Kilmer D D, Abresch R T, McCrory M A et al 1995 Profiles of neuromuscular diseases – facioscapulohumeral muscular dystrophy. American Journal of Physical Medicine and Rehabilitation 74(5):S131–S139

Kilmer D D, Aitkens S G, Wright N C et al 2000 Simulated work performance tasks in persons with neuropathic and myopathic weakness. Archives of Physical Medicine and Rehabilitation 81(7):938–943

Kilmer D D, Wright N C, Aitkens S 2005 Impact of a home-based activity and dietary intervention in people with slowly progressive neuromuscular diseases. Archives of Physical Medicine and Rehabilitation 86(11):2150–2156

Kim C, Eng J J 2003 The relationship of lower extremity muscle torque to locomotor performance in people with stroke. Physical Therapy 83:49–57

Kinne S, Patrick D L, Maher E J 1999 Correlates of exercise maintenance among people with mobility impairments. Disability and Rehabilitation 21:15–22

Kurillo G, Zupan A, Bajd T 2004 Force tracking system for the assessment of grip force control in patients with neuromuscular diseases. Clinical Biomechanics 19(10):1014–1021

Kwakkel G, Kollen B, Lindeman E 2004a Understanding the pattern of functional recovery after stroke: facts and theories. Restorative Neurology and Neuroscience 22(3–5):281–299

Kwakkel G, van Peppen R, Wagenaar R C et al 2004b Effects of augmented exercise therapy time after stroke – a meta-analysis. Stroke 35(11):2529–2536

Lewitt P A, Bharucha A, Chitrit I et al 1994 Perceived exertion and muscle efficiency in Parkinson's disease – L-dopa effects. Clinical Neuropharmacology 17(5):454–459

Lim I, van Wegen E, de Goede C et al 2005 Effects of external rhythmical cueing on gait in patients with Parkinson's disease: a systematic review. Clinical Rehabilitation 19(7): 695–713

Lin F M, Sabbahi M 1999 Correlation of spasticity with hyperactive stretch reflexes and motor dysfunction in hemiplegia. Archives of Physical Medicine and Rehabilitation 80(5):526–530

Lin S I 2005 Motor function and joint position sense in relation to gait performance in chronic stroke patients. Archives of Physical Medicine and Rehabilitation 86(2):197–203

Lindeman E, Leffers P, Spaans F et al 1995 Strength training in patients with myotonic-dystrophy and hereditary motor and sensory neuropathy – a randomized clinical-trial. Archives of Physical Medicine and Rehabilitation 76(7):612–620

Lindeman E, Leffers P, Reulen J et al 1998 Quadriceps strength and timed motor performances in myotonic dystrophy, Charcot–Marie–Tooth disease, and healthy subjects. Clinical Rehabilitation 12(2):127–135

Lord S, Wade D T, Halligan P W 1998 A comparison of two physiotherapy treatment approaches to improve walking in MS: a pilot randomised controlled study. Clinical Rehabilitation 2(6):477–486

Lun V, Pullan N, Labelle N et al 2005 Comparison of the effects of a self-supervised home exercise program with a physiotherapist-supervised exercise program on the motor symptoms of Parkinson's disease. Movement Disorders 20 (8):971–975

McCarthy M, Beaumont J G, Thompson R et al 2005 Modality-specific aspects of sustained and divided attentional performance in multiple sclerosis. Archives of Clinical Neuropsychology 20(6):705–718

McCool F D, Tzelepis G E 1995 Inspiratory muscle training in the patient with neuromuscular disease. Physical Therapy 75(11):1006–1014

McCrory M A, Kim H R, Wright N C et al 1998 Energy expenditure, physical activity, and body composition of ambulatory adults with hereditary neuromuscular disease. American Journal of Clinical Nutrition 67(6):1162–1169

McDonald C M 2002 Physical activity, health impairments, and disability in neuromuscular disease. American Journal of Physical Medicine and Rehabilitation 81(11 Suppl):S108–S120

McDonald C M, Abresch R T, Carter G T et al 1995a Profiles of neuromuscular diseases: Becker's muscular dystrophy. American Journal of Physical Medicine and Rehabilitation 74(5):S93–S103

McDonald C M, Johnson E R, Abresch R T et al 1995b Profiles of neuromuscular diseases – limb-girdle syndromes. American Journal of Physical Medicine and Rehabilitation 74(5):S117–S130

MacKay-Lyons M J, Makrides L 2004 Longitudinal changes in exercise capacity after stroke. Archives of Physical Medicine and Rehabilitation 85(10):1608–1612

Macko R F, Katzel L I, Yataco A et al 1997 Low-velocity graded treadmill stress testing in hemiparetic stroke patients. Stroke 28(5):988–992

Macko R F, Ivey F M, Forrester L W et al 2005 Treadmill exercise rehabilitation improves ambulatory function and cardiovascular fitness in patients with chronic stroke – a randomized, controlled trial. Stroke 36(10):2206–2211

Mercier C, Bourbonnais D 2004 Relative shoulder flexor and handgrip strength is related to upper limb function after stroke. Clinical Rehabilitation 18(2):215–221

Miyai I, Fujimoto Y, Ueda Y et al 2000 Treadmill training with body weight support: its effect on Parkinson's disease. Archives of Physical Medicine and Rehabilitation 81(7):849–852

Miyai I, Fujimoto Y, Yamamoto H et al 2002 Long-term effect of body weight-supported treadmill training in Parkinson's disease: a randomized controlled trial. Archives of Physical Medicine and Rehabilitation 83(10):1370–1373

Mochizuki-Kawai H, Kawamura M, Hasegawa Y et al 2004 Deficits in long-term retention of learned motor skills in patients with cortical or subcortical degeneration. Neuropsychologia 42(13):1858–1863

Moreland J D, Goldsmith C H, Huijbregts M P et al 2003 Progressive resistance strengthening exercises after stroke: a single-blind randomized controlled trial. Archives of Physical Medicine and Rehabilitation 84(10):1433–1440

Morris S L, Dodd K J, Morris M E 2004 Outcomes of progressive resistance strength training following stroke: a systematic review. Clinical Rehabilitation 18(1):27–39

Mostert S, Kesselring J 2002 Effects of a short-term exercise training program on aerobic fitness, fatigue, health perception and activity level of subjects with multiple sclerosis. Multiple Sclerosis 8(2):161–168

Nadeau S, Arsenault A B, Gravel D et al 1999a Analysis of the clinical factors determining natural and maximal gait speeds in adults with a stroke. American Journal of Physical Medicine and Rehabilitation 78(2):123–130

Nadeau S, Gravel D, Arsenault A B et al 1999b Plantarflexor weakness as a limiting factor of gait speed in stroke subjects and the compensating role of hip flexors. Clinical Biomechanics (Bristol, Avon) 14(2):125–135

Nallegowda M, Singh U, Handa G et al 2004 Role of sensory input and muscle strength in maintenance of skill gait and posture in Parkinson's disease – a pilot study. American Journal of Physical Medicine and Rehabilitation 83(12):898–908

Ng A V, Miller R G, Kent-Braun J A 2000 Intramuscular metabolic responses to voluntary isometric exercise in multiple sclerosis are consistent with central neuronal fatigue – Reply. Journal of Applied Physiology 89(5):2106

Ng A V, Miller R G, Gelinas D et al 2004 Functional relationships of central and peripheral muscle alterations in multiple sclerosis. Muscle and Nerve 29(6):843–852

Nogaki H, Kakinuma S, Morimatsu M 1999 Movement velocity dependent muscle strength in Parkinson's disease. Acta Neurologica Scandinavica 99(3):152–157

Nogues M A, Roncoroni A J, Benarroch E 2002 Breathing control in neurological diseases. Clinical Autonomic Research 12(6):440–449

Noth J 1997 Clinical pattern and clinical neurophysiology of spasticity. 2. Clinical pattern and clinical neurophysiology. Aktuelle Neurologie 24(5):188–193

Ohkubo T, Asayama K, Kikuya M et al 2004 Prediction of ischaemic and haemorrhagic stroke by self-measured blood pressure at home: the Ohasama study. Blood Pressure Monitoring 9(6):315–320

Olgiati R, Jacquet J, Di Prampero P E 1986 Energy cost of walking and exertional dyspnea in multiple sclerosis. American Review of Respiratory Disease 134(5):1005–1010

Olgiati R, Burgunder J M, Mumenthaler M 1988 Increased energy cost of walking in multiple sclerosis: effect of spasticity, ataxia, and weakness. Archives of Physical Medicine and Rehabilitation 69(10):846–849

Olsen D B, Orngreen M C, Vissing J 2005 Aerobic training improves exercise performance in facioscapulohumeral muscular dystrophy. Neurology 64(6):1064–1066

Paasuke M, Mottus K, Ereline J et al 2002 Lower, limb performance in older female patients with Parkinson's disease. Aging Clinical and Experimental Research 14(3):185–191

Pang M, Eng J J, Daweson A S, Gylfadottir S 2006 The use of aerobic exercise training in improving aerobic capacity in individuals with stroke: a meta-analysis. Clinical Rehabilitation 20:97–111

Pentland B, Barnes M P, Findley L J et al 1992 Parkinson's disease – the spectrum of disabilities. Journal of Neurology, Neurosurgery and Psychiatry 55:32–35

Petajan J H, Gappmaier E, White A T et al 1996 Impact of aerobic training on fitness and quality of life in multiple sclerosis. Annals of Neurology 39(4):432–441

Petrof B J 1998 The molecular basis of activity-induced muscle injury in Duchenne muscular dystrophy. Molecular and Cellular Biochemistry 170:111–123

Philips B A, Mastaglia F L 2000 Exercise therapy in patients with myopathy. Current Opinion in Neurology 13:547–552

Piemonte M E, Faeli G P, Capato T T et al 2004 Motor learning in Parkinson's disease and Huntington disease: improvement of performance in a new motor skill after brief training. Movement Disorders 19:S38

Pollock A, Baer G, Pomeroy V, Langhorne P 2003 Physiotherapy treatment approaches for the recovery of postural control and lower limb function following stroke. The Cochrane Database of Systematic Reviews, John Wiley, Chichester. UK DOI: 10.1002/14651858.CD001920

Ponichtera J A, Rodgers M M, Glaser R M et al 1992 Concentric and eccentric isokinetic lower-extremity strength in persons with multiple-sclerosis. Journal of Orthopaedic and Sports Physical Therapy 16(3):114–122

Ponichtera-Mulcare J A 1993 Exercise and multiple sclerosis. Medicine and Science in Sports and Exercise 25(4):451–465

Reuter I, Engelhardt M 2002 Exercise training and Parkinson's disease – placebo or essential treatment? Physician and Sportsmedicine 30(3):43–50

Rietberg M B, Brooks D, Uitdehaag B M J et al 2005 Exercise therapy for multiple sclerosis. Cochrane Database of Systematic Reviews (1)

Rimmer J H 2005 Exercise and physical activity in persons aging with a physical disability. Physical Medicine and Rehabilitation Clinics of North America 16(1):41–56

Rimmer J H, Riley B, Wang E et al 2004 Physical activity participation among persons with disabilities: barriers and facilitators. American Journal of Preventive Medicine 26(5):419–425

Rochester L, Hetherington V, Jones D et al 2004 Attending to the task: interference effects of functional tasks on walking in Parkinson's disease and the roles of cognition, depression, fatigue, and skill. Archives of Physical Medicine and Rehabilitation 85(10):1578–1585

Rodgers A, MacMahon S, Yee T et al 1998 Blood pressure, cholesterol, and stroke in eastern Asia. Lancet 352(9143):1801–1807

Romberg A, Virtanen A, Aunola S et al 2004 Exercise capacity, disability and leisure physical activity of subjects with multiple sclerosis. Multiple Sclerosis 10(2):212–218

Saltin B, Landin S 1975 Work capacity, muscle strength and SDH activity in both legs of hemiparetic patients and patients with Parkinson's disease. Scandinavian Journal of Clinical and Laboratory Investigation 35(6):531–538

Saunders D H, Greig C A, Young A et al 2004 Physical fitness training for stroke patients. Cochrane Database Systematic Reviews (1): CD003316

Scandalis T A, Bosak A, Berliner J C et al 2001 Resistance training and gait function in patients with Parkinson's disease. American Journal of Physical Medicine and Rehabilitation 80(1):38–43

Schenkman M, Cutson T M, Kuchibhatla M et al 1998 Exercise to improve spinal flexibility and function for people with Parkinson's disease: a randomized, controlled trial. Journal of the American Geriatrics Society 46(10):1207–1216

Schenkman M, Morey M, Kuchibhatla M 2000 Spinal flexibility and balance control among community-dwelling adults with and without Parkinson's disease. Journal of Gerontology Series. Biological Sciences and Medical Sciences 55(8):M441–M445

Schiemanck S K, Post M W M, Kwakkel G et al 2005 Ischemic lesion volume correlates with long-term functional outcome and quality of life of middle cerebral artery stroke survivors. Restorative Neurology and Neuroscience 23(3–4):257–263

Schulz K H, Gold S M, Witte J et al 2004 Impact of aerobic training on immune-endocrine parameters, neurotrophic factors, quality of life and coordinative function in multiple sclerosis. Journal of the Neurological Sciences 225(1–2):11–18

Scott O M, Hyde S A, Vrbrova G, Dubowitz V 1985 Effects of chronic low frequency electrical stimulation on normal human tibialis anterior muscle. Journal of Neurology, Neurosurgery and Psychiatry 48:774–781

Selles R W, Li X Y, Lin F et al 2005 Feedback-controlled and programmed stretching of the ankle plantarflexors and dorsiflexors in stroke: effects of a 4-week intervention program. Archives of Physical Medicine and Rehabilitation 86(12): 2330–2336

Sharp S A, Brouwer B J 1997 Isokinetic strength training of the hemiparetic knee: effects on function and spasticity. Archives of Physical Medicine and Rehabilitation 78(11):1231–1236

Shinton R, Sagar G 1993 Lifelong exercise and stroke. British Medical Journal 307(6898):231–234

Smidt N, de Vet H C W, Bouter L M et al 2005 Effectiveness of exercise therapy: a best-evidence summary of systematic reviews. Australian Journal of Physiotherapy 51(2):71–85

Solari A, Filippini G, Gasco P et al 1999 Physical rehabilitation has a positive effect on disability in multiple sclerosis. Neurology 52:57–62

Soliveri P, Brown R G, Jahanshahi M et al 1997 Learning manual pursuit tracking skills in patients with Parkinson's disease. Brain 120:1325–1337

Spector S A, Lemmer J T, Koffman B M et al 1997 Safety and efficacy of strength training in patients with sporadic inclusion body myositis. Muscle and Nerve 20(10):1242–1248

Stoquart G G, Detrembleur C, Nielens H et al 2005 Efficiency of work production by spastic muscles. Gait and Posture 22(4):331–337

Sutherland G, Andersen M B 2001 Exercise and multiple sclerosis: physiological, psychological, and quality of life issues. Journal of Sports Medicine and Physical Fitness 41(4):421–432

Swinnen S P, Debaere F, Puttemans V et al 2002 Coordination deficits on the ipsilesional side after unilateral stroke: the effect of practice on nonisodirectional ipsilateral coordination. Acta Psychologica 110(2–3):305–320

Teixeira-Salmela L F, Olney S J, Nadeau S et al 1999 Muscle strengthening and physical conditioning to reduce impairment and disability in chronic stroke survivors. Archives of Physical Medicine and Rehabilitation 80(10):1211–1218

Thompson A J 2001 Symptomatic management and rehabilitation in multiple sclerosis. Journal of Neurology, Neurosurgery and Psychiatry 71:II22 II27

Tiavassalo T, De Stefano N, Chen J et al 1999 Short-term aerobic training response in chronic myopathies. Muscle and Nerve 22:1239–1243

Trost S G, Owen N, Bauman A E et al 2002 Correlates of adults' participation in physical activity review and update. Medicine and Science in Sport and Exercise 2002(34): 1996–2001

Van den Berg M, Newman M, Dawes H, Wade D 2005 A randomised crossover trial: the effects of aerobic treadmill training on gait characteristics, walking speed and endurance and fatigue in individuals with multiple sclerosis (abstract). Gait and Posture 21(Suppl 1):S135

Van der Kooi E L, Lindeman E, Riphagen I et al 2004 Strength training and albuterol in facioscapulohumeral muscular dystrophy. Neurology 63(4):702–708

Van Peppen R P, Kwakkel G, Wood-Dauphinee S et al 2004 The impact of physical therapy on functional outcomes after stroke: what's the evidence? Clinical Rehabilitation 18(8):833–862

White L J, Dressendorfer R H 2004 Exercise and multiple sclerosis. Sports Medicine 34(15):1077–1100

White L J, Dressendorfer R H 2005 Factors limiting maximal oxygen uptake in exertional monoparesis. Multiple Sclerosis 11(2):240–241

Wiles C, Newcombe R G, Fuller K J et al 2001 Controlled randomised crossover trial of the effects of physiotherapy on mobility in chronic multiple sclerosis. Journal of Neurology, Neurosurgery and Psychiatry 70:174–179

Willen C, Sunnerhagen K S, Ekman C et al 2004 How is walking speed related to muscle strength? A study of healthy persons and persons with late effects of polio. Archives of Physical Medicine and Rehabilitation 85(12):1923–1928

Wineinger M A, Walsh S A, Abresch T 2002 Muscle fatigue in animal models of neuromuscular disease. American Journal of Physical Medicine and Rehabilitation 81(11):S81–S98

Winer W J, Goetz C G (ed) 1999 Neurology for the non neurologist. Lippincott Williams & Wilkins, London

Winkler G, Zifko U, Nader A et al 2000 Dose-dependent effects of inspiratory muscle training in neuromuscular disorders. Muscle and Nerve 23(8):1257–1260

Winogrodzka A, Wagenaar R C, Booij J et al 2005 Rigidity and bradykinesia reduce interlimb coordination in Parkinsonian gait. Archives of Physical Medicine and Rehabilitation 86(2):183–189

Wright N C, Kilmer D D, McCrory M A et al 1996 Aerobic walking in slowly progressive neuromuscular disease: effect of a 12-week program. Archives of Physical Medicine and Rehabilitation 77:64–69

Yamanaka H, Kawahira K, Arima M et al 2005 Evaluation of skilled arm movements in patients with stroke using a computerized motor-skill analyser for the arm. International Journal of Rehabilitation Research 28(3):277–283

Yates J S, Studenski S, Gollub S et al 2004 Bicycle ergometry in subacute-stroke survivors: feasibility, safety, and exercise performance. Journal of Aging and Physical Activity 12(1):64–74

Yogev G, Giladi N, Peretz C et al 2005a Dual tasking, gait rhythmicity, and Parkinson's disease: which aspects of gait are attention demanding? European Journal of Neuroscience 22(5):1248–1256

Yogev G, Giladi N, Springer S et al 2005b The effect of mental loading on gait asymmetry in patients with Parkinson's disease and idiopathic fallers. Journal of the American Geriatrics Society 53(4):S191–S191

Yogev G, Giladi N, Springer S et al 2005c Mental loading increases gait asymmetry and stride-to-stride variability in patients with Parkinson's disease. Movement Disorders 20:S119–S119

Zamparo P, Pagliaro P 1998 The energy cost of level walking before and after hydro-kinesi therapy in patients with spastic paresis. Scandinavian Journal of Medicine and Science in Sports 8(4):222–228

Zhang Z, Roman G C 1993 Worldwide occurrence of Parkinson's disease: an updated review. Neuroepidemiology 12:195–208

Ziv I, Avraham M, Michaelov Y et al 1998 Enhanced fatigue during motor performance in patients with Parkinson's disease. Neurology 51(6):1583–1586

Further reading

Websites

http://www.stroke.org.uk/information/all_about_stroke/index.html
http://www.headway.org.uk
http://www.parkinsons.org.uk/
http://www.nationalmssociety.org/
http://www.muscular-dystrophy.org/
http://www.inclusivefitness.org/

Books

American College of Sports Medicine (ACSM) 1995 Guidelines for exercise testing and prescription. Lea and Febiger, Philadelphia

American College of Sports Medicine (ACSM) 2002 ACSM's guidelines for exercise testing and prescription. Guidelines for graded exercise testing and training. Lippincott Williams & Wilkins, Philadelphia

Barnes P R J, Hilton-Jones D, Dalakas M C et al 2003 Myopathies in clinical practice. Martin Dunitz; Taylor and Francis, London

Enoka R M 2002 Neuromechanics of human movement. Human Kinetics, London

Fuller G, Manford M R 1999 Neurology: an illustrated colour text. Elsevier Health Sciences, Oxford

Key reviews

Gordon N F, Gulanick M, Costa F et al 2004 Physical activity and exercise recommendations for stroke survivors – An American Heart Association scientific statement from the Council on Clinical Cardiology, Subcommittee on Exercise, Cardiac Rehabilitation, and Prevention; the Council on Cardiovascular Nursing; the Council on Nutrition, Physical Activity, and Metabolism; and the Stroke Council. Stroke 35(5):1230–1240

Reuter I, Engelhardt M 2002 Exercise training and Parkinson's disease – placebo or essential treatment? Physician and Sportsmedicine 30(3):43–50

Rietberg M B, Brooks D, Uitdehaag B M J et al 2005 Exercise therapy for multiple sclerosis. Cochrane Database of Systematic Reviews (1)

Van der Kooi E L, Lindeman E, Riphagen I 2005 Strength training and aerobic exercise training for muscle disease (Review). The Cochrane Collaboration (2):1–20

White L J, Dressendorfer R H 2004 Exercise and multiple sclerosis. Sports Medicine 34(15):1077–1100

Chapter **10**

Spinal cord injury

Nick Webborn and Victoria Goosey-Tolfrey

CHAPTER CONTENTS

Learning objectives   309
The spinal cord – structure and
   function   310
The autonomic nervous system   312
Spinal cord injury   312
Types of incomplete spinal injuries   315
Spinal cord trauma – epidemiology   315
   Incidence/Prevalence   315
   Age/Sex distribution   316
Physical activity and spinal cord
   injury   318
Benefits of exercise in SCI   320

Aerobic capacity   322
Types of exercise and suitability for
   SCI groups   324
Exercise volume: manipulations of
   intensity and duration   325
Monitoring training intensity   326
Cautions   327
Future research requirements   330
Key points   331
References   332
Further reading   334

LEARNING OBJECTIVES

After studying this chapter, you should be able to:

1. Understand the basic structure and function of the spinal cord.
2. Understand the pathophysiology of spinal cord injury.
3. Understand the epidemiology and incidence of spinal cord injury.
4. Evaluate the links between physical activity and fitness as predisposing factors to spinal cord injury.
5. Identify key terminology relating to spinal cord injury.
6. Identify the differences between an incomplete and complete spinal cord injury.
7. Distinguish between the different types of incomplete spinal cord injuries.
8. Understand the age and sex distribution and common causes of spinal cord injury.
9. Understand the potential health benefits of physical activity for people with spinal cord injury.
10. Identify studies that have provided evidence that exercise training can be a safe form of exercise for most people with spinal cord injury.
11. Describe the factors that need to be considered when designing an effective exercise training programme.

12. Understand the potential risks of exercise in people with spinal cord injury.
13. Critically evaluate the evidence that shows people with spinal cord injury are able to demonstrate significant gains in fitness following exercise.
14. Critically appraise where future research projects might focus when considering physiological trainability in spinal cord injury.

THE SPINAL CORD – STRUCTURE AND FUNCTION

The spinal cord is the main pathway for information connecting the brain and peripheral nervous system. It lies inside the bony spine within the vertebral foramen and is made up of 31 segments: 8 cervical, 12 thoracic, 5 lumbar, 5 sacral and 1 coccygeal (Fig. 10.1). A pair of spinal nerves exits from each segment of the spinal cord to transmit and receive information to and from the peripheral nervous system. It is cylindrical in shape and starts as an extension of the lower part of the brainstem. It is protected by the spinal column, the spinal meninges, the cerebrospinal fluid and the vertebral ligaments. The spinal cord is approximately 45 cm long in men and 43 cm long in women. It is much shorter than the length of the bony spinal column as it extends down only to the level around the thoracolumbar junction. The nerves that form the lumbar and sacral nerves actually run within the vertebral canal for a distance before they exit the vertebral column. This collection of nerves is called the *cauda equina* or 'horse's tail'.

In cross-section there are two distinct regions (Fig. 10.2). Firstly the grey matter which is shaped like a butterfly's wings and contains the nerve cell bodies. Surrounding that is the white matter, which consists of axons running up and down the spinal

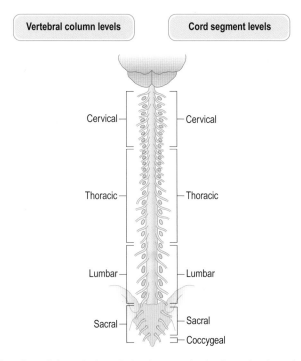

| Vertebral column levels | Cord segment levels |

Cervical — Cervical

Thoracic — Thoracic

Lumbar — Lumbar

Sacral — Sacral

— Coccygeal

Figure 10.1 Drawing of the spinal cord showing vertebral column levels and cord segmental levels.

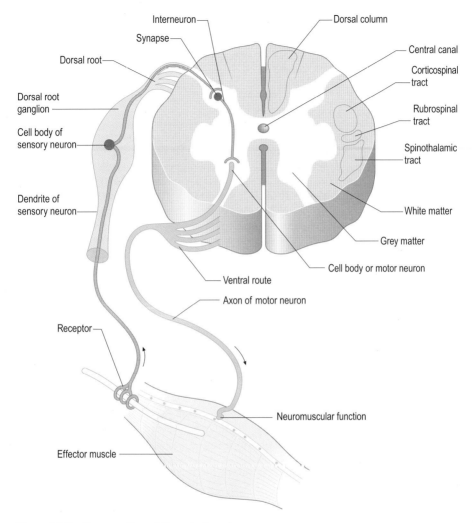

Figure 10.2   Cross-section of the spinal cord.

cord. Throughout the cord, the dorsal grey matter (dorsal horn) deals with sensory perception, and receives information from the periphery through the dorsal root. The ventral horns contain the alpha-motor neurons, whose axons exit the cord via the ventral roots and travel directly to supply the muscles. The ventral horns are larger in the cervical and lumbar segments of the cord as they contain the motor neurons that control movement of the arms (cervical segment) and legs (lumbar segment). In the thoracic section there is an extra cell column called the intermediate horn, or the intermediolateral cell column. It is the source of all of the sympathetic neurons in the body and occurs only in thoracic sections (see under 'The autonomic nervous system').

The axons in the different regions of the cord relate to different information being relayed to and from the brain and periphery. For example, information regarding deep touch, vibration and proprioception (balance) are carried in the dorsal (posterior) column at the back of the cord whereas pain and temperature information is carried more laterally in the spinothalamic tract. Information on voluntary motor function is carried anteriorly. As a result, when different areas of the cord are damaged in an incomplete injury, different consequences occur; these will be discussed later.

THE AUTONOMIC NERVOUS SYSTEM

The autonomic nervous system is so named as it 'autonomously' runs bodily functions without our awareness or control but may be influenced by other factors. There are two systems working together with often opposing actions which together constitute the autonomic nervous system: the sympathetic and parasympathetic systems. Their functions are illustrated in Figure 10.3. The sympathetic system typically, in extreme situations, evokes 'fight-or-flight' responses; for example, pupils dilate, muscle vasculature dilates, the heart rate increases, and the digestive system is put on hold. The parasympathetic system has many specific functions including slowing the heart, constricting the pupils, and stimulating the gut and salivary glands. The state of the body at any given time represents a balance between these two systems.

SPINAL CORD INJURY

A spinal cord injury (SCI) is one of the most significant injuries someone can endure, with implications for multiple body systems arising from damage to just a small area of the body. The injury can result from a wide range of different mechanisms leading to tissue damage in the cord:

- destruction of spinal cord neurons from direct trauma
- compression by bone fragments, haematoma or intervertebral disc
- ischaemia from damage to or compression of the spinal arteries that supply the cord
- swelling (oedema) of the cord tissue following one of the above.

The damage to the spinal cord can result in a variety of motor, sensory or autonomic functions of the body depending on the extent and level of the injury. The International Standards for Neurological and Functional Classification of Spinal Cord Injury describe the level and the extent of the injury based on an examination of motor and sensory neurological function:

- tetraplegia (formerly called quadriplegia) – injury to the spinal cord in the cervical region with associated loss of muscle strength in all four extremities
- paraplegia – injury to the spinal cord in the thoracic, lumbar or sacral segments, including the cauda equina and conus medullaris, with strength-loss in the legs.

Traditionally, people would be classified as having a 'complete' spinal cord injury by having no voluntary motor or conscious sensory function below the injury site. However, this definition can be difficult to apply in a variety of situations; for example, a common situation is for someone to have some function below the level of the injury for a few segments but then no motor or sensory function below this level. Most clinicians would regard an injury as complete if the person has any level below which no function is present. The American Spinal Injury Association (Fig. 10.5) decided to take this criterion to its logical limit, i.e. if the person has any spinal level

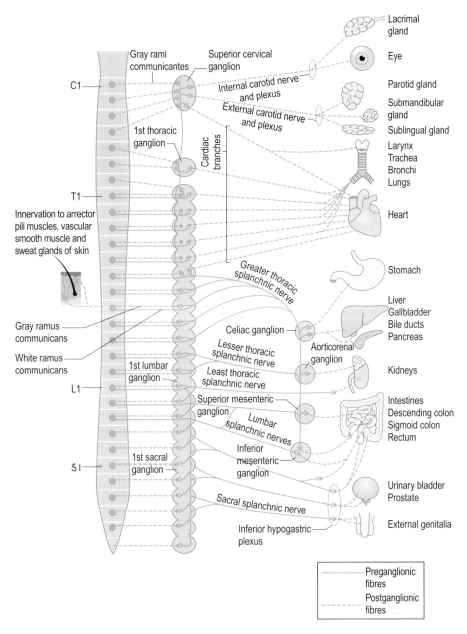

Figure 10.3   The autonomic nervous system.

below which there is no neurological function, that person would be classified as having a 'complete' injury. This translates into a simple definition of 'complete' spinal cord injury: a person is spoken of as a 'complete' if they do not have motor and sensory function in the anal and perineal region representing the lowest sacral cord (S4–S5). Thus:

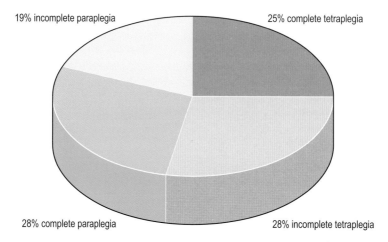

Figure 10.4 Incidence of spinal cord injury by type of lesion and completeness. (Source: Spinal Cord Injury: Definition, Epidemiology, Pathophysiology – www.emedicine.com/pmr/ topic182.htm.)

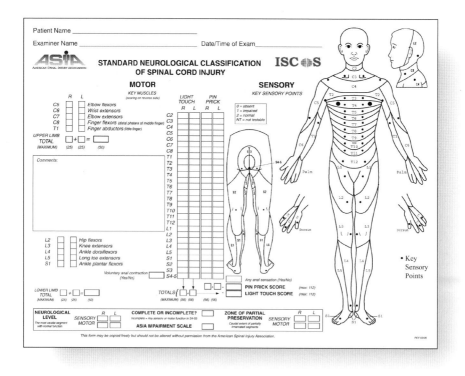

Figure 10.5 American Spinal Injury Association assessment form (with thanks to ASIA www. asia-spinalinjury.org).

- complete – absence of sensory and motor functions in the lowest sacral segments.
- incomplete – preservation of some sensory or motor function below the level of the injury, including the lowest sacral segments.

It is important to have an awareness of the potential consequences of incomplete lesions when advising on physical activity because of different capabilities and risks. Incomplete spinal injuries will differ from one person to another because the amount of damage to each person's nerve fibres is different, and so an individual approach is important.

TYPES OF INCOMPLETE SPINAL INJURIES

The effects of incomplete lesions depend upon the area of the cord (front, back, side, etc.) affected. The part of the cord damaged depends on the forces involved in the injury.

- Anterior cord syndrome occurs when the damage is towards the front of the spinal cord; it may cause the loss or impairment of ability to sense pain, temperature and touch below the level of injury. Pressure and joint sensation may be preserved.
- Central cord syndrome occurs when the damage is in the centre of the cervical spinal cord. This typically results in the loss of function in the arms, but some leg movement may be preserved. Some control over the bowel and bladder may also be preserved. It is possible for some recovery from this type of injury, usually starting in the legs and gradually progressing upwards.
- Posterior cord syndrome occurs when the damage is towards the back of the spinal cord. This type of injury may leave the person with good muscle power, pain and temperature sensation; however, they may experience difficulty in coordinating movement of their limbs.
- Brown-Séquard syndrome occurs when damage is towards one side of the spinal cord. This results in impairment or loss of movement on the injured side, but pain and temperature sensation may be preserved. The opposite side of injury will have normal movement, but pain and temperature sensation there will be impaired or lost.
- *Cauda equina* lesion: As noted above, the spinal cord ends at L1 and L2, at which point a bundle of nerves travel downwards through the lumbar and sacral vertebrae. Injury to these nerves will cause partial or complete loss of movement and sensation.

SPINAL CORD TRAUMA – EPIDEMIOLOGY
Incidence/Prevalence

- Incidence – the relative frequency of occurrence, e.g. number of new cases per year.
- Prevalence – the number of people with the condition in the given population.

The International Campaign for Cures of Spinal Cord Injury Paralysis (ICCP) describes SCI as a global epidemic (http://www.campaignforcure.org/globalsum.htm#_edn1):

> Based on conservative average annual incidence of 22 people/million population in the western and developing world it is estimated that over 130 000 people each year survive a traumatic spinal cord injury and begin a 'new and different life' bound to a wheelchair for 40 years or more.

Table 10.1   Incidence and prevalence of SCI in different countries

Country	Population (millions)	Injuries/annum	Injuries/million population	Population estimated living with SCI
USA	260	10 000	40	250 000
Canada	30	843	27	30 000
UK	59	700	12	35 000
Australia	17	241	13.2	10 000

Source: The International Campaign for Cures of Spinal Cord Injury Paralysis (ICCP) (www.campaignforcure.org/globalsum.htm).

This rather evocative statement does, however, illustrate that it is a relatively common condition and that there will be a significant number of people living within a community with SCI who require physical activity for health. For example, Table 10.1 gives an estimate of 35 000 people in the UK currently living with SCI. In the UK approximately 2 to 3 people every day become paralysed through SCI, although these figures may not reflect all SCIs as incomplete injuries may be treated by general hospitals instead of a specialist spinal injuries unit and it is from the latter that these figures come.

Age/Sex distribution

Figure 10.6 shows the distribution of ages at the time of injury. It is clearly most common in young adults, often as a result of risk-taking behaviour such as driving recklessly, alcohol-related incidents and sports. It is relatively rare in young children but when it does occur 72–79% of injuries are caused by either a fall or being struck by a vehicle and about 20% are sports-related injuries (Cirak et al 2004).

The male to female ratio is 4 to 1 (Jackson et al 2004). This ratio may be explained by the higher proportion of males driving motorcycles, poorer driving habits possibly combined with alcohol consumption, and greater participation in sports or other dangerous activities. The male to female ratio is smaller in people older than 65, in whom falls are a more common cause of injury. This may occur in the early morning and is associated with prior taking of alcohol or medications, such as hypnotics, which cause drowsiness and impaired coordination (National Spinal Cord Injury Statistical Center 2005).

The causes of spinal cord injury are much the same worldwide but the relative frequency of the causes will depend upon the individual nation. For example, countries with lower proportions of motor vehicles in use have reduced risk from this cause. Countries where firearms are commonly used have a higher risk of SCIs from gunshots (Velmahos et al 1995). The type of sports or activities undertaken will influence the frequency of injury from sports.

In general it is accepted that motor vehicle accidents are the most common cause of SCI, with estimates varying between 50% and 75% of cases. These account for a large proportion of the injuries occurring in young people, whereas a greater proportion of injuries occur due to falls in the elderly. With regard to road traffic accidents, 20% of deaths are contributed to or caused by severe cervical SCI (Jackson et al 2004).

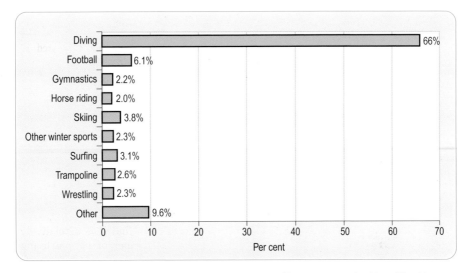

Figure 10.6   Age at time of injury of spinal cord injury. (Source: www.skyaid.org/Skyaid%
20Org/Medical/spinal_cord_injury.htm.)

Sporting activities are a reasonably common cause of SCI; however, caution should be applied to interpretation of some data. For example, Figure 10.6 shows percentage occurrence by sports activity from data from the USA and shows a 66% incidence from diving (National Spinal Cord Injury Statistical Center 2005). Diving in this context is not a sport but the activity the person was undertaking at the time of injury. Diving into shallow water is the commonest cause of injury and the individual may also be under the influence of alcohol at the time. Estimated rates of people sustaining their SCI from any cause while under the influence of alcohol vary between 17% and 49%. The sport of diving in an appropriate pool and under instruction does not carry anywhere near the same degree of risk as diving injuries occurring outside this controlled environment.

Other national variations due to sporting causes will vary according to participation levels in different sports. For example, rugby football has been associated with quite a high incidence of injury but has major participation in only a small number of nations. 'Football' in Figure 10.6 refers to American football rather than 'soccer' (the term used for 'football' by the rest of the world). Motor sports (cycle and car) are a major cause of spinal injury in sport and have a cross-over in statistics with 'motor vehicle accidents'.

Clearly the role of the sporting community is to help identify causes of injuries in sports to try and reduce their incidence. This may result in changes in regulation of the sport or changes in equipment. For example, the collapse of the scrummage in rugby football was deemed to be a major cause of SCI and laws were introduced to reduce the risk (Silver & Stewart 1994). Changes in helmet design and neck supports in motor racing have helped reduce the risk of injury. In technical sports such as gymnastics, trampolining, etc., coaching and appropriate supervision are key factors in injury prevention (Silver 1993).

It would be helpful if data collected on sporting-related activities more clearly identified if the injuries occurred in organized sport or recreational activity. For example, children trampolining unsupervised in the garden may be at a higher

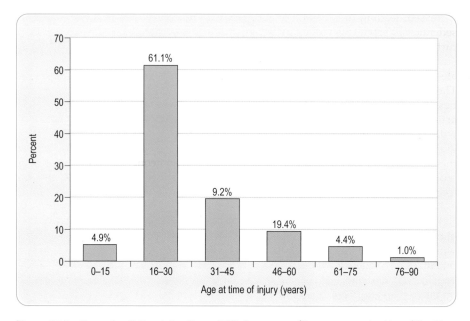

Figure 10.7 Type of activity at the time of SCI from sport. (Source: www.skyaid.org/Skyaid% 200rg/Medical/spinal_cord_injury.htm.)

risk than those in a supervised class but the relative degrees of risk are not known.

Approximately 13% of SCI cases are the result of accidents relating to occupational activity, with almost half of these occurring in the construction industry:

- 50% = falls
- 19% = falling objects
- 19% = motor vehicle accidents.

In examining the causes of SCI detailed above, it will be clear that there is no association with physical activity in most cases, e.g. those involving road traffic accident or injuries due to violence. Sporting activities usually relate to technical factors, e.g. gymnastics, or possibly muscle strength, e.g. scrummage collapse. The cause that may have most relation to levels of physical activity is that of falls in the elderly, and there is strong evidence that muscle strengthening, balance training and exercises that focus on balance and agility, such as tai chi, are most effective at reducing older adults' fall risk (Janssen et al 2004, Sattin et al 2005, Suzuki et al 2004). There are strong associations between fall risk, proprioception, strength and developing tetraplegia in the elderly. Therefore programmes that reduce fall risk will reduce the number of SCIs in the older population.

PHYSICAL ACTIVITY AND SPINAL CORD INJURY

There is a significant public health problem of the development of chronic diseases, e.g. coronary heart disease, diabetes and obesity, facing the nation as the result of decreasing levels of physical activity. The management of the complications of spinal cord injury has improved such that the longevity of these patients has increased, leading to exposure to more chronic disease processes as a result of a sedentary lifestyle, which in turn will result in health service resources being further stretched. The current recommendations for physical activity for the general population as a minimum are for the accumulation of 30 minutes of moderate-intensity exercises on at least 5 days per week (Department of Health, 2004). The challenge for people with SCI is to find safe and beneficial physical activities that are appropriate to their disability. The principles of increasing physical activity or training are exactly the same, although some issues relating to recovery will be discussed later. Training is an adaptation response to gradual and progressive overload. The duration, intensity and frequency of the activity govern the response to that training stimulus. The key for someone with SCI is to find a mode of activity that is compatible with their disability and that is intense enough to give specific health benefits while taking account of potential adverse effects of exercise.

Historically there have been several reasons why people with SCI have less frequently been able to maintain an active lifestyle. Parental over-protection of a child with an SCI is perhaps understandable but it is important that parents are aware of potential downsides of a continued sedentary lifestyle and understand the potential benefits of improved self-esteem and self-efficacy as well as better general health by integration and inclusion within a physical activity programme. Part of the problem, however, has resulted from medical over-protection (Patel & Greydanus 2002, Sargent 1983, Thomasgard & Metz 1997). The lack of education in medical undergraduate and postgraduate programmes regarding the benefits of physical activity in general is well known. This applies even more when dealing with people with SCI, and the view that 'perhaps it's safer not to' may be born out of ignorance. Generally within specific spinal cord injury centres there is an acknowledgement of the importance of physical activity for health, and sport is commonly used in rehabilitation. However, community healthcare workers have limited knowledge about SCI and exercise.

The leading cause of death in patients following SCI is pneumonia and other respiratory conditions, followed by heart disease, subsequent trauma, and septicaemia (Soden et al 2000). Suicide and alcohol-related deaths are also major causes of death in patients with SCI. The suicide rate is 10 times higher among the SCI population who are younger than 25 years than among their age equivalent without SCI (Hartkopp et al 1998, Rish et al 1997). Regular physical activity has mental health benefits in reducing depression and anxiety as well as generally improving self-esteem and self-efficacy. Recreational activities and sports also provide social support and can have a positive impact on mental health.

It appears that people with SCI who are more physically active make fewer visits to physicians and tend to have fewer medical complications and hospitalizations than their sedentary counterparts (Curtis et al 1986). A further study showed that paraplegic athletes were more successful than non-athletes in avoiding major medical complications of spinal cord injury (Stotts 1986). A study comparing the prevalence of shoulder pain in wheelchair athletes and non-athletic wheelchair users showed that the odds of having shoulder pain were twice as high among non-athletes. However, it is clear that further research in this whole area is required. A consensus statement regarding research on physical activity and health among people with disabilities stated that as people with disabilities live longer, the need for addressing long-term health issues and risk of secondary disability must receive greater attention (Cooper et al 1999).

There are many desirable outcomes from increased physical activity. These include increased cardiovascular fitness, muscle strength, range of joint motion and flexibility, increased bone density and psychological and social benefits. This list is not exhaustive but when considering giving advice one needs to take into account the potential for gain in each of these areas with regard to the individual's disability. For optimum health all of these components are desirable but possibly in different proportions. For example, for someone with paraplegia, regular workouts in a wheelchair or swimming will have beneficial effects on the cardiovascular system and increase muscle strength in the upper limbs. However, the absence of weight-bearing activity will limit maintenance of bone density and so the use of a standing frame may still be appropriate to stimulate osteoblastic activity while not per se being seen as physical activity.

As described earlier, physical inactivity in many SCI participants is of great concern. Some authors have even suggested that in the majority of long-term SCI patients, peak oxygen uptake ($\dot{V}O_2$ peak) is only marginally sufficient to meet the tasks involved for daily living (Janssen et al 1994). Exercise, therefore, must be viewed as an essential part of the therapy during the rehabilitation process following SCI. However, many factors may limit SCI participants' ability to exercise, such as autonomic nervous system dysfunction and motor dysfunction. The concept of exercise and its benefits for SCI populations is more complex than for able-bodied participants. Initially there is a prolonged period of bed rest that causes a decreased exercise tolerance. This period discourages individuals with SCI from engaging in a regular physical fitness programme or maintaining a rehabilitation programme when discharged from hospital.

From a health perspective, regular exercise can help make everyday living easier and more enjoyable. The many benefits of exercise include increased fitness, better muscle strength, weight control and improved coordination and balance (Department of Health 2004). If exercise programmes are implemented correctly and the modalities appropriately selected for SCI populations, then they can also have wider health benefits, as they may help in the prevention and management of secondary health complications (Fig. 10.8). These include muscle atrophy, osteoporosis, decubitus ulcers, and a host of cardiopulmonary disorders (Janssen & Hopman 2005).

People with SCI use a considerably smaller amount of muscle mass compared to their able-bodied counterparts. It has been shown that there is limited effect on the cardiorespiratory system from daily activities (Janssen et al 1994), so in order to prevent a debilitative cycle we need to help SCI participants to understand the benefits of exercise training in maintaining and improving their physical capacity. Strength and endurance capacity are also two important concepts that contribute to functional capacity in those with SCI. Ellenburg et al (1989) suggested that rehabilitation personnel should emphasize continued endurance exercise regimens both for psychological well-being and for cardiovascular health benefits.

BENEFITS OF EXERCISE IN SCI

Prevention of obesity, diabetes and coronary heart disease: It has been shown that exercise training can stimulate changes in body composition. Exercise helps keep weight under control, which is important for everyone with SCI. However, in the SCI population, reduced basal metabolic rate due to skeletal muscle wasting and

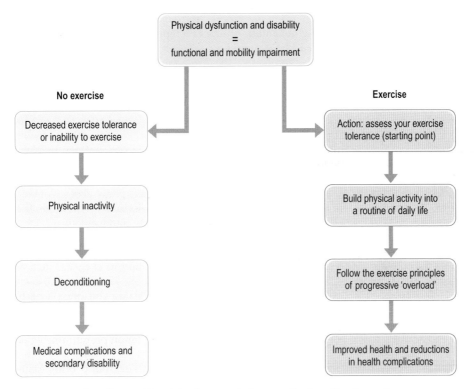

Figure 10.8   The effects of inactivity (no exercise) versus the benefits of exercise.

lower daily energy expenditure due to physical inactivity may lead to gains in body fat. Thus, excessive bodyweight, which can also contribute to cardiovascular risks as well as making daily living more stressful, may be counterbalanced by increased physical activity. This has been demonstrated by Midha et al (1999), who reported significant changes in percentage lean bodyweight and adiposity following a period of exercise in SCI patients. Not surprisingly there has been much debate in the literature concerning measurement of body composition. It has been demonstrated that underwater weighing techniques can be employed although the residual lung volume (RV) must be measured directly, as RV is elevated in SCI participants (particularly in tetraplegic patients). Anthropometric specific equations have been reported and the limitations are discussed in detail in the review by Wells & Hooker (1990). They highlight that despite prediction equations being derived for these populations, errors associated with this technique may arise from differences in SCI participants' degree of injury, duration of injury, degree of spasticity (which influences lean body mass (LBM)), bone demineralization of the spine and lower limbs, body fluid shifts due to loss of LBM and extent of training. Moreover, they recommend that if skinfold techniques are utilized then triceps, subscapular and suprailiac sites should be measured and the sum of the three sites reported. Surprisingly, researchers in the area of interest have either opted not to report any measure of body composition or reported the sum of four values including the aforementioned sites along with the skinfold measurement taken from the biceps. The suggestion of a fourth site by Wells & Hooker (1990), using the anterior thigh as a representation of the fat deposition in the lower limbs, should be explored.

Finding a suitable technique to quantify the active muscle mass within this specific population is difficult. This may be important as the use of body mass as a scaling denominator assumes implicitly that the proportion of whole body mass comprised by active muscle mass is constant across the participants – perhaps unlikely in a heterogeneous SCI sample. Although as mentioned earlier, some studies with SCI athletes have included skinfold measurements taken from sites traditionally employed with able-bodied groups, it is recognized that the estimation of percentage total body fat from these measurements has not been validated in an SCI population. Future studies might wish to include a more direct measurement of active muscle mass using techniques such as magnetic resonance imaging (MRI) or dual energy X-ray absorptiometry (DEXA). Until then, we recommend that simple measures of skinfolds be taken as a covariate to account partially for sample heterogeneity in body composition.

It has been shown that immobilization following SCI results in a reduction of high-density lipoprotein (HDL) (Hoffman 1986), which is associated with increased risk for coronary heart disease (CHD). Dearwater et al (1986) found that HDL was lower in sedentary SCI patients when compared to SCI patients reported to be active. This implies that exercise is important for SCI populations in order to gain a favourable lipid profile, particularly in view of the estimation that based upon average HDL-C levels, sedentary SCI individuals are at 60% increased risk of CHD relative to the general population. Work from the Dutch research centres on 'Physical Strain, Work Capacity and Mechanisms of Restoration of Mobility in the Rehabilitation of Persons with SCI' has focused on the effects of lipid profiles, rehabilitation and sport involvement; however, longitudinal studies examining the relationship between cardiovascular fitness and lipid profiles within this specific population are still warranted.

The rate of type 2 diabetes has been reported to be four times higher in SCI patients than in the general population (Bauman 2004). Regular exercise has been shown to increase insulin sensitivity and maintain low levels of plasma insulin (de Groot et al 2003), resulting in a decreased risk of obesity, diabetes and CHD. Exercise training studies of 10 weeks' duration have demonstrated that both glucose and insulin levels decline with training. The effects of training intensity on both the lipid profile and insulin sensitivity in early rehabilitation of SCI individuals will be discussed later.

AEROBIC CAPACITY

As the above paragraphs clearly indicate, spinal cord injured people typically encounter similar problems to those of having a sedentary lifestyle. An associated problem is a low aerobic capacity, which can be further complicated in some cases by a loss of sympathetic neural regulation of the heart and vasomotor tone. It is believed that SCI patients benefit from endurance exercise training. However, during the rehabilitation process the main focus tends to be on activities of daily living and chair transfers involved in daily living, as opposed to longer duration activities that may form part of an endurance exercise regimen. Some studies have shown that SCI participants who have a lesion level of T6 and below can achieve central training effects. This results in an increased capacity to circulate blood and lower resting heart rate. On the other hand, Lockette & Keyes (1994) stated that:

> *with a complete SCI above T6, you may not be able to achieve central cardiovascular training because sympathetic nervous system dysfunction and limited active muscle mass prevent you from reaching target heart rates and from stressing the central circulation. (p. 102)*

Therefore, for these individuals, hybrid training methods described later may be one approach to enable them to achieve target heart rates that could result in central adaptations. Alternatively, training at a raised but restricted heart rate during continuous aerobic activity should be sufficient to prevent declines in aerobic capacity and see gains at a peripheral level (Janssen & Hopman 2005).

It is important to consider the individual's lesion level and the completeness of the lesion in order to make any judgement on the effectiveness of that particular training programme. Furthermore, it is also important to consider the onset of disability and previous training history, as this would influence the degree of adaptation that may take place through training.

Longitudinal profiles observed from trained wheelchair basketball players showed a 7% improvement in $\dot{V}O_2$ peak across a 2-year period (Goosey-Tolfrey 2005); this may be considered small when comparisons are made with the findings of Miles and co-workers (1982), also studying wheelchair exercisers, who demonstrated a 26% improvement in $\dot{V}O_2$ peak after only 8 weeks of training. However, the larger improvement was most likely the result of a relatively low initial level of aerobic fitness. Monitoring of aerobic training becomes a little more complex for SCI participants who have a lesion at T6 or above; this will be discussed later.

If exercise programmes are put into practice correctly, and the type of exercise is selected appropriately, then they can help prevent any long-term effects that may result from the SCI debilitative cycle. Performing daily activities alone is not sufficient for people with SCI to improve their fitness levels. All too often, people with SCI assume that exercise opportunities are not open to them and that their options are limited (or exposure to recreational activities as a child becomes limited for reasons mentioned earlier). This is not necessarily the case. Many reviews published over the past decade have described a variety of exercise options with positive results in terms of improving independence and quality of life (Jacobs & Nash 2004). Physiological outcome parameters in exercise training studies with SCI populations have included heart rate, peak oxygen uptake ($\dot{V}O_2$ peak), maximal power output (POmax), gross mechanical efficiency (GME), lactic acid (blood lactate), lipid-lipoproteins and adipose tissue. Other research-design outcome parameters have included activities of daily living, often referred to as ADLs. The following section will focus primarily on which exercise modalities for SCI individuals may help reduce the secondary health complications that arise following SCI. The various combinations of training intensity, duration and frequency that have been proposed in the literature for people with SCI in order to improve fitness will also be discussed.

From a physical perspective, it is imperative to develop or maintain the components of fitness. Certainly the exercise training principles utilized with able-bodied populations apply but with some modification. There is strong evidence to suggest that people with SCI gain similar health benefits and exercise training adaptations to their able-bodied counterparts through aerobic and anaerobic (muscle strength and power) conditioning. However, the degree of improvement will differ considerably between individuals. Therefore, when monitoring the effectiveness of exercise, differences in SCI characteristics and previous training history need to be considered. Moreover, the effects of training are very much dependent upon the available muscle mass during the selected exercise modality (e.g. arm cranking involves the upper body whereas hand cycling involves the recruitment of more muscle groups through the involvement of the trunk. In order to develop and implement safe and effective exercise programmes it is important that the trainer/adviser has a basic understanding of the disability and its exercise implications as described earlier.

TYPES OF EXERCISE AND SUITABILITY FOR SCI GROUPS

There are a number of types of exercise which can be used by SCI patients for improving fitness and helping maintain functional independence, such as aerobics, ambulation with crutches, arm cranking, hand cycling, hybrid exercise (which involves electrical stimulation of the lower body combined with arm cranking), rowing, swimming, strength training using weights, medicine balls and/or elasticated resistance bands, wheelchair propulsion on rollers, free wheeling, and wheelchair sports. The main choice will depend upon availability, but key in the first instance should be specificity.

The main advantage of wheelchair exercise is its specificity for SCI wheelchair users. It is essential that participation in exercise does not result in the early onset of pain in the shoulder region and cause long-term musculoskeletal problems. Recent studies suggest that people with a SCI have musculoskeletal problems that are similar to the general population but more frequent and possibly more severe because they use their upper extremities for weight-bearing, mobility, and in awkward or extreme positions (van der Woude et al 2001). These concerns may challenge us when looking into the suitability of exercise modalities. Hence the exercises must be varied on a weekly basis. Careful planning of recovery sessions within the exercise routine is essential. Moreover, hand cycling or swimming may be more favourable and may provide the participant with a well-rounded exercise programme. Training studies in the past have used wheelchair and arm crank ergometers, with manipulations in exercise volume (frequency, intensity and duration), in order to evaluate physiological changes objectively. Recent work has focused on circuit training with resistance training, functional electrical stimulation (FES) and hybrid systems which involve a combined arm crank ergometer and electrical stimulation of the legs (FES-LCE). The hybrid training is becoming popular at a rehabilitation level, as larger muscle groups can be recruited, reactivating the muscle pump of the legs. The reduced venous pooling in the lower limbs improves venous return, stroke volume and cardiac output. As a result, higher cardiac volume load is achieved, which promotes a central training effect. These benefits, however, do come with a cost (labour and materials); technical assistance and qualified personnel are also required. There may be some discomfort from muscle spasm, particularly if the person has an incomplete lesion and can feel pain.

As with anyone undertaking exercise training, the programme must be based on the overload principle. In general, the literature tends to suggest that for SCI populations, a positive cardiovascular stimulus is around 70–80% of peak HR (Tolfrey et al 2001). However, it is important to note that there is a smaller margin between an effective stimulus and over-training. For SCI participants with a complete lesion above T6, interval-based endurance sessions may be more suitable than continuous exercise. In this case, the kind of pattern recommended might be 2 to 5 minutes of aerobic activity followed by 1 minute of rest in order to delay muscular fatigue. For SCI exercise participants whose injury level is below T6, endurance training strategies may include steady-state exercise, fartlek-based and/or interval-based sessions (Goosey-Tolfrey 2004).

Training studies of SCI exercise participants typically utilize an exercise frequency of three times per week. However, Hicks et al (2003) did find physical benefits of training only twice a week for 9 months. The main thrust of the research into exercise and physiological adaptations and SCI has focused on different exercise type or the manipulation of intensity and duration. As a general principle, habitually performing some exercise on most days of the week should be the goal.

EXERCISE VOLUME: MANIPULATIONS OF INTENSITY AND DURATION

Training to improve aerobic capacity   In the literature, exercise duration has ranged from 4 to 36 weeks, with a frequency of two to three sessions per week. The American College of Sports Medicine (ACSM) (1997) recommends moderate aerobic training for non-athletic SCI populations that is based upon 50–80% HR peak/$\dot{V}O_2$ peak, 3 to 5 days a week for 20 to 60 minutes. For individuals with SCI, the magnitude of improvement in $\dot{V}O_2$ peak has been found to be inversely related to the level of spinal cord injury, and the absolute aerobic capacity is dependent upon the available active muscle mass (Jacobs & Nash 2004). Davis and co-workers (1991) investigated four manipulations of exercise volume: (1) high intensity: long duration (40 minutes at 70% $\dot{V}O_2$ peak); (2) high intensity: short duration (20 minutes at 70% $\dot{V}O_2$ peak); (3) low intensity: long duration (40 minutes at 50% $\dot{V}O_2$ peak); and (4) low intensity: short duration (20 minutes at 50% $\dot{V}O_2$ peak) for three sessions per week. Although training varied inversely to intensity, the only condition that did not result in a significant increase in $\dot{V}O_2$ peak was condition (4), the low intensity and short duration. Hence the exercise duration needs to be 40 minutes if SCI participants exercise at 50% $\dot{V}O_2$ peak. If a shorter exercise period is warranted then an exercise intensity of 70% $\dot{V}O_2$ peak must be maintained for any training benefits. An obvious issue relating to the effectiveness of Davies et al's (1991) work is that the subjects were elderly; hence they were unaccustomed to any form of structured activity. Bizzarini et al (2005) agreed with the findings of Davies et al (1991) and suggested that intensity threshold of exercise should be set at 70% of HRmax. However, it should be noted that the use of % peak HR as a proxy measure for % $\dot{V}O_2$ peak, as originally endorsed by the ACSM, is only suitable for those with a lesion level of T6 and below. (Monitoring training and the use of HR are discussed below.)

It is not the intention here to review the many exercise volume combinations within the research designs of SCI training studies, but to highlight the main points of interest. Other studies designed to establish the minimum exercise thresholds during varying exercise modalities have adopted a similar approach to Davies et al (1991). As mentioned earlier, exercise can have a favourable effect on lipid profiles and insulin sensitivity, but by comparing exercise regimens of high versus low volume, we can begin to establish the threshold required. De Groot et al (2003) found that when different arm-training exercise intensities were employed (high, 70–80% HR reserve versus low, 40–50% HR reserve) the improvements in physical capacity and lipid profiles were more pronounced in response to high-intensity training.

The major goal of aerobic exercise training should be long-term adherence to the routine. Therefore, it is advisable to be on the conservative side with respect to intensity and duration and it would be prudent to mix other modes of physical activity within a session. The recent work by Jacobs and co-workers summarized in Jacobs & Nash (2004), which focuses on circuit training, is one way to achieve this. The circuit training (CRT) exercise incorporated periods of low-intensity high-paced movements interposed within activities performed at a series of resistance training stations. The CRT comprised three circuits of six resistance stations encompassing three pairs of agonist/antagonist movements and three 2-minute periods of free-wheeling arm cranking performed between the resistance manoeuvres. Three 45-minute sessions were performed each week. After 12 weeks of CRT training (described above), the SCI exercisers who were over 40 years of age had improved their endurance, strength and anaerobic power. Following 16 weeks of CRT training, younger SCI exercise participants increased their $\dot{V}O_2$ peak by 29%, with 13–40% improvement in strength (depending upon exercise measured). Moreover, after the CRT programme the participants' total LDL-C was lowered and HDL-C increased by around 10%. Since these studies, Jacobs & Nash (2004) have suggested that strength training should be recommended twice weekly and consist of three sets of 8–12 repetitions.

Training to improve strength   The findings from research investigating whether resistance exercise improves muscle strength necessary for daily activities are limited. We know that there is a need to build resistance training into an exercise routine to enable participants to accommodate body transfer activities, wheelchair propulsion uphill, etc. Although research in this area has been limited to small sample sizes, there is evidence to suggest that there are strength benefits for those unaccustomed to resistance training, as noted in the earlier study by Hicks et al (2003). This particular study employed two sets, at 50% 1-RM (one repetition maximum) then progressed to three sets at 70–80% 1-RM. The load was reassessed every 6 weeks to accommodate any development in strength. Other forms of exercise such as seated rowing have been shown to be beneficial in improving scapular retractor activity and cardiorespiratory fitness (Olenik et al 1995). The dose–response relationship between training frequency and strength gains must be kept in mind when discussing the effectiveness of strength training, and warrants further attention.

MONITORING TRAINING INTENSITY

When developing aerobic exercise training programmes, an effective training intensity may be more difficult to set. The methods for monitoring exercise intensity in the SCI population (athletic and non-athletic groups) have included the use of top speed, HR, ratings of perceived exertion (RPE), blood lactate threshold points and power output. When laboratory testing is not available the easiest methods to administer are percentages of HR and RPE.

HR monitors have become more widely used as an exercise training aid. However, it has been noted that the training principles employed for able-bodied populations are not directly transferable to SCI participants (Jacobs & Nash 2004, Tolfrey et al 2001). This is because SCI populations have unique physiological responses during upper limb exercise resulting from possible vascular insufficiency of the lower extremities and adrenergic dysfunction. As a result, if exercise training programmes are prescribed on the basis of target heart rates (HR peak or HR reserve), they may not be suitable for specific SCI populations. For those unaware of the specific details of these physiological limitations, the following discussion must be taken into consideration.

It is important to note that after a lesion above the sixth thoracic vertebra (T6), the heart will be affected and HR will remain low during exercise. Therefore the age-predicted maximal heart rate used in many gyms (220 – chronological age) needs to be adjusted to 190 – age (Lockette & Keyes 1994). The potential influence of certain medications on HR will also need to be considered, particularly since medication use is more common in this group than the average population.

It appears that when trained male SCI subjects work at moderate HR exercise intensities (85% or lower), relative percentages of $\dot{V}O_2$ peak are slightly underestimated (Tolfrey et al 2001). One explanation for this is that venous blood pooling may have resulted in higher submaximal $\dot{V}O_2$–HR ratios for the SCI subjects when compared to the former able-bodied guidelines (Tolfrey et al 2001). However, at the upper end of the exercise intensity continuum, the continued use of HR monitors based upon the able-bodied (ACSM) guidelines as a proxy measure of exercise intensity is recommended.

For those with a high spinal cord lesion, at the level of T1 or above, adaptations will need to be made in setting heart rate responses. The absence of sympathetic cardiac innervation produces a depressed maximal heart rate. Maximal heart rates of between 110 and 130 beats per minute have been observed and are determined by intrinsic sino-atrial node activity. This reduction in heart rate reserve means that standard guidelines for heart rate responses to activity and threshold levels cannot be followed. Thus, the use of HR monitors is not recommended for tetraplegic patients. Instead, ratings of perceived exertion (RPE; ratings of effort of the workout; Borg scale) should be used. When using this method, several trials will need to be employed to ensure that the individual is aware of the different levels of effort when exercising, and that they become familiar with the Borg scale. Alternatively percentage of peak power output is a recent recommendation in the literature for this SCI subgroup (McLean et al 1995), but it is difficult to measure during some exercise modalities. During hand cycling it is possible to use a commercially available power hub device to measure power output; work is currently being conducted in this area.

To summarize, it is appears difficult to come to any firm aerobic exercise guidelines as the use of HR and the use of maximal power output achieved or the Borg scale require further attention.

CAUTIONS

When advising someone with a disability about modes of physical activity, it is the motor limitations that are uppermost in the exercise prescriber's mind. However, there are many other considerations. In general terms there are relatively few absolute contraindications to participation. The general principles of gradual and progressive increase in training are followed and improvement in cardiovascular fitness can be made in a variety of disabilities. However, there is increasing awareness that sudden deaths occurring in the young are mostly due to cardiac abnormalities. Certain diseases and syndromes will be associated with an increased incidence of cardiac disease and this may require evaluation if strenuous participation is intended.

Some activities such as competitive basketball or hand cycling will have an increased risk of injury for obvious reasons, while in contact sports such as wheelchair rugby or ice sledge hockey there is danger of collision. Secondary to immobilization there will be a reduction of bone mineral density in the paralysed limbs with increased risk of fracture. Thought will be needed with regard to collision potential in certain sports and protective equipment may be required.

People with disabilities taking part in regular physical activity are no less susceptible to overuse injuries than their able-bodied counterparts; however, the pattern of injuries may be different. Biomechanical factors are known to predispose towards certain injuries and different disabilities will provide different biomechanical challenges. Technical factors of particular sports are contributory sources of injury and it may not be possible for someone with a disability to achieve 'perfect technique' for a variety of reasons including coordination difficulties, poor flexibility or muscle contractures. Shoulder pain is one of the most commonly reported problems in wheelchair users, and may limit activity levels and have an impact on the ability to perform activities of daily living, particularly in the ageing person (Fullerton et al 2003). There is some debate about whether this is more prevalent in active or sedentary people with SCI, i.e. does regular physical activity have a protective or causative effect? Also, although shoulder pain is a common presenting symptom in wheelchair users, this does not automatically mean that the shoulder is the source of the pain. In the first author's experience in elite sportsmen treated at Paralympic Games, the pain was more commonly referred from the cervical and thoracic spine. Specific factors in sports such as swimming or racket sports are common causes of shoulder pain independent of disability, resulting in injury to the rotator cuff. However, the act of propelling the chair does not place the shoulder into a position of sub-acromial impingement, which is the most common position for injury to the rotator cuff. Spinal stiffness, scoliosis and habitual posture may alter the scapular position and muscle imbalance may occur through poor training habits, but a balanced programme of aerobic conditioning, good postural control and resistance training to correct muscle imbalance will have a positive effect (Burnham et al 1993). Neglecting any of these factors is more likely to result in pain.

Other common injuries include blisters (from repetitive push motion) and skin lacerations and abrasions. The abrasions may be in areas of skin without sensation and may go undetected if not looked for. The new exerciser should be educated to look for areas of skin that may be subject to abrasion by a new action and its repetitive nature.

The repetitive and forceful hand movements and pressure with the heel of the hand on the push rim of the chair may result in peripheral nerve entrapments causing symptoms of hand weakness or numbness. The median nerve at the carpal tunnel is most frequently affected, followed by the ulnar nerve at the wrist and forearm.

The loss of autonomic control may cause a person with a spinal cord injury to lose bladder and bowel function. The loss of bladder control means that the person does not have control of voiding urine and must manage this by intermittent catheterization of the bladder, an indwelling catheter or condom drainage into a urine collection bag, usually on the leg. Apart from predisposing to urinary tract infection, renal or bladder stones and hypertension, bag use also has a practical effect in that leakage of urine may occur particularly with effort that raises intra-abdominal pressure. This may make the individual wary of exercising or cause them to withdraw from an exercise session. Discussing this with the person at the start of any exercise programming will display an understanding of the challenges faced and allow adaptations to be made to the programme if necessary. This applies similarly to bowel incontinence, where the passage of wind or bowel contents may occur during exercise.

The impaired autonomic control also has implications for the cardiovascular system. In general those without any renal disease, and particularly with a higher level spinal lesion, will tend to have a lower than average resting blood pressure with the absence of the muscle pump in the lower limbs and inability to make changes in vascular tone. As a result, a lowering of blood pressure (hypotension) can occur post-activity and a gentle warm-down and fluid replacement is recommended.

Furthermore, the loss of autonomic control in those with injuries at about the level of T6 or above can result in a condition called autonomic dysreflexia. A painful stimulus below the level of the spinal cord injury may initiate reflex sympathetic activity. Absence of higher control over such activity, due to the cord injury, is the main problem but additional factors such as supersensitivity of adrenoreceptors have also been implicated. Systemic hypertension occurs, which is not controlled by feedback of the parasympathetic system but causes flushing of the skin above the level of the lesion, vascular headache and nasal congestion. Autonomic dysreflexia has been regarded as a medical emergency because of the severe rises in blood pressure that can occur, with systolic pressures of 300 mmHg sometimes attained. In a tetraplegic person a rise from their normal systolic pressure of 90 mmHg by even 20–40 mmHg may be significant. Reported complications include seizures, cerebral haemorrhage and cardiac arrhythmias resulting in death. The stimulus may be something as simple as an ingrown toe-nail or a blocked catheter causing bladder distension. The exercise adviser should consult the person about the occurrence of previous episodes of dysreflexia to look for susceptibility. It may be that chafing of the skin in a new exercise mode could cause this to occur. Removal of the source of the problem, e.g. kinked catheter, is important where possible but management also includes:

1. calling for medical assistance for the non-medically trained
2. reducing the blood pressure by placing the patient in a sitting position and/or raising the head
3. recording the blood pressure – know the normal resting pressure for that individual
4. nifedipine – the person may carry sublingual nifedipine 10 mg in capsule form, which should be pierced, bitten or chewed for rapid absorption in the mouth.

Environmental issues are also important as the ability to gain or lose heat is accelerated with certain disabilities. For those with a spinal cord injury there will be reduction in the functioning peripheral receptor and heat loss mechanism below the level of the lesion. Paraplegic and tetraplegic individuals exercising in a hot environment will have an increased susceptibility to heat-related illness (Webborn et al 2005). There is a basal sweat rate below the level of the spinal lesion; however, above the level of the lesion, sweat rates of up to sixfold above normal have been observed (Petrofsky 1992). Instead of evaporation and cooling taking place, the sweat may drip off. Regular intake of fluids during exercise in a warm environment is imperative and appropriate cooling (Hagobian et al 2004, Webborn et al 2005), clothing or recovery period should be used. Conversely rapid cooling can occur in cold environments and there may be circulatory disorders associated with the disability, which will need consideration with regard to appropriate clothing, headgear and exposure. The individual may not be aware of the falling core temperature until a dangerous level is reached because of a lack of peripheral receptor input.

There are several practical issues that the inexperienced practitioner may face when administering exercise programmes for SCI participants. Some key examples are noted below:

- It is important that the trainer is aware of the participant's trunk balance and handgrip ability before they participate in any new exercises. Generally, the higher the level of SCI the greater the functional impairment. Experiment with different types and different positioning of strapping – this may improve the individual's trunk stability and subsequent exercise performance. If the individual does have impaired gripping ability then consider using gripping aids such as strapped gloves to enable arm cranking to be performed.
- Some exercise participants will have impaired temperature regulation. Ensure that they maintain adequate hydration during exercise, so as to aid renal function and thermoregulation.
- Some exercisers develop muscle imbalances due to prolonged sitting. They need to stretch affected areas but be careful with recommending exercises that may have a negative impact on a person's functional abilities (e.g. an over-stretched back can make it more difficult to maintain upright posture).
- For some participants, problems occur with muscular endurance. Thus, there may be a need to reduce the number of exercises and/or provide additional recovery periods.
- Tetraplegic patients will usually display low heart rates during exercise; it is not uncommon to find maximal heart rate as low as 120 beats/minute.

FUTURE RESEARCH REQUIREMENTS

In summary, there is no need to debate the importance of physical activity and exercise training to SCI populations. However, in the authors' view it is desirable that SCI patients begin physical activity as soon after injury as possible. When working with SCI patients it is important to understand the exercise implications and to individualize exercise training programmes accordingly.

Exercise programmes for this specific population employ the same underpinning training principles as for able-bodied participants with some subtle but significant alterations. It is generally acknowledged that SCI participants will demonstrate significant improvements in strength, mechanical efficiency and $\dot{V}O_2$ peak following exercise training, but no consensus exists on the type, intensity and frequency of the training programmes for SCI. The key question that still remains to be answered is how much exercise? Remarkably few studies have attempted to define a minimum effective intensity and duration of exercise training following SCI. However, whether the minimum exercise threshold varies with exercise mode is a topic that warrants further investigation. It is quite clear that there is high variability in the training responses of people with SCI. This may be due to the type of exercise combined with the person's SCI characteristics. Hence, it is important that research articles provide details about these characteristics in the SCI sample studied.

Body composition deteriorates markedly during the first 6 months after SCI (Wells & Hooker 1990). Longitudinal body composition studies in people with SCI are few, missing time points, and small in numbers. Several studies have used cross-sectional designs to compare body composition changes in response to exercise training. However, because people with SCI may be more obese than the able-bodied population, the measurement techniques need to be explored and further validated for this specific population. Moreover, strategies for innovative interventions aimed at reducing the relative decrease in lean tissue and increase in adiposity should be considered.

The research literature to date does allow us to draw some conclusions regarding exercise prescription. However, the use of heterogeneous SCI samples with respect to lesion level, incomplete or complete, onset of disability and previous trained status casts doubt upon the validity of these assumptions. If conclusions concerning deconditioning and reconditioning in SCI exercise participants are to be reached, then studies of homogeneous SCI groups are essential. It should be clear that in order to monitor exercise training we need to understand the disability and lesion characteristics of the individual. It should also be noted that the use of % peak HR as a proxy measure for % $\dot{V}O_2$ peak, as originally endorsed by the ACSM, may not be suitable for all SCI subjects (Tolfrey et al 2001).

Finally, arm ergometry is an effective form of exercise when use of the lower limbs is either impossible or problematic. This is the most common form of exercise, but does limit the cardiopulmonary load. The need to find a suitable mode of exercise for the maintenance of cardiovascular health and the prevention of disease, particularly in wheelchair-dependent individuals, presents a challenge to the practitioner. The use of a wheelchair allows people with physical incapacities the independence to move around. However, wheelchair propulsion is an inefficient form of locomotion, carries a high risk of overuse injuries and may be deemed unsuitable in the winter months for pushing outdoors. For these reasons, and to enable wheelchair-dependent individuals further options for aerobic training, other exercise forms have been discussed above. It is anticipated that in future years there will be an emerging evidence base focusing on hand cycling and FES-induced leg exercise. These exercise alternatives enable the participant to activate larger muscle mass, and when combined (hybrid training) the evidence suggests that both central and peripheral training effects are gained (Janssen & Hopman 2005).

KEY POINTS

1. SCI is a relatively common condition resulting in various levels of impairment which affect the ability to exercise.
2. Physical activity has a key role in health maintenance of people with SCI.
3. Spinal cord injury directly alters body composition due to the loss of voluntary control in the major muscle mass of the body. Assessment of body composition is complex.
4. Aerobic capacity depends upon total active muscle mass.
5. For lesions above the sixth thoracic vertebra (T6), heart rate is affected (typically found to be lower during maximal exercise).
6. The use of the normal age-predicted maximal heart rate becomes problematic for exercise prescription of SCI participants.
7. The use of HR monitors for tetraplegic individuals is not recommended. Instead, use ratings of perceived exertion (RPE) for the workout.
8. SCI participants have an impaired thermoregulatory capacity and are more susceptible to thermal stress when compared to their able-bodied counterparts.
9. In some settings, electrically stimulated muscle contractions can recruit sufficient muscle mass to significantly increase aerobic capacity.
10. Studies have demonstrated improvements in body composition and lipid profiles as consequences of regular exercise.
11. Even within well-controlled studies the heterogeneous nature of the typical sample makes data interpretation difficult.

12. There is scope to investigate the long-term benefits of exercise in SCI populations with larger groups, assessing the role of exercise intensity on key physiological outcome parameters.

13. The minimum exercise intensity threshold for different types of exercise suitable for SCI populations needs to be examined.

References

ACSM 1997 ACSM's exercise management for persons with chronic diseases and disabilities. Human Kinetics, Champaign, IL

Bauman W A, Waters R L 2004 Aging with a spinal cord injury. In: Aging with a disability: what the clinician needs to know. Johns Hopkins University Press, Baltimore, MD, pp 153–174

Bizzarini E, Saccavini M, Lipanje F et al 2005 Exercise prescription in subjects with spinal cord injuries. Archives of Physical Medicine and Rehabilitation 86:1170–1175

Burnham R S, May L, Nelson E et al 1993 Shoulder pain in wheelchair athletes. The role of muscle imbalance. American Journal of Sports Medicine 21(2):238–242

Cirak B, Ziegfeld S, Knight V M et al 2004 Spinal injuries in children. Journal of Pediatric Surgery 39(4):607–612

Cooper R A, Quatrano L A, Axelson P W et al 1999 Research on physical activity and health among people with disabilities: a consensus statement. Journal of Rehabilitation Research and Development 36:142–154

Curtis K A, McClanahan S, Hall K M et al 1986 Health, vocational, and functional status in spinal cord injured athletes and nonathletes. Archives of Physical Medicine Rehabilitation 67:862–865

Davis G, Plyley M J, Shephard R J 1991 Gains of cardiorespiratory fitness with arm-crank training in spinally disabled men. Canadian Journal of Sport Sciences 16:64–72

Dearwater S R, Laporte R E, Robertson R J et al 1986 Activity in the spinal cord-injured patient: an epidemiologic analysis of metabolic parameters. Medicine and Science in Sports and Exercise 18:541–544

de Groot P C E, Hjeltnes N, Heijboer A C et al 2003 Effect of training intensity on physical capacity, lipid profile and insulin sensitivity in early rehabilitation of spinal cord injured individuals. Spinal Cord 41:673–679

Department of Health 2004 At least five a week – physical activity, health improvement and prevention. London

Ellenberg M, MacRitchie M, Franklin B et al 1989 Aerobic capacity in early paraplegia: implications for rehabilitation. Paraplegia 27:261–268

Fullerton H D, Borckardt J J, Alfano A P 2003 Shoulder pain: a comparison of wheelchair athletes and nonathletic wheelchair users. Medicine and Science in Sports and Exercise 35(12):1958–1961

Goosey-Tolfrey V L 2004 Optimising physical training: paralympic athletes. Faster Higher Stronger 22:26–27

Goosey-Tolfrey V L 2005 Physiological profiles of elite wheelchair basketball players in preparation for the 2000 Paralympic Games. Adapted Physical Activity Quarterly 22:57–66

Hagobian T A, Jacobs K A, Kiratli J et al 2004 Foot cooling reduces exercise-induced hyperthermia in men with spinal cord injury. Medicine and Science in Sports and Exercise 36:411–417

Hartkopp A, Bronnum-Hansen H, Seidenschnur A M et al 1998 Suicide in a spinal cord injured population: its relation to functional status. Archives of Physical Medicine and Rehabilitation 79(11):1356–1361

Hicks A L, Martin K A, Ditor D S et al 2003 Long-term exercise training in persons with spinal cord injury: effects on strength, arm ergometry performance and psychological well-being. Spinal Cord 41:34–43

Hoffman M D 1986 Cardiorespiratory fitness and training in quadriplegics and paraplegics. Sports Medicine 3:312–330

Jackson A B, Dijkers M, Devivo M J et al 2004 A demographic profile of new traumatic spinal cord injuries: change and stability over 30 years. Archive of Physical Medicine and Rehabilitation 85(11):1740–1748

Jacobs P L, Nash M S 2004 Exercise recommendations for individuals with spinal cord injury. Sports Medicine 34:727–751

Janssen T W J, Hopman M T E 2005 Spinal cord injury. In: Skinner J S (ed) Exercise testing and exercise prescription for special cases: theoretical basis and clinical applications. Lippincott Williams & Wilkins, Baltimore, pp 203–219

Janssen T W J, Oers C A J M, Hollander A P et al 1994 Relationship between physical strain during standardised ADL tasks and physical capacity in men with spinal cord injury. Paraplegia 32:844–859

Janssen H C, Samson M M, Meeuwsen I B et al 2004 Strength, mobility and falling in women referred to a geriatric outpatient clinic. Experimental Aging Research 16(2):122–125

Lockette K F, Keyes A M 1994 Conditioning with physical disabilities. Human Kinetics, Champaign, IL, pp 91–116

McLean K P, Jones P P, Skinner J S 1995 Exercise prescription for sitting and supine exercise in subjects with quadriplegia. Medicine and Science in Sports and Exercise 27:15–21

Midha M, Schmitt J K, Sclater M 1999 Exercise effect with the wheelchair aerobic fitness trainer on conditioning and metabolic function in disabled persons: a pilot study. Archives of Physical Medicine and Rehabilitation 80:258–261

Miles D, Sawka M N, Wilde S et al 1982 Pulmonary function changes in wheelchair athletes subsequent to exercise training. Ergonomics 25:239–246

National Spinal Cord Injury Statistical Center 2005 Annual statistical report. University of Alabama, Birmingham

Olenik L M, Laskin J J, Burnham R 1995 Efficacy of rowing, backward wheeling and isolated scapular retractor exercise as remedial strength activities for wheelchair users: application of electromyography. Paraplegia 33:148–152

Patel D R, Greydanus D E 2002 The pediatric athlete with disabilities. Pediatric Clinics of North America 49(4):803–827

Petrofsky J S 1992 Thermoregulatory stress during rest and exercise in heat in patients with a spinal cord injury. European Journal of Applied Physiology and Occupational Physiology 64(6):503–507

Rish B L, Dilustro J F, Salazar A M et al 1997 Spinal cord injury: a 25-year morbidity and mortality study. Military Medicine 162(2):141–148

Sargent J 1983 The sick child: family complications. Journal of Developmental and Behavioural Pediatrics 4(1):50–56

Sattin R W, Easley K A, Wolf S L et al 2005 Reduction in fear of falling through intense tai chi exercise training in older, transitionally frail adults. Journal of the American Geriatrics Society 53(7):1168–1178

Silver J R 1993 Spinal injuries in sports in the UK. British Journal of Sports Medicine 27(2):115–120

Silver J R, Stewart D 1994 The prevention of spinal injuries in rugby football. Paraplegia 32(7):442–453

Soden R J, Walsh J, Middleton J W et al 2000 Causes of death after spinal cord injury. Spinal Cord 38(10):604–610

Stotts K M 1986 Health maintenance: paraplegic athletes and nonathletes. Archives of Physical Medicine and Rehabilitation 67:109–114

Suzuki T, Kim H, Yoshida H et al 2004 Randomized controlled trial of exercise intervention for the prevention of falls in community-dwelling elderly Japanese women. Journal of Bone and Mineral Metabolism 22(6):602–611

Thomasgard M, Metz W P 1997 Parental overprotection and its relation to perceived child vulnerability. American Journal of Orthopsychiatry 67(2):330–335

Tolfrey K, Goosey-Tolfrey V L, Campbell I G 2001 The oxygen uptake–heart rate relationship in elite wheelchair racers. European Journal of Applied Physiology 86:174–178

van der Woude L H, Veeger H E, Dallmeijer A J et al 2001 Biomechanics and physiology in active manual wheelchair propulsion. Medical Engineering and Physics 23:713–733

Velmahos G C, Degiannis E, Hart K et al 1995 Changing profiles in spinal cord injuries and risk factors influencing recovery after penetrating injuries. Journal of Trauma 38(3):334–337

Webborn N, Price M J, Castle P C et al 2005 Effects of two cooling strategies on thermoregulatory responses of tetraplegic athletes during repeated intermittent exercise in the heat. Journal of Applied Physiology 98:2101–2107

Wells C L, Hooker S P 1990 The spinal cord injured athlete. Adapted Physical Activity Quarterly 7:265–285

Further reading

Janssen T W J, Hopman M T E 2005 Spinal cord injury. In: Skinner J S (ed) Exercise testing and exercise prescription for special cases: theoretical basis and clinical applications. Lippincott Williams & Wilkins, Baltimore, pp 203–219

Lockette K F, Keyes A M 1994 Conditioning with physical disabilities. Human Kinetics, Champaign, IL, pp 91–116

Webborn A D J 2001 Sports in children with physical disabilities; medical problems of disabled child athletes. In: Maffulli N et al (eds) Sports medicine for specific ages and abilities. Churchill Livingstone, Edinburgh

Webborn N 2001 Delivering an exercise prescription for patients with disabilities. In: Young A, Harries M (eds) Physical activity for patients: an exercise prescription. Royal College of Physicians, London

Index

A

abdominal obesity
  diabetes risk, 26
  myocardial infarction risk, 28
  see also waist circumference
accelerometers, 11
  obesity–inactivity association studies,
    30, 31, 32
active listening, 6
activity theory of ageing, 168
adipocytokines, 27
adiponectin, 27
adolescents
  asthma, 107, 112
  low back pain, 140
  menarche, 250
  obesity, 29
  peak bone mineral density
    enhancement, 234, 240
  physical inactivity–weight gain
    association, 31, 32
aerobic endurance, 3
aerobic fitness *see* fitness,
  cardiorespiratory
aerobic power *see* maximal aerobic
  power (VO$_2$max)
aerobic/aerobic endurance exercise
  arthritis, 125–7, 128
  chronic low back pain, 148–9
    with active rest periods, 148
  chronic obstructive pulmonary disease,
    110–11
  coronary heart disease
    primary prevention, 59–61
    secondary prevention/
      rehabilitation, 62, 63–4
  energy expenditure for weight loss, 39
  heart failure, 72–3
    interval approach, 72, 73

patients with implantable
    cardioverter defibrillators, 75
  intensity measurement, 12–13
  multiple sclerosis, 284–5
  neuromuscular disorders, 288
  older people, 162, 180
  Parkinson's disease, 280–1
  postmenopausal women, 264
  spinal cord injury, 320, 322
  stroke, 276
aerobics
  bone health enhancement, 183, 234
  spinal cord injury, 324
Aerobics Centre Longitudinal Study, 33
age-adjusted maximal heart rate
  arthritis, 127
  cardiovascular disease, 81, 87
  exercise testing end-point, 81–2
  spinal cord injury, 327
ageing, 161–210
  activity theory, 168
  biological theories, 167–8
  body fat increase, 170
  cardiovascular system effects, 170–1
  continuity theory, 169
  definitions, 163–4
  endocrine system effects, 176–7
  functional performance impact, 170–8
  genetic effects, 167, 168
  musculoskeletal system effects, 171–4
  nervous system effects, 174–6, 177
  primary, 164
  processes, 164–6
    heterogeneity, 163
  psychological function effects, 178
  psychological theories, 168
  quantitative aspects, 166–7
  rate, 166
  respiratory system effects, 170–1
  secondary, 164

ageing (*Continued*)
  slowing, 169–70
  sociological theories, 168–9
  successful, 169
  see also older people
airway obstruction
  asthma, 103, 104
  chronic obstructive pulmonary disease,
    100
Allied Dunbar National Fitness Survey
  (ADNFS), 171
alpha-motor neurons, 311
amenorrhoea, 251–2, 254
  athletic, 252
    bone health, 238, 256–8
    female athlete triad, 253, 254–6, 258
aminoglycosides, 176
amiodarone, 78
amlodipine, 77
angina pectoris, 53, 54, 79
  exercise testing, 83
  postural changes triggering, 80
  see also unstable angina
angiotensin-converting-enzyme (ACE)
  inhibitors, 77, 80
  heart failure management, 71
  skeletal muscle function effects, 71–2
ankle, ageing-related range of motion
  decline, 174, 175
anorexia nervosa, 256, 257
anterior cord syndrome, 315
anti-arrhythmics, 77
antiplatelet agents, 77
anti-thrombotics, 77, 78
appetite, hormonal regulation, 23, 25
aquatic exercise
  arthritis, 121, 125, 126
    resistance training, 137–9
  multiple sclerosis, 284
  older people, 200
    flexibility improvement, 184
arm cranking
  gripping aids, 330
  spinal cord injury, 324, 326, 331
arteries
  ageing-related changes, 170
  nitric oxide response in heart failure,
    71–2
arthritis, 119–39, 153–4
  benefits of exercise, 120
  categories, 120
  economic burden, 120
  gait changes, 177
  intensity of exercise, 126, 127, 133, 136
  key points, 153–4

management principles, 153
obesity association, 40
older people, 174, 175
proprioceptive exercise, 131–3
psychological considerations, 152
resistance training
  isometric, 135
water-based, 137–9
see also osteoarthritis; rheumatoid
    arthritis
aspirin, 77, 78, 176
asthma, 98
  aerobic fitness levels, 98
  bronchoconstriction, 103, 104, 112
  chronic obstructive pulmonary disease
    co-morbidity, 104
  diagnosis, 103
  dynamic lung hyperinflation, 103–4
  dyspnoea, 103
    levels of perception, 109
  in elite athletes, 98, 107, 108
  epidemiology, 98
  exercise limitation, 98, 103, 104
    respiratory effort, 104
  exercise training
    evidence-based guidance, 112–13
    inspiratory muscle training, 108–9
    monitoring, 112
    precautions, 112
    pulmonary rehabilitation, 107–9
  key points, 113, 114
  pathophysiology, 103–4
  symptoms, 103
  see also exercise-induced asthma
atherosclerotic plaque (atheroma), 53–4
  cardioprotective mechanisms of
    physical activity, 63, 64
  rupture, 54
  stability, 54
    exercise-related enhancement,
      56, 61
athletic amenorrhoea *see* amenorrhoea;
    female athlete triad
autonomic dysreflexia, 329
autonomic nervous system, 312

B

balance, 4, 16–17
  ageing-related decline, 175, 177
    pre-exercise assessment, 192
  arthritis, 128
  neuromuscular disorders, 288
  stroke/traumatic brain injury, 274

balance training
    avoidance in pregnancy, 262
    coronary heart disease
        primary prevention, 61–2
        secondary prevention/
            rehabilitation, 65
    heart failure, 74
    knee arthritis, 130
    older people, 162, 199, 201
        falls prevention, 185, 186, 318
        nervous system effects, 184
        safety, 200
ballistic stretching, 16
barriers to physical activity, 5
    neurological/neuromuscular disorders,
        271
    older people, 204, 205
    strategies for overcoming, 9
        client-centred approach, 7–8
basketball
    bone health enhancement, 234
    spinal cord injury, 323
        cautions, 327
Becker's muscular dystrophy, 286
behaviour change, 5
    older people, 204–5
    relapse prevention, 9–10
    stages, 6
benefits of physical activity, 2
    arthritis, 120–1, 125–6, 180
    bone health, 231–4
        children/adolescents, 240
    cardiac arrhythmias, 74, 76
    cardiovascular risk, 36–7, 56, 180
    chronic obstructive pulmonary disease,
        102, 109
    diabetes, 36–7, 40, 180
    heart failure, 72
    joint range of motion enhancement,
        61–2
    low back pain, 120–1
    low-density lipoproteins, 263, 326
    older people, 4, 179, 180–8
    osteoporosis, 4, 180, 184
    postmenopausal women, 263
    psychological, 10, 125–6, 319
    spinal cord injury, 319–20,
        321–2, 323
beta-blockers, 77, 80
    exercise capacity effects, 78
    exercise testing, 82
    patients with implantable cardioverter
        defibrillators, 75
bisphosphonates, 230, 263
blood pressure, 3

measurement in cardiovascular
        patients, 83, 85
    older people, 170
        aerobic training response, 181
    spinal cord injury, 329
    autonomic dysreflexia, 329
    see also hypertension
body fat
    ageing-related increase, 170
    measurement in spinal cord injury
        patients, 322
body mass index (BMI)
    obesity, 22, 27
        accuracy, 27, 29, 41
        in children (BMI for age), 28, 29
    older people, 189
    overweigtht, 22
    postmenopausal women, 262, 263
bodyweight exercises
    older people, 182
    resistance training with arthritis, 134
bone
    age-related changes, 173–4, 228, 231
        prevention, 231
    cortical, 226, 228
    fractures see fracture risk
    peak mass, 173, 228
        maximization in childhood, 231
    remodelling, 227–8
        hormonal regulation, 228
        mechanical loading response, 231
        oestrogen effects, 257
    structure, 226–7
    trabecular, 226, 227, 228
        osteogenic response to strain, 234
bone health, 225–42
    adverse effects of progesterone-only
        contraception, 238–9
    amenorrhoeic athletes, 238, 256–8
    benefits of physical activity,
        231–4, 240
        weight-bearing exercise, 231–2
    case study, 241–2
    dietary advice, 240–1
    exercise dose response, 234–7
        frequency/intensity/duration,
            236–7
        mode, 235–6
    exercise training
        children/adolescents, 240
        older people, 183–4
        postmenopausal women, 264
        practical issues, 238–9
        principle of diminishing returns, 238
        progressive overload, 237

bone health (*Continued*)
    reversibility, 237–8
    specificity, 237
  key points, 242
  osteoporosis markers, 231
  Wolff's law, 231
  see also bone loss; bone mineral density
Bone Loading History Questionnaire, 233
bone loss
  age-related, 179, 228, 256
  female athlete triad, 256, 258
  immobilization-related, 179
  low-dose oestradiol/progesterone-only
      contraception effects, 239
  menstrual dysfunction-related, 238
  perimenopausal, 228, 239, 257
  postmenopausal, 173, 174, 263
    back strengthening exercises, 184
    bone loading exercises, 183
  risk in spinal cord injury patients, 327
bone mineral density
  age-related decline, 164, 173
  amenorrhoeic athletes, 238, 257, 258
  genetic factors, 233
  increase through exercise, 229, 233
    cardiac rehabilitation, 65
    children/adolescents, 240
    older people, 182, 183–4
    training principles, 183
  low-dose oestradiol oral contraception
      effects, 239
  measurement
    broadband ultrasound, 231
    computed tomography, 231
    dual energy X-ray absorptiometry,
      229, 231, 257
  menopause-related decrease, 239
  osteopenia, 229
  osteoporosis, 174, 229
  progesterone-only contraception
      effects, 238–9
  reversibility of augmentation, 237–8
  spinal cord injury patients, 327
bone-specific alkaline phosphatase, 227,
  231
Borg rating scales, 13, 110, 127, 136, 203,
  262, 327
brain injury *see* traumatic brain injury
brain natriuretic peptide, 66, 74
breathing retraining, chronic obstructive
  pulmonary disease, 111–12
breathlessness
  asthma, 103
  chronic obstructive pulmonary disease,
    98, 99, 100, 106, 110

  heart failure, 66
    inspiratory muscle training, 73
broadband ultrasound attenuation of
  calcaneus, 231
bronchitis, chronic, 98
  see also chronic obstructive pulmonary
    disease
Brown-Séquard syndrome, 315
Bruce protocol, 85
Brugada syndrome, 56
bulimia nervosa, 256

C

calcitonin, 228
  osteoporosis therapy, 230
calcium channel blockers, 77, 80
calcium, dietary, 240
calcium supplementation
  bone health in children, 240–1
  female athlete triad, 258
  osteoporosis, 230
  premenstrual syndrome, 259
cancer, obesity association, 40
cardiac abnormalities, neuromuscular
  disorders, 286–7
cardiac arrest
  exertion-related, 55
  non-exercise-related, 56
cardiac arrhythmias, 53, 79
  benefits of exercise, 74, 76
  exercise-induced, 74
    heart failure patients, 69–71
  older people, 191
cardiac conduction abnormalities, 52, 53
cardiac events
  exertion-related, 55–6
  prevention through regular exercise,
    55, 56
  see also myocardial infarction; unstable
    angina
cardiac mass, aerobic training response
  in older people, 181
cardiac output
  older people, 170
  in pregnancy, 260
cardiovascular disease, 51–88
  co-morbidity, 79
    chronic obstructive pulmonary
      disease, 102, 110
  cool-down exercise, 79–80
  diabetes type 2 association, 40
  epidemiology, 53
  exercise testing, 81–4

cardiovascular disease (*Continued*)
  fitness change assessment protocols,
    87
  functional assessment, 84–6
    performance, 84–5
    physiological responses, 85–6
  key points, 87
  medications, 77–9, 80, 81
    exercise capacity effects, 78–9
  myocardial ischaemia prevention
    during daily activities, 81
  postural change effects, 80
  practical considerations for exercise,
    79–81
    equipment hazards, 81
  secondary prevention, 53
  spinal cord injury patients, 319, 320
  warm-up exercise, 79–80
cardiovascular risk, 52
  athletic/secondary amenorrhoea, 254
  beneficial effects of physical activity,
    36–7, 56
    older people, 180
  cardiorespiratory fitness relationship,
    59–60
  diabetes, 36–7, 40, 52, 53, 61, 68
  modification, 53
  neuromuscular disorders, 286
  obesity, 52, 53, 61
  physical inactivity, 54–5
  postmenopausal women, 262, 263, 264
  secondary prevention, 54
  spinal cord injury, 322
  stroke, 274
cardiovascular system
  ageing effects, 170–1
    exercise training influence, 180–1
  pregnancy-related changes, 260
carotid artery disease, 274
catecholamines, 79, 80
cauda equina, 310
  lesions, 315
central cord syndrome, 315
central processing of information, ageing
    effects, 174, 175
  noisy processing, 178
chair rise, older people, 172
Charcot–Marie–Tooth disease, 286
children
  asthma, 98
    exercise training, 107, 112
  bone growth, 228
  bone health
    calcium supplementation, 240–1
    exercise programme, 240

diabetes prevalence, 29–30
    type 2, 30
  obesity
    exercise in management, 36
    prevalence, 28–9
  peak bone mass maximization, 231
    jumping, 234
    physical activity recommendations,
      234, 240
  physical inactivity–weight gain
      association, 31–2
  spinal cord injury, 316, 317–18, 319
chronic obstructive pulmonary disease
    (COPD), 98
  aetiology, 98
  associated muscular dysfunction, 98,
    99–100
  beneficial effects of exercise, 102, 109
  chronic inspiratory muscle loading,
    100–1
    muscle fibre type changes, 99, 101
  co-morbidity, 98, 102, 110
    asthma, 104
    congestive heart failure, 67, 68
  dynamic lung hyperinflation, 100, 110
  dyspnoea, 98, 99, 100, 110
    health-related quality of life, 106
  epidemiology, 98
  exercise limitation, 98, 99, 100, 102
    training-related improvement,
      105–6
    ventilatory work demand, 102, 106
  exercise training guidance, 109–12
  inspiratory muscle weakness, 100,
    101, 102
  key points, 113–14
  pathophysiology, 99–102
  psychosocial aspects, 102
  pulmonary rehabilitation, 102, 104–7
    inspiratory muscle training, 105,
      106–7
    outcome measures, 105
    reversibility of training effects, 112
  systemic manifestations, 99
  weight loss, 99, 100
client-centred approach, 5–10
  decisional balance, 6–7
  goal-setting, 8–9
  overcoming barriers to activity, 7–8
  relapse prevention, 9–10
  self-efficacy enhancement, 9
  self-monitoring, 8–9
  social support, 8
  stages of change, 6
clopidogrel, 78, 81

cognitive behavioural strategies, 5
cognitive disuse, 178, 184
cognitive function, ageing effects, 178
  benefits of exercise, 184–5, 186
communication skills, 6
computed tomography, bone mineral
  density, 231
confidence enhancement, 5, 7
congenital cardiomyopathies, 67
congestive heart failure *see* heart failure
connective tissue disorders, 120
continuity theory of ageing, 169
contraceptive implants, 238–9, 251
cool-down exercise
  cardiovascular rehabilitation, 79–80
  heart failure patients
    exercise-induced arrhythmias
      prevention, 69
    with implantable cardioverter
      defibrillators, 75
  neurological/neuromuscular disorder
    patients, 289
  older people, 202
coordination, 4, 16–17
  impairment
    multiple sclerosis, 283
    neuromuscular disorders, 288
    Parkinson's disease, 279
    stroke/traumatic brain injury,
      274
coordination exercises
  coronary heart disease
    primary prevention, 61–2
    secondary prevention/
      rehabilitation, 65
  heart failure, 74
  multiple sclerosis, 285
  neuromuscular disorders, 289
  Parkinson's disease, 281
  stroke, 277
core stability exercises *see* spinal
  stabilization exercise
coronary angioplasty, 62, 78
coronary arteries
  cardioprotective mechanisms of
    physical activity, 63–4
  warm-up exercise response, 79
coronary artery bypass surgery, 62, 78
coronary heart disease, 6, 7, 52
  co-morbidity
    chronic obstructive pulmonary
      disease, 110
    diabetes type 2, 40
    heart failure, 71
    obesity, 40, 58

epidemiology, 53
exercise in primary prevention,
    56–62
  aerobic endurance exercise,
    59–61
  balance/proprioceptive/
    coordination exercise, 61–2
  muscular strength/endurance
    exercise, 61
exertion-related cardiac events,
    55–6, 71
  older people, 188
pathophysiology, 53–4
physical activity relationship,
    54–5, 56
physical inactivity relationship,
    58
  associated mortality, 58–9
secondary prevention/rehabilitation,
    62–6
  aerobic endurance exercise,
    62, 63–4
  balance/proprioceptive/
    coordination exercise, 65
  muscular strength/endurance
    exercise, 64–5
spinal cord injury patients, 322
prevention, 321
stroke risk, 274
therapeutic interventions, 66–7
corpus luteum, 251, 253
cortisol
  ageing-related changes, 176, 178
    response to exercise, 185
  female athlete triad, 254, 256
cross-training, arthritis patients, 126
cycle ergometer, 81
  cardiorespiratory testing
    cardiovascular patients, 87
    chronic obstructive pulmonary
      disease patients, 111
    older people, 191
cycling, 235
  arthritis, 121, 125, 127
  asthma, 107
  chronic obstructive pulmonary disease,
    105
  diabetes type 2, 40
  low back pain, 121
    acute, 142
    chronic, 148
  multiple sclerosis, 284
  older people, 200
  Parkinson's disease, 281
  stroke, 276

D

Da Qing Impaired Glucose Tolerance and Diabetes Study, 34, 39
daily living activities
    aerobic training effect in heart failure patients, 72
    energy expenditure, 1–2, 60
    muscular strength requirements, 73
    myocardial ischaemia prevention, 81
    obesity–inactivity association, 30–1
    older people, effects of muscle weakness, 172
    physical activity measurement, 11
    spinal cord injury, 322, 323
dance
    bone health enhancement, 234
        bone mineral density, 183
        children/adolescents, 240
    felxibility improvement in older people, 184
    musculoskeletal disorders, 121
decisional balance, 6–7
depot medroxyprogesterone acetate (DMPA), 238–9
diabetes insipidus, 25
diabetes mellitus, 21–42
    aetiology, 25–7
    benefits of physical activity, 36–7, 40, 180
    cardiovascular risk, 36–7, 40, 52, 53, 61
        heart failure, 68
    children, 29–30
        exercise-related hypoglycaemia, 40
    co-morbidity, 40–1
    gestational, 260
    hyperglycaemia, 25–6, 27
    older people, 29, 180
    prevalence, 29–30
    spinal cord injury patients, 321, 322
    stroke risk, 274
    treatment, 26
    type 1 (insulin-dependent), 25, 26, 29–30, 32, 36, 40, 123
    type 2 (non-insulin-dependent), 6, 25, 26, 29, 30, 52, 53
        barriers to physical activity, 7
        exercise prescription, 39–40
        exercise-related acute glycaemic reactions, 7, 41
        life expectancy impact, 40
        obesity association, 26–7, 30, 39
        physical activity in management, 36–8, 41
        physical activity in risk reduction, 32–5
        postmenopausal women, 263
        risk factors, 33
diabetic neuropathy, 40, 270
diaphragm breathing, 112
dietary intervention
    bone health, 240–1
    obesity prevention/management, 39
digitalis, 77
diltiazem, 77
diuretics, 77
dizziness, older people, 175–6
dorsal (posterior) column, 312
dorsal root, 311
doubly labelled water technique, 11, 30
drop-outs from exercise programmes, 5
dual energy X-ray absorptiometry
    body composition measurement in spinal cord injured patients, 322
    bone mineral density measurement, 229, 231, 257
duration of exercise, 11
    bone mineral density response, 236–7
    cardiovascular benefit, 58
    chronic obstructive pulmonary disease, 110
    heart failure, 72
    neurological/neuromuscular disorders, 290
    spinal cord injury, 325–6
dynamic lung hyperinflation, chronic obstructive pulmonary disease, 100, 110
dysmenorrhoea, 252, 259
    treatment, 259
dyspnoea *see* breathlessness

E

eating, disordered, female athlete triad, 253, 256, 258
elasticated resistance bands
    older people, 182
    spinal cord injury, 324
electrogoniometry, 16
empathy, 6
    emphysema, 98
    see also chronic obstructive pulmonary disease (COPD)
endochondral ossification, 228

endocrine system, ageing effects, 176–7
    benefits of exercise, 185
energy availability, athletic amenorrhoea
    relationship, 255
energy expenditure
    cardiovascular benefit, 57–8, 59, 60
        threshold level, 57, 61
    obesity aetiology, 22
        inactivity association evaluation,
            30–1
    weight loss, 39
enjoyment, 5
epiphyseal plates, 228
Epstein–Barr virus, 123
ergometers, 81
    multiple sclerosis, 284
    spinal cord injury, 324
Erlangen Fitness Osteoporosis Prevention
    Study, 239, 264
European Prospective Investigation into
    Cancer Questionnaire, 233
exercise, definition, 2
exercise dose, 10–11
    monitoring, 11
    muscular strength training, 15
    optimal, 11
    see also intensity of physical activity
exercise ECG testing, cardiovascular
    patients, 83, 84
    functional assessment, 85
exercise prescription
    asthma, 112–13
    chronic obstructive pulmonary disease,
        110–12
    coronary heart disease
        primary prevention, 62
        secondary prevention/
            rehabilitation, 64–5
    neurological/neuromuscular disorders,
        289–92
    obesity prevention/management, 38–9
    older people, 194–8
exercise testing
    cardiovascular patients, 81–4
        aims, 81, 82
        end-points, 81–2
    neurological/neuromuscular disorders,
        289–90
    older people, 191–2
exercise-induced arrhythmias, 74
    heart failure, 69–71
exercise-induced asthma
    exercise training programmes, 107–8,
        112–13
    refractory period, 113

exertion-related cardiac events, 74, 78
    prevention, 79, 81
        regular exercise, 55, 56
exertion-related myocardial infarction, 74
exertion-related physical symptoms, 3
expiratory flow
    chronic obstructive pulmonary disease,
        100
    older people, 171
expiratory muscle training, multiple
    sclerosis, 285

F

facioscapulohumeral muscular dystrophy,
    286, 289
falls
    arthritic patients, 128
    cardiac disease relationship, 65
    long-lie complications, 177
    older people, 177–8
        pre-exercise risk assessment, 192,
            193
        prevention, 162, 182, 183, 185–6,
            318
    postmenopausal women, 264
    risk factors, 73
    risk reduction, 17, 162
        exercise training response, 74, 182,
            183, 185–6
    spinal cord injury, 316, 318
    stroke/traumatic brain injury,
        273, 274
fartlek-based exercise sessions
    older people, 203
    spinal cord injury, 325
fasting, 22–3
fatigue, 3
    multiple sclerosis, 282, 284, 292
    neuromuscular disorders, 286, 287
    Parkinson's disease, 278, 279
female athlete triad, 253–8
    amenorrhoea, 253, 254–5
    diordered eating, 253, 256
    osteopenia, 257
    osteoporosis, 253, 256–8
    physical activity guidelines, 258
    treatment, 258
female exercise participants, 249–65
    key points, 265
    physiology, 250–3
    femoral neck fracture, 174, 229
    see also hip fracture
fetal response to exercise, 261

field sports, bone mineral density response, 183.
Finnish Diabetes Prevention Study, 34, 39
fitness
  benefits of improvement, 2, 58
  cardiorespiratory
    asthma, 98, 104
    coronary artery narrowing relationship, 54
    coronary heart disease prevention, 59–60
    coronary heart disease rehabilitation, 62, 63–4
    metabolic syndrome risk reduction, 58
    multiple sclerosis, 282
    neuromuscular disorders, 286–7
    Parkinson's disease, 278
    stroke, 273
    traumatic brain injury, 273
  cardiovascular risks of low level, 52
  components, 2–4
  diabetes co-morbidity prevention, 36–7
  older people, 171
fixed weight machines
  low back pain exercise programme development, 146–47
  resistance training in arthritis, 134
flexibility, 4
  ageing-related decline, 174
  multiple sclerosis, 283
  older people, 184
  Parkinson's disease, 279
  stroke/traumatic brain injury, 274
flexibility exercises, 15–16
  arthritis, 121, 127–30
  implantable cardioverter defibrillator patient rehabilitation, 75
  low back pain, 121, 148
  modes of training, 16
  multiple sclerosis, 285
  neuromuscular disorders, 289
  older people, 199
  Parkinson's disease, 281
  in pregnancy, 262
  stroke patients, 277
fluoride, osteoporosis therapy, 230
follicle-stimulating hormone, 250, 251
food intake, obesity aetiology, 22–3
foot problems, older people, 175
football
  bone health enhancement, 234
  contribution to arthritis development, 125

forced expiratory volume in one second (FEV1), older people, 171
fracture risk
  ageing effects, 173–4
  female athlete triad, 257, 258
  osteoporosis/osteopenia, 229
  postmenopausal women, 264
  spinal cord injury, 327
Framington Study, 67
free weight training
  arthritis, 134
  older people, 182
frequency of exercise, 11
  arthritis, 128, 133, 135–6
  bone mineral density response, 236–7
  neurological/neuromuscular disorders, 290
  spinal cord injury, 325
Friedreich's ataxia, 286
Fullerton Advanced Balance (FAB) Scale, 192
functional assessment, cardiovascular patients, 84–6
  performance changes, 84–5
  physiological response changes, 85–6
functional electrical stimulation (FES), 324, 331
Functional Fitness Framework, 192
furosemide, 176

G

gait abnormalities, arthritis, 128
gas exchange impairment, chronic obstructive pulmonary disease, 102
gender differences
  bone loss, 173, 228
  life expectancy, 167
  osteoporosis, 229
  see also female exercise participants
genetic factors
  ageing, 167, 168
  bone mineral density, 233
  obesity, 23
  osteoporosis, 230–1
  rheumatoid arthritis, 123
gestational diabetes, 260
glomerular filtration rate, ageing-related decline, 164
glucose tolerance
  exercise-related improvement, 35
  postmenopausal women, 262
goal-setting, client-centred approach, 8–9

gonadotrophin-releasing hormone, 250, 254
gonadotrophins, 250, 252, 253
gripping aids, 330
growth hormone
   ageing-related changes, 176–7
      exercise effects, 185
   female athlete triad, 256
gymnastics
   asthma exercise training programmes, 107
   bone health enhancement, 234
      children/adolescents, 240

H

hand cycling, spinal cord injury, 324, 327, 331
   cautions, 327
head injury *see* traumatic brain injury
Health Professionals Follow-Up Study, 26
heart failure, 53, 66–74, 79
   diagnosis, 66
   epidemiology, 66–7
   exercise
      aerobic endurance, 72–3
      balance/proprioceptive/
         coordination, 74
      muscular strength/endurance, 73
      primary prevention, 68
      secondary prevention/
         rehabilitation, 68–74
   exercise-induced arrhythmias, 69–71
      preventive precautions, 69, 71
   implantable cardioverter defibrillators, 71
   activity-based rehabilitation, 74–6
   secondary muscle dysfunction/
      functional capacity reduction, 71–2
      beneficial effects of exercise, 72
   severity categories
      functional aerobic capacity, 72
      New York Heart Association
         (NYHA), 66, 67
   symptoms, 66
heart rate
   older people
      aerobic training response, 181
      exercise-induced increase, 170, 178, 202–3
      reserve, 13, 202, 203
   in pregnancy, 261

see also age-adjusted maximal heart rate;
   heart rate monitoring; maximal
   heart rate
heart rate monitoring, 11, 13
   neurological/neuromuscular disorders, 290
   older people, 202–3
   spinal cord injury, 323, 325, 326–7, 330
heart transplant patients, 71
heat-related illness, spinal cord injury, 329
hereditary motor and sensory neuropathy
   type I and II, 286
high-density lipoproteins
   atherosclerotic plaque stability
      enhancement, 54
   benefits of physical activity
      older people, 181
      postmenopausal women, 263
   spinal cord injury, 322, 326
hip fracture
   age-related bone quality, 174
   osteoporosis, 229
   prevention during exercise training, 200
hip joint
   ageing-related range of motion decline, 174
   osteoarthritis, 123
hip protectors, 200
home-based exercise programmes
   neuromuscular disorders, 288, 289
   older people, 185–6, 204
hormone replacement therapy, 263, 274
   osteoporosis management, 230
human chorionic gonadotrophin, 253
hybrid exercise, spinal cord injury, 324
hydrotherapy
   multiple sclerosis, 285
   stroke/traumatic brain injury, 276, 277
hypertension
   atherosclerotic plaque stability
      influence, 54
   congestive heart failure, 67–8
   diabetes type 2 association, 40
   obesity association, 40
   postmenopausal women, 263
   stroke risk, 274, 275
hypothalamic hormones, ageing effects, 176
hypothalamic–pituitary axis, 250, 251
   athletic amenorrhoea, 254–5

I

implantable cardioverter defibrillators, 71
  electrical-lead failure, 75
  exercise-based rehabilitation, 74–6
inactivity *see* sedentary lifestyle
inclinometers, 31
incremental performance tests, chronic obstructive pulmonary disease, 105
indirect calorimetry, 30
individualized exercise programmes, 5
  chronic low back pain, 148
  heart failure, 72
inspiratory capacity, older people, 171
inspiratory muscle training
  heart failure, 73
  Parkinson's disease, 281
  pulmonary rehabilitation
    asthma, 108–9, 112
    chronic obstructive pulmonary disease, 105, 106–7, 111
inspiratory muscle weakness, chronic obstructive pulmonary disease, 100, 101, 102
inspiratory muscle work
  asthma, 103, 104
  chronic obstructive pulmonary disease, 100–1, 106
insulin deficiency, 25
insulin resistance, 275–6
  obesity, 26–7
  type 2 diabetes, 25
insulin sensitivity
  exercise-related improvement, 35, 64
    type 2 diabetes, 38, 40
  in pregnancy, 259, 260
  spinal cord injury patients, 322, 325
insulin treatment, 26
insulin-like growth factor (IGF–1), 177, 185, 239, 257
insulin-like growth factor-binding protein–1, 256
intellectual performance, ageing effects, 175
intensity of exercise, 10–11, 12
  aerobic activities, 12
  arthritis, 126, 127, 133, 136
  bone mineral density response, 236–7
  cardiovascular benefit relationship, 57, 58, 59
    coronary heart disease primary prevention, 62
    coronary heart disease secondary prevention/rehabilitation, 66
  chronic obstructive pulmonary disease, 110–11
  exercise-related myocardial infarction, 74
  heart failure, 72
    exercise-induced arrhythmias prevention, 69
  implantable cardioverter defibrillator patient rehabilitation, 75
  neurological/neuromuscular disorders, 290–1
  older people, 202–3
  in pregnancy, 261
  relative versus absolute, 12
  spinal cord injury, 325–7
INTERHEART study, 27, 28
intermediolateral cell column, 311
International Physical Activity Questionnaire (IPAQ), 233
interval training
  arthritis, 126
  chronic low back pain, 148
  chronic obstructive pulmonary disease, 110
  older people, 180, 200, 203
  spinal cord injury, 325
intramembranous ossification, 228
isokinetic activity, 14, 15
isometric activity, 14, 15
  arthritis, 135
  older people, 202
isotonic activity, 14–15
  arthritis, 135

J

jogging, bone mineral density response, 183, 236
joint range of motion
  ageing-related decline, 174
    response to exercise, 184
  arthritis, 127–8, 129, 130
    aerobic exercise effects, 126–7
  benefits of enhancement, 61–2
  flexibility exercise effects, 16
  measurement of change, 16
  see also flexibility; flexibility exercises
joint stability
  osteoarthritis, 122
  proprioceptive exercise in arthritis patients, 130
joint trauma, 16

jumping
    bone mineral density response, 234,
        236, 237, 239
        children/adolescents, 240
    contribution to arthritis development,
        125

K

Karvonen range, 13
    exercise testing end-point, 82
Kegel exercises, 262
knee joint
    ageing-related range of motion decline,
        174
    arthritis, 123
        exercise, 128, 130, 131–2

L

lactate, cool-down exercise in
    cardiovascular patients, 80
lactate threshold, 3
    chronic obstructive pulmonary disease,
        110
    spinal cord injury, 326
lactic acidosis, chronic obstructive
    pulmonary disease, 100
left ventricular dysfunction, 66, 67
    exercise-induced arrhythmia risk, 71
    see also heart failure
left ventricular ejection fraction, 66, 72
leg exercise
    chronic obstructive pulmonary disease,
        105
    implantable cardioverter defibrillator
        patients, 75–6
leptin, 23, 239
    deficiency, 23
        leptin therapy response, 23, 24
    female athletic triad, 256
levodopa, 278
life expectancy, 166–7
    enhancement, 170
lifespan, 166
ligaments
    flexibility exercise effects, 16
    laxity with osteoarthritis, 122
limb-girdle syndrome, 286
lipid management agents, 77
lipid profiles
    heart failure, 68
    spinal cord injury, 322, 325, 326
London Transport Company study, 56

low back pain, 119–20, 139–54
    acute, 140, 141
        case study, 142–57, 151
        physical activity response, 148
    benefits of exercise, 120–1
    chronic, 140, 141
        aerobic exercise, 148–9
        exercise dose response, 149
        psychosocial issues, 141, 148
        resistance training case study,
            150–1
        spinal stabilization exercise (core
            stability), 148, 149
    economic burden, 120
    epidemiology, 139–40
    key points, 153–4
    management principles, 153
    pathophysiology, 140–1
    in pregnancy, 260
    psychological considerations, 151–2
        graded exposure, 151
    referral to lower limbs, 140
low-density lipoproteins
    aerobic training response in older
        people, 181
    atherosclerotic plaque stability, 54
    benefits of physical activity, 263, 326
    cardiovascular risk, 52
    postmenopausal women, 262, 263
    spinal cord injury, 326
lung function
    older people, 171
    see also respiratory system
luteinizing hormone, 250, 251, 254

M

magnetic resonance imaging, body
    composition measurement, 322
Malmö Feasibility Study, 33–4
Maslow's hierarchy of needs, 168
mastery experience, 9
maximal aerobic power (VO$_2$max),
    2–3, 58
    ageing-related decline, 164, 171, 179
        training response, 180
    measurement, 12
        in clinical populations, 12–13
        maximal testing protocol, 12
        surrogates, 13
        VO$_2$ peak, 13
        VO$_2$ reserve, 13
    in pregnancy, 260
    spinal cord injury, 322–4

maximal aerobic power (VO$_2$max)
(*Continued*)
    monitoring, 326, 327
    training for improvement, 325–6
maximal heart rate, 13
  exercise intensity measurement
    arthritis patients, 127
    older people, 202
  in pregnancy, 260
  spinal cord injury, 327, 331
maximum voluntary contraction (MVC),
15
medication effects
  cardiovascular patients, 77–9, 82
  older people
    cardiorespiratory testing, 191
    vestibular adverse effects, 176
  Parkinson's disease, 278
  spinal cord injury, 327
menarche, 250, 251, 254
menopause, 251, 252–3
  bone loss, 257
  see also postmenopausal women
menses, 250, 251
  painful, 252
menstrual cycle, 250–2
  follicular phase, 250
  luteal phase, 250
    energy requirements, 255
    maintenance in exercising women,
    255–6
metabolic equivalents (METs)
  cardiovascular patients, 82, 85
  exercise intensity measurement, 13
  older people
    cardiorespiratory testing, 191
    exercise monitoring, 203
metabolic function, 3
metabolic syndrome, 58
modelling, 9
monitoring exercise, 11–12
  asthma, 112
  older people, 202–3
  self-monitoring, 8–9
  spinal cord injury, 326–7, 331
motion picture sampling, 30
motivation
  behaviour change, 6
  goal-setting, 8, 9
  physical activity
    obesity management, 35
    older people, 204–6
  psychological benefits of exercise,
    10
  self-monitoring, 8

motor units, ageing-related remodelling,
172
movement control, 16–17
  measurement methods, 17
multiple sclerosis, 270, 282–5
  cardiorespiratory fitness, 282
  clinical course, 282
  co-morbidity, 293–4
  coordination/skills, 283
  exercise, 283–5
    cardiorespiratory training, 284–5
    coordination/skills training, 285
    flexibility, 285
    intensity, 290
    muscular strength/power/
      endurance, 285
  fatigue, 282, 284, 292
  motor control reduction, 283
  muscle endurance, 283
  muscle weakness, 283
  pathophysiology, 282
  spasticity, 283
  symptoms, 284
muscle
  ageing effects, 171–3
    denervation/reinnervation, 175
  contraction speed
    Parkinson's disease, 279
    stroke/traumatic brain
      injury, 274
muscle atrophy
  ageing-related, 171–2, 175
    motor unit remodelling, 172
    strength training response, 182
  heart failure, 73
  immobilization-related, 179
  neuromuscular disorders, 286
  rheumatoid arthritis, 124
  spinal cord injury, 320
muscle fibre type changes
  ageing-related, 173
  chronic obstructive pulmonary disease,
    99, 101
  heart failure, 71
  multiple sclerosis, 283
  neuromuscular disorders, 287
muscular dysfunction
  chronic obstructive pulmonary disease,
    98, 99–100
  heart failure, 71–2
muscular dystrophies, 270, 286
muscular endurance, 4
  multiple sclerosis, 283
  stroke, 273
  traumatic brain injury, 273

muscular endurance training, 14–15
  chronic obstructive pulmonary disease,
    105
  coronary heart disease
    primary prevention, 61
    secondary prevention/
      rehabilitation, 64–5
  exercise prescription, 15
  functional goals, 15
  heart failure, 73
  multiple sclerosis, 285
  neuromuscular disorders, 288–9
  Parkinson's disease, 281
  in pregnancy, 262
  stroke, 276
muscular power training
  bone mineral density response, 236
    postmenopausal women, 264
  multiple sclerosis, 285
  neuromuscular disorders, 288–9
  Parkinson's disease, 281
  stroke, 276
muscular strength, 3
  ageing-related, 172–3, 175, 182
  immobilization-related, 179
  Parkinson's disease, 279
  stroke, 274
  traumatic brain injury, 274
muscular strength training, 14–15
  arthritis, 121, 134–7
    joint range of motion augmentation,
      129
  chronic obstructive pulmonary disease,
    111
  coronary heart disease
    primary prevention, 61
    secondary prevention/
      rehabilitation, 64–5
  exercise prescription, 15
  functional goals, 15
  heart failure, 73
  low back pain, 121, 148
  multiple sclerosis, 285
  neurological disorders, 271
  neuromuscular disorder, 271, 288–9
  older people, 162, 180, 181–2, 200
    bone mineral density response, 183
    falls prevention, 186, 318
    rest/recovery, 203
  Parkinson's disease, 281
  in pregnancy, 262
  spinal cord injury, 320, 324, 326
  stroke, 276
muscular weakness
  ageing-related, 172

multiple sclerosis, 283
  neuromuscular disorders, 286, 287
  Parkinson's disease, 279
musculoskeletal disorders, spinal cord
  injury, 324, 328
musculoskeletal system, ageing effects,
  171–4
  benefits of exercise training, 181–4
myocardial changes, older people, 170
  exercise training response, 181
myocardial energy metabolism, 64
myocardial infarction, 53
  atherosclerotic plaque rupture, 54
  chronic obstructive pulmonary disease
    co-morbidity, 102
  congestive heart failure, 67, 68
  exertion-related, 55, 74
  obesity-related risk, 27–8
  secondary prevention/rehabilitation,
    62
  myocardial pumping dysfunction,
    52, 53, 66
  see also heart failure
myotonic dystrophy, 286, 289

N

National Health Service frameworks, 59
National Service Framework for Older People,
  162
negative learning in older people, 178
nervous system, ageing effects,
  174–6, 177
  benefits of exercise, 184–5
netball, bone health enhancement, 234
neurological disorders, 269–96
  barriers to physical activity, 272
  co-morbidities, 292–6
  exercise, 289–92
    dose, 289–90
    duration, 290
    frequency, 290
    intensity, 290–1
    mode, 289
    overload, 291
    specificity, 291
  incidence/prevalence, 272
  key points, 296
neuromuscular atrophies, 286
neuromuscular disorders, 270, 286–96
  balance/coordination, 287
  cardiorespiratory fitness, 286–7
  co-morbidities, 292, 295–6
  exercise, 287–92

neuromuscular disorders (*Continued*)
cardiorespiratory training, 288
coordination/skills training, 289
dose, 289–90
duration, 290
flexibility, 289
frequency, 290
intensity, 290–1
mode, 289
muscular strength/endurance,
288–9
overload, 291
specificity, 291
general fitness, 286
key points, 296
muscle fatigue, 287
muscle weakness, 287
pathophysiology, 286
symptoms, 288
nifedipine, 329
nitrates, 77, 80
nitric oxide
arterial endothelial response in heart
failure, 71–2
atherosclerotic plaque stability, 54
myocardial perfusion effects, 64
non-exercise activities thermogenesis
(NEAT), 30–1
non-verbal communication, 6
Nurses Health Study, 26, 33, 263

O

obesity, 21–42
aetiology, 22–3
physical inactivity, 22, 58, 60
cardiovascular risk, 52, 53, 61
myocardial infarction, 27–8
children, 36
co-morbidity, 1, 40
coronary heart disease, 58
diabetes type 2, 26, 30, 39
definition, 22, 41
exercise prescription, 38–9
concurrent dietary intervention, 39
genetic factors, 23, 24
monogenic syndromes, 23–4
response to exercise, 36
insulin resistance, 26–7
key points, 41
life expectancy impact, 40
neuromuscular disorder patients, 286
physical activity benefits, 35–6, 180
prevention, 30–2, 41

prevalence, 27–9
adolescents, 29
children, 28–9
older people, 29
spinal cord injury patients, 330
stroke risk, 274
weight regain following loss, 35, 39
oedema, heart failure, 66
oestradiol, 250–1
oestrogen, 250
bone health, 233, 256, 257
cyclic exposure in women, 251
female athlete triad, 256
in pregnancy, 253, 259
oestrogen deficiency
athletic amenorrhoea, 254
bone loss, 173, 228, 239
menopausal/postmenopausal,
173, 252, 262, 263
Old Order Mennonites study, 31–2
older people, 16–17, 161–210
age categories, 163
assessment, 188–93
ability to exercise, 191–2
cardiorespiratory testing, 191–2
physical activity levels, 192
principles, 189–91
barriers to physical activity, 204, 205
bone loss minimization, 231
chronic disease, 169, 178–9, 180, 188
compression of morbidity, 169
demographic trends ('greying' of
population), 167
diabetes, 29, 180
exercise sessions
cool-down, 202
group programmes, 204
home-based programmes,
185–6, 204
induction session, 206
monitoring intensity, 202–3
observation/interpretation, 203–4
rest/recovery, 203
warm-up, 202
exercise training benefits, 4, 180–8
cardiovascular, 180–1
endocrine, 185
functional independence, 180
musculoskeletal, 181–4
nervous system, 184–5
psychological, 186–8
respiratory, 180–1
exercise training guidelines, 193–206
exercise prescription, 194–8
injury prevention, 199–200

older people (*Continued*)
  progressive overload, 201–2
  specificity, 200–1
 falls, 177–8
  prevention, 185–6, 318
 foot problems, 175
 functional ability, 164, 166
  evaluation, 192–3
  mobility-specific exercises, 182
  strength training effects, 182
 heart failure, 67
 key points, 207–10
 motivation for exercise, 204–6
  support strategies, 206
 muscular strength requirements for
    daily activities, 73
 obesity
  prevalence, 29
  prevention, 31
 osteoarthritis, 121
 physical activity effects, 163, 180–8
 pre-activity screening, 189–91
  contraindications, 190
 proprioceptive sensitivity, 130, 175
 quality of life, 16–17, 163, 167, 169,
    178, 180, 188
 sedentary lifstyle effects, 178–9
 sleep patterns, 169, 176
 spinal cord injury, 318
 stereotypes/myths, 205–6
 vestibular abnormalities, 175–6, 177
 visual impairment, 176, 177
 see also ageing; postmenopausal
    women
oligomenorrhoea, 251
one-repetition-maximum lift (1-REP),
  3, 15
 measurement, 15
 resistive training intensity for arthritic
    client, 136
optimization selective compensation,
  168
oral contraception, 251, 259, 274
 bone health effects, 239
ossification, 228
osteoarthritis, 120, 121–3
 aerobic activity, 125–7, 128
 benefits of exercise, 120–1
  older people, 180
  secondary prevention, 125
 clinical assessment, 124, 129
 epidemiology, 12–122
 flexibility exercise, 127–30
 management principles, 153
 movement impairment, 123

pain
 degenerative changes relationship,
    121, 122
 during exercise, 135–6
 pathophysiology, 122–3
 periods of disease inactivity, 127
 physical activity in aetiology, 124–5
 primary, 123
 progressive nature, 121–2
 proprioceptive exercise, 130–3
  exercise programme, 131–3
 resistance training, 134–5, 137
  frequency, 135–6
  intensity, 136
  isometric, 135
  isotonic, 135
  repetitions, 136–7
  water-based, 137–9
 secondary, 123
 soft tissue changes, 122–3
 tertiary, 123
osteoarthrosis, 123
osteoblasts, 227
osteocalcin, 227, 231
osteoclasts, 227, 228
osteoid calcification, 227
osteonectin, 227
osteopenia, 228–31
 amenorrhoeic athletes, 238, 257
 bone mineral density, 229
 fracture risk, 229
 postmenopausal, 263, 264
 risk factors, 230
osteoporosis, 7, 228–31
 amenorrhoeic athletes, 238
  female athlete triad, 253, 256–8
 assessment, 231
 benefits of physical activity, 4,
    180, 184
 bone markers, 231
 bone mineral density, 174, 229
 cardiac rehabilitation exercises, 65
 diagnosis (T-score), 229
 fracture risk, 229
 gait changes, 177
 genetic factors, 230–1
 key points, 242
 older people, 180, 184
  exercise programmes, 184
 pharmacological treatment, 230
 postmenopausal, 263, 264
 prevention, 230, 231
  exercise training in youth, 238
 risk factors, 73, 230
  dietary, 241

osteoporosis (*Continued*)
spinal cord injury patients, 320
overload
bone osteogenic response, 237
chronic obstructive pulmonary disease
rehabilitation, 110–11
neurological/neuromuscular disorders,
291
older people, 201–2
spinal cord injury, 324
see also intensity of exercise
overweigtht
definition, 22
prevalence, 27
ovulation, 250, 251, 252

P

Paffenbarger Physical Activity
Questionnaire, 233
pannus, 124
paraplegia, 312, 329
general health of athletes, 319–20
see also spinal cord injury
parasympathetic nervous system, 312
parathyroid hormone
ageing-related changes, 174
calcium metabolism regulation, 228
osteoporosis therapy, 230
Parkinson's disease, 270, 278–81
activity limitation, 278
cardiorespiratory fitness, 278
co-morbidity, 294–5
coordination, 279
exercise, 279–81
cardiorespiratory, 280–1
coordination/skills training, 281
flexibility training, 281
intensity, 291
muscle strength/endurance training,
281
in primary prevention, 279
flexibility, 279
muscle endurance, 279
muscle strength/speed, 279
pathophysiology, 278
symptoms, 279, 280
treatment, 278
parvovirus, 123
peak bone mass, 173, 228
maximization in childhood, 231
pedometers, 12
cardiovascular patient assessment, 87
pelvic floor exercises, 262

peripheral neuropathies, 286
gait changes, 177
physical activity
ageing rate influence, 166
bone health benefits, 231–4
dose response, 234–7
cardioprotective mechanisms, 63
coronary heart disease, 54–5
primary prevention, 56–62
definition, 1
diabetes
management, 36–8
type 2, risk reduction, 32–5, 41
frequency, 11
increasing/maintaining, 4–5
intensity, 10–11
relative versus absolute, 12
misperceptions, 10–11
monitoring, 11–12
obesity
management, 35–6
risk reduction, 30–2, 41
older people, 170, 179
assessment, 192
spinal cord injury patients, 319–20
volume, 11
physical activity diaries/questionnaires, 12
Physical Activity Readiness Medical
Examination (PARmed-X) for
Pregnancy Questionnaire, 261
Physical Activity Readiness Questionnaire
(PAR-Q), 191
Physical Activity Scale for the Elderly
(PASE), 192
physical inactivity *see* sedentary lifestyle
Physician-based Assessment and
Counseling for Exercise (PACE), 192
Physicians' Health Study, 33
physiological response to exercise, 9
Pima Indians, 32
pituitary hormones, ageing effects, 176
placental hormones, 253
plyometrics, bone health enhancement, 234
children/adolescents, 240
posterior cord syndrome, 315
post-event stretching, 15, 16
postmenopausal women, 262–4
benefits of physical activity, 263
osteoporosis/oestopenia risk, 263
physical activity guidelines, 263–4
postural changes, exercise in
cardiovascular patients, 80
postural hypotension prevention, 80, 81
postural stability, older people, 175
pre-event stretching, 15, 16

pre-exercise screening
    older people, 189–91
        balance, 192
    in pregnancy, 261
pregnancy, 253, 259–62
    cardiorespiratory changes, 260
    physical activity
        following delivery, 262
        guidelines, 261–2
    pre-exercise screening, 261
    response to exercise, 260–1
        fetal, 261
    weight gain, 259–60
premenses, 250
premenstrual syndrome, 252, 259
    diagnosis, 259
progesterone, 250, 251
    in pregnancy, 253, 259
progesterone-only contraception, bone
    health adverse effects, 238–9
proprioception, 4, 16–17
    ageing effects, 175, 177
proprioceptive exercise
    arthritis, 130–3
    coronary heart disease
        primary prevention, 61–2
        secondary prevention/
            rehabilitation, 65
    heart failure, 74
proprioceptive neuromuscular facilitation
    (PNF), 16
prostaglandin inhibitors, 259
protein intake, bone health, 241
psychological benefits of exercise, 10
    arthritis, 125–6
    spinal cord injury, 319
psychological factors
    goal-setting, 8
    low back pain, 151–2
        graded exposure approach, 151, 152
    maintainance of physical activity, 5
    participation in exercise, 5
    successful ageing, 168
psychological function, ageing effects,
    178
    benefits of exercise, 186–8
psychological theory of ageing, 168
psychosocial development stages, 168
psychosocial issues
    chronic low back pain, 141, 148
    chronic obstructive pulmonary disease,
        102
pulmonary function testing,
    cardiovascular patients, 84
pulmonary hypertension, 68

pulmonary rehabilitation, 104
    asthma
        children, 107
        evidence-based guidance, 112–13
        exercise training, 107–9
        inspiratory muscle training, 108–9
    chronic obstructive pulmonary disease,
        102, 104–7
        evidence-based guidance, 109–12
        inspiratory muscle training, 105,
            106–7
        outcome measures, 105–6
        reversibility of training effects, 112
    components of programme, 104
    goals, 104

Q

qigong, 181
quality of life, 10
    balance/proprioceptive/coordination
        exercise, 74
    muscular strength requirements for
        daily activities, 73
    older people, 16–17, 163, 167, 169, 178,
        180, 188
    pulmonary rehabilitation in chronic
        obstructive pulmonary disease,
        106
questionnaires, 30, 31
quinine, 176

R

racket sports
    bone mineral density response, 183
        specificity, 237
    shoulder pain, 328
radius fracture, 229
raloxifene, 263
rate pressure product (RPP), 83–4
ratings of perceived exertion (RPE)
    aerobic exercise intensity measurement,
        13
    arthritis patients, 127
    cardiovascular patients, 85
    older people, 203
    in pregnancy, 262
    spinal cord injury, 326, 327
reaction time, ageing effects, 174, 177
relapse
    high-risk situations, 10
    prevention training, 9–10
        older people, 206

relaxin, 253, 262
resistance bands
    arthritis patients, 134
    older people, 202
resistance training
    arthritis, 134–5, 137
        frequency, 135–6
        intensity, 136
        isometric, 135
        isotonic, 135
        repetitions, 136–7
        water-based, 137–9
    bone health benefits, 183, 184, 233,
        236, 239
    chronic low back pain, 150–1
    chronic obstructive pulmonary disease,
        105
    neuromuscular disorders, 288–9
    older people, 180, 181, 182, 199, 201–2
        bone mineral density response,
            183, 184
        endocrine system benefit, 185
        falls prevention, 186
        psychological function benefit,
            187–8
    Parkinson's disease, 281
    spinal cord injury, 324, 326
    stroke, 276
resistin, 27
respiratory disorders, 97–114
    key points, 113–14
    neuromuscular disease, 286–7
    pulmonary rehabilitation
        see pulmonary rehabilitation
    spinal cord injury patients, 319, 320
    therapeutic effect of exercise, 104
respiratory muscle weakness
    chronic obstructive pulmonary disease,
        99–100, 101, 102
    heart failure, 71
    multiple sclerosis, 282
respiratory system
    ageing effects, 170–1
        exercise training influence, 180–1
    pregnancy-related changes, 260
    sympathetic stimulation, 3
reversibility of training effect
    bone mineral density gains, 183,
        237–8
    chronic obstructive pulmonary disease,
        112
rheumatoid arthritis, 120
    aerobic activity, 125–7, 128
    benefits of exercise, 120–1
        secondary prevention, 125
    clinical assessment, 124, 129
    epidemiology, 123–4
    flexibility exercise, 127–30
    genetic factors, 123
    management principles, 153
    pain during exercise, 135–6
    pannus, 124
    pathophysiology, 124
    periods of disease inactivity, 127
    physical activity in aetiology, 124–5
    proprioceptive exercise, 130–3
        exercise programme, 131–3
    resistance training, 134–5, 137
        frequency, 135–6
        intensity, 136
        isometric, 135
        isotonic, 135
        repetitions, 136–7
        water-based, 137–9
    rest during exacerbations, 136
    stength training, 134–7
    variants, 124
right ventricular wall myopathy, 56
rowing, 235
rowing ergometer, 81
    low back pain, 149
    spinal cord injury, 324, 326
running
    asthma exercise training programme,
        107
    bone mineral density response,
        183, 235
        children/adolescents, 240
        specificity, 237
    contribution to arthritis development,
        125

S

seated arm exercise, implantable
    cardioverter defibrillator patients, 75
sedentary lifestyle, 2, 58
    asthma patients, 98
    cardiovascular risk, 52
    chronic morbidity relationship, 1, 54
    chronic obstructive pulmonary disease,
        99
    coronary heart disease relationship,
        58–9
    musculoskeletal disorders, 120, 121
    neuromuscular disorders, 286
    obese patients, 22, 23, 30, 58, 59
    older people
        age-related decline influence, 178–9

sedentary lifestyle (*Continued*)
  ageing rate influence, 166
  gait changes, 177
  osteoarthritis, 123
  spinal cord injured patients,
    319, 320
  stroke risk, 274
selective oestrogen receptor modulators
  (SERMs), 230, 263
self-efficacy, 5, 9
  exercise in older peope, 186, 188, 205
  successful ageing determinants, 168
self-esteem
  benefits of exercise, 186
  successful ageing determinants, 168
self-image, 2
self-management, arthritis patients,
  127
self-monitoring, 8–9
Senior Fitness Test (SFT), 192
shoulder
  osteoarthritis, 123
  pain, spinal cord injured wheelchair
    users, 324, 328
sickle cell disease, 274
sit-to-stand activities, arthritis patients,
  132
skeletal muscle perfusion, warm-up
  exercise, 79
skipping, bone health enhancement, 234,
  239
  children/adolescents, 240
sleep apnoea, 56
sleep pattern, older people, 169, 176
  physical activity benefits, 180
SMARTER (goal-setting), 8, 9
smoking, 52, 54, 98, 169
social support
  physical activity participation, 5, 8
  successful ageing determinants, 169
spasticity
  multiple sclerosis, 283
  stroke, 274, 276
spinal cord, 310–12
  grey matter, 310
  motor pathways, 312
  segments, 310
  sensory pathways, 311–12
  white matter, 310–11
spinal cord injury, 309–32
  aerobic capacity, 322–4
  age/sex distribution, 316
  autonomic nervous system dysfunction,
    328–9
  autonomic dysreflexia, 329

bladder/bowel problems, 328
  blood pressure, 329
  cardiac effects, 322, 323, 327
  body composition measurement,
    321–2
  active muscle mass, 322
  skinfold measurements, 321, 322
  causes, 316–18
  sports, 317
  classification, 312–13
  complete, 312, 315
  daily living activities, 322, 323
  exercise, 330–1
  aerobic capacity improvement,
    325–6
  duration, 325–6, 330
  frequency, 325
  intensity, 325–6, 330
  muscular strength improvement,
    326
  overload principle, 324
  physiological outcome parameters,
    323
  practical issues, 329–30
  training intensity monitoring, 326–7,
    331
  types, 324–5, 330
  exercise benefits, 319–20, 321–2, 323
  incidence/prevalence, 315–16
  incomplete, 315
  types, 315
  key points, 331–2
  mechanisms, 312
  muscle spasms, 324
  older people, 318
  physical activity, 319–20
  cautions, 327–30
  health outcomes, 320
  nerve entrapment symptoms, 328
  overuse injuries, 328
  psychosocial aspects, 319
  shoulder pain, 324, 328
  skin abrasions, 328
  temperature regulation
    abnormalities, 329, 330
  secondary health complications, 310,
    320, 323
spinal muscular atrophy, 286
spinal nerves, 310
spinal stabilization exercise, 121
  chronic low back pain, 148, 149
spine, ageing-related range of motion
  decline, 174
spinothalamic tract, 312
sports-related spinal cord injury, 317–18

stability balls, 149
stair climbing
    bone mineral density response, 183
    chronic obstructive pulmonary disease,
        105, 111
stair descent, perceptual errors with visual
    impairment, 176
static stretching, 16
statins, 77
step testing, cardiovascular patient
    assessment, 87
steroid-induced myopathy, 99
Stockholm Weight Development Study
    (SWEDES), 32
strength exercise *see* muscular strength
    training
stretching exercises
    arthritis, 128–9
        duration of stretch, 129
    multiple sclerosis, 285
    see also flexibility exercises
stroke, 16, 270, 271, 273–7
    balance/coordination, 274
    cardiorespiratory fitness, 273
    co-morbidity, 293
    diabetes type 2, 40
    epidemiology, 53
    exercise, 276–7
        cardiorespiratory training, 276
        coordination/skill training, 277
        flexibility training, 277
        intensity, 290, 291
        muscular strength/endurance
            training, 276
        in primary prevention, 274–5
    flexibility, 274
    haemorrhagic, 271, 275
    hand dexterity, 274
    ischaemic, 271
        risk factors, 274
    motor deficits, 274
    muscle contraction speed, 274
    muscle strength/endurance deficits, 274
    obesity association, 40
    pathophysiology, 271
    recovery process, 273
    recurrent cerebrovascular event risk,
        275
    secondary prevention, 275–6
    spasticity, 274, 276
    symptoms, 275
sudden death, 327
    exercise-related myocardial infarction,
        74
    heart failure patients, 71

swimming, 235, 240
    asthma, 107
    diabetes mellitus type 2, 40
    low back pain, 148
    older people, 200
    in pregnancy, 262
    shoulder pain, 328
    spinal cord injury, 324
sympathetic nervous system, 312
synovitis, 122

T

tai chi, 74
    bone mineral density response, 183
    falls prevention, 186, 318
    joint range of motion augmentation,
        129
    multiple sclerosis patients, 285
    musculoskeletal disorders, 121, 129
    older people, 181, 186, 199
        balance improvement, 199
        flexibility improvement, 184
        nervous system effects, 184
temperature regulation abnormalities,
    spinal cord injury, 329, 330
tendons
    ageing-related changes, 172
    flexibility exercise effects, 16
tennis, bone health enhancement, 234
    specificity of response, 237
tetraplegia, 312, 329
    maximal heart rate, 327, 330
    see also spinal cord injury
throwing, contribution to arthritis
    development, 125
thyroid function, 177
timed walks
    cardiovascular patients, 87
    chronic obstructive pulmonary disease,
        105
transient ischaemic attack, 271, 274
    recurrent cerebrovascular
        events, 275
transtheoretical model
    decisional balance, 6–7
    self-efficacy, 9
    stages of change, 6
traumatic brain injury, 16, 270,
    271, 273–7
    balance/coordination, 274
    cardiorespiratory fitness, 273
    co-morbidity, 293
    exercise

traumatic brain injury (*Continued*)
  cardiorespiratory training, 276
    duration, 290
    intensity, 291
    muscular strength, 276
  flexibility, 274
  hand dexterity, 274
  muscle contraction speed, 274
  muscle endurance/strength, 273, 274
  pathophysiology, 273
  symptoms, 275
treadmills, 81
  cardiorespiratory testing in older
      people, 191
  cardiovascular patient assessment, 87
  low back pain exercise programme
      development, 146–7
  multiple sclerosis, 284
  neurological/neuromuscular disorders,
      271, 289
  Parkinson's disease, 281
  stroke, 276
tri-iodothyronine, 256, 257
triglycerides, 52
trunk core stability exercises *see* spinal
    stabilization exercise
twin studies, obesity, 23
type of physical activity, 11

U

unstable angina
  atherosclerotic plaque rupture, 54
  chronic obstructive pulmonary disease
      co-morbidity, 102
upper limb training, chronic obstructive
    pulmonary disease, 105, 111
US Diabetes Prevention Program, 34, 35,
    39

V

valve replacement, 78
valvular heart disease, 52, 53
  congestive heart failure, 67, 68
ventral root, 311
ventricular assist devices, 71
ventricular exertion-related arrhythmias,
    55
ventricular fibrillation
  heart failure patients, 67
    exercise-induced, 71
  implantable cardioverter defibrillator
      patient rehabilitation, 75

ventricular tachycardia
  heart failure patients, 67
    exercise-induced, 71
  implantable cardioverter defibrillator
      patient rehabilitation, 75
verapamil, 77
verbal persuasion, 9
verbal skills, ageing effects, 175
vertebral fracture
  age-related bone quality relationship,
      174
  osteoporosis, 229
vestibular abnormalities, older people,
    175–6, 177
visual impairment, older people,
    176, 177
vital capacity, older people, 171
vitamin D
  ageing-related changes, 174
  bone health, 241
vitamin D deficiency, 241
  older people, 177
vitamin D supplementation
  female athlete triad management,
      258
  older people, 177
  osteoporosis therapy, 230
vitamin intake, bone health, 241
volleyball, bone health enhancement,
    234

W

waist circumference, 41
  childhood obesity assessment, 29
  see also abdominal obesity
waist-to-hip ratio *see* abdominal obesity
walking, 12, 15
  ageing-related gait changes, 177
  arthritis, 125, 126
  bone mineral density response, 183,
      234–5
  chronic obstructive pulmonary disease,
      105, 111
  diabetes mellitus type 2, 40
  energy expenditure for weight loss,
      39
  heart failure, 72
  joint range of motion augmentation,
      129
  low back pain, 148
  multiple sclerosis, 282
  musculoskeletal disorders, 121, 129
  neuromuscular disorders, 287, 288

walking (*Continued*)
    older people, 171, 180–1, 193, 200
        bone health, 234–5
        falls prevention, 185
    Parkinson's disease, 281
    postmenopausal women, 264
    in pregnancy, 262
    stroke, 274, 276
    traumatic brain injury, 274
warfarin, 78, 81
warm-up exercise
    cardiovascular rehabilitation, 79–80
    exercise-induced asthma refractory
        period, 113
    heart failure patients
        exercise-induced arrhythmias
            prevention, 69
        implantable cardioverter
            defibrillator patients, 75
    neurological/neuromuscular disorders,
        289
    older people, 202
water-based exercise *see* aquatic exercise
weight loss, bone mineral density
    relationship, 233–4

weight-bearing exercise, bone health,
    183, 231–2
weighted belt exercises, older people, 182
weightlifting
    bone mineral density response, 240
    contribution to arthritis development,
        125
wheelchair exercise, spinal cord injury,
    324, 331
    shoulder pain, 324, 328
    sports, 324
        cautions, 327
whole body vibration, 183–4
wobble-board exercises, 130, 132, 133
Wolff's law, 231

Y

yoga
    arthritis, 129
    joint range of motion augmentation,
        129, 184
    multiple sclerosis, 285
    older people, 184, 199